# Access Your Online Resources

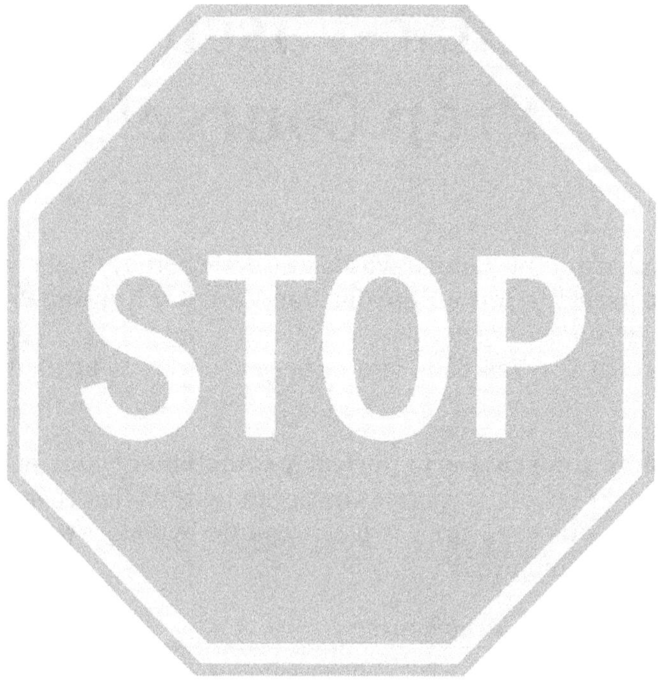


**Don't miss out on the Online Resources included with your purchase!**

Your purchase of this product unlocks access to our Online Resources page. Elevate your study experience with our **interactive practice test interface**, along with all of the additional resources that we couldn't include in this book.

**Flip to the Online Resources section at the end of this book to find the link and a QR code to get started!**

Mometrix TEST PREPARATION

# Cardiac/Vascular Nurse Exam

# Secrets

## Study Guide

Your Key to Exam Success

Mometrix

TEST PREPARATION

Written and edited by the Mometrix Nursing Certification Test Team

Mometrix offers volume discount pricing to institutions. For more information or a price quote, please contact our sales department at sales@mometrix.com or 888-248-1219.



Paperback
ISBN 13: 978-1-60971-239-6
ISBN 10: 1-60971-239-0

Ebook
ISBN 13: 978-1-62120-483-1
ISBN 10: 1-62120-483-9

Hardback
ISBN 13: 978-1-5167-0564-1
ISBN 10: 1-5167-0564-5

# Dear Future Exam Success Story

First of all, **THANK YOU** for purchasing Mometrix study materials!

Second, congratulations! You are one of the few determined test-takers who are committed to doing whatever it takes to excel on your exam. **You have come to the right place.** We developed these study materials with one goal in mind: to deliver you the information you need in a format that's concise and easy to use.

In addition to optimizing your guide for the content of the test, we've outlined our recommended steps for breaking down the preparation process into small, attainable goals so you can make sure you stay on track.

We've also analyzed the entire test-taking process, identifying the most common pitfalls and showing how you can overcome them and be ready for any curveball the test throws you.

Standardized testing is one of the biggest obstacles on your road to success, which only increases the importance of doing well in the high-pressure, high-stakes environment of test day. Your results on this test could have a significant impact on your future, and this guide provides the information and practical advice to help you achieve your full potential on test day.

**Your success is our success**

**We would love to hear from you!** If you would like to share the story of your exam success or if you have any questions or comments in regard to our products, please contact us at **800-673-8175** or **support@mometrix.com**.

Thanks again for your business and we wish you continued success!

Sincerely,
The Mometrix Test Preparation Team

**Need more help? Check out our flashcards at:**
**http://mometrixflashcards.com/CardiacVascular**

# TABLE OF CONTENTS

# Introduction

**Thank you for purchasing this resource!** You have made the choice to prepare yourself for a test that could have a huge impact on your future, and this guide is designed to help you be fully ready for test day. Obviously, it's important to have a solid understanding of the test material, but you also need to be prepared for the unique environment and stressors of the test, so that you can perform to the best of your abilities.

For this purpose, the first section that appears in this guide is the **Secret Keys**. We've devoted countless hours to meticulously researching what works and what doesn't, and we've boiled down our findings to the five most impactful steps you can take to improve your performance on the test. We start at the beginning with study planning and move through the preparation process, all the way to the testing strategies that will help you get the most out of what you know when you're finally sitting in front of the test.

We recommend that you start preparing for your test as far in advance as possible. However, if you've bought this guide as a last-minute study resource and only have a few days before your test, we recommend that you skip over the first two Secret Keys since they address a long-term study plan.

If you struggle with **test anxiety**, we strongly encourage you to check out our recommendations for how you can overcome it. Test anxiety is a formidable foe, but it can be beaten, and we want to make sure you have the tools you need to defeat it.

# Secret Key #1 – Plan Big, Study Small

There's a lot riding on your performance. If you want to ace this test, you're going to need to keep your skills sharp and the material fresh in your mind. You need a plan that lets you review everything you need to know while still fitting in your schedule. We'll break this strategy down into three categories.

## Information Organization

Start with the information you already have: the official test outline. From this, you can make a complete list of all the concepts you need to cover before the test. Organize these concepts into groups that can be studied together, and create a list of any related vocabulary you need to learn so you can brush up on any difficult terms. You'll want to keep this vocabulary list handy once you actually start studying since you may need to add to it along the way.

## Time Management

Once you have your set of study concepts, decide how to spread them out over the time you have left before the test. Break your study plan into small, clear goals so you have a manageable task for each day and know exactly what you're doing. Then just focus on one small step at a time. When you manage your time this way, you don't need to spend hours at a time studying. Studying a small block of content for a short period each day helps you retain information better and avoid stressing over how much you have left to do. You can relax knowing that you have a plan to cover everything in time. In order for this strategy to be effective though, you have to start studying early and stick to your schedule. Avoid the exhaustion and futility that comes from last-minute cramming!

## Study Environment

The environment you study in has a big impact on your learning. Studying in a coffee shop, while probably more enjoyable, is not likely to be as fruitful as studying in a quiet room. It's important to keep distractions to a minimum. You're only planning to study for a short block of time, so make the most of it. Don't pause to check your phone or get up to find a snack. It's also important to **avoid multitasking**. Research has consistently shown that multitasking will make your studying dramatically less effective. Your study area should also be comfortable and well-lit so you don't have the distraction of straining your eyes or sitting on an uncomfortable chair.

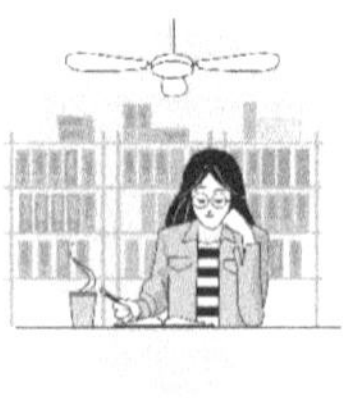

The time of day you study is also important. You want to be rested and alert. Don't wait until just before bedtime. Study when you'll be most likely to comprehend and remember. Even better, if you know what time of day your test will be, set that time aside for study. That way your brain will be used to working on that subject at that specific time and you'll have a better chance of recalling information.

Finally, it can be helpful to team up with others who are studying for the same test. Your actual studying should be done in as isolated an environment as possible, but the work of organizing the information and setting up the study plan can be divided up. In between study sessions, you can discuss with your teammates the concepts that you're all studying and quiz each other on the details. Just be sure that your teammates are as serious about the test as you are. If you find that your study time is being replaced with social time, you might need to find a new team.

# Secret Key #2 – Make Your Studying Count

You're devoting a lot of time and effort to preparing for this test, so you want to be absolutely certain it will pay off. This means doing more than just reading the content and hoping you can remember it on test day. It's important to make every minute of study count. There are two main areas you can focus on to make your studying count.

## Retention

It doesn't matter how much time you study if you can't remember the material. You need to make sure you are retaining the concepts. To check your retention of the information you're learning, try recalling it at later times with minimal prompting. Try carrying around flashcards and glance at one or two from time to time or ask a friend who's also studying for the test to quiz you.

To enhance your retention, look for ways to put the information into practice so that you can apply it rather than simply recalling it. If you're using the information in practical ways, it will be much easier to remember. Similarly, it helps to solidify a concept in your mind if you're not only reading it to yourself but also explaining it to someone else. Ask a friend to let you teach them about a concept you're a little shaky on (or speak aloud to an imaginary audience if necessary). As you try to summarize, define, give examples, and answer your friend's questions, you'll understand the concepts better and they will stay with you longer. Finally, step back for a big picture view and ask yourself how each piece of information fits with the whole subject. When you link the different concepts together and see them working together as a whole, it's easier to remember the individual components.

Finally, practice showing your work on any multi-step problems, even if you're just studying. Writing out each step you take to solve a problem will help solidify the process in your mind, and you'll be more likely to remember it during the test.

## Modality

*Modality* simply refers to the means or method by which you study. Choosing a study modality that fits your own individual learning style is crucial. No two people learn best in exactly the same way, so it's important to know your strengths and use them to your advantage.

For example, if you learn best by visualization, focus on visualizing a concept in your mind and draw an image or a diagram. Try color-coding your notes, illustrating them, or creating symbols that will trigger your mind to recall a learned concept. If you learn best by hearing or discussing information, find a study partner who learns the same way or read aloud to yourself. Think about how to put the information in your own words. Imagine that you are giving a lecture on the topic and record yourself so you can listen to it later.

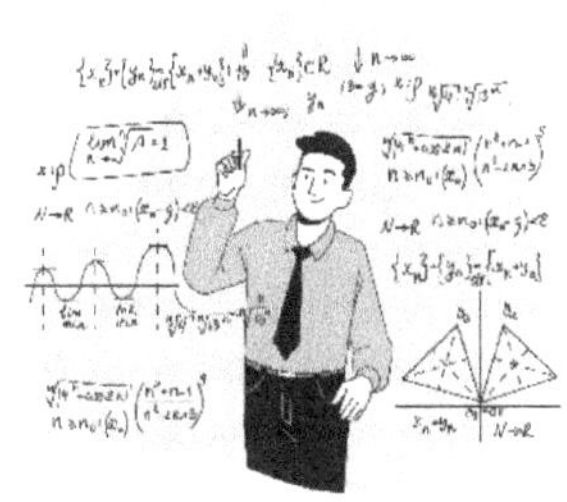

For any learning style, flashcards can be helpful. Organize the information so you can take advantage of spare moments to review. Underline key words or phrases. Use different colors for different categories. Mnemonic devices (such as creating a short list in which every item starts with the same letter) can also help with retention. Find what works best for you and use it to store the information in your mind most effectively and easily.

# Secret Key #3 – Practice the Right Way

Your success on test day depends not only on how many hours you put into preparing, but also on whether you prepared the right way. It's good to check along the way to see if your studying is paying off. One of the most effective ways to do this is by taking practice tests to evaluate your progress. Practice tests are useful because they show exactly where you need to improve. Every time you take a practice test, pay special attention to these three groups of questions:

- The questions you got wrong
- The questions you had to guess on, even if you guessed right
- The questions you found difficult or slow to work through

This will show you exactly what your weak areas are, and where you need to devote more study time. Ask yourself why each of these questions gave you trouble. Was it because you didn't understand the material? Was it because you didn't remember the vocabulary? Do you need more repetitions on this type of question to build speed and confidence? Dig into those questions and figure out how you can strengthen your weak areas as you go back to review the material.

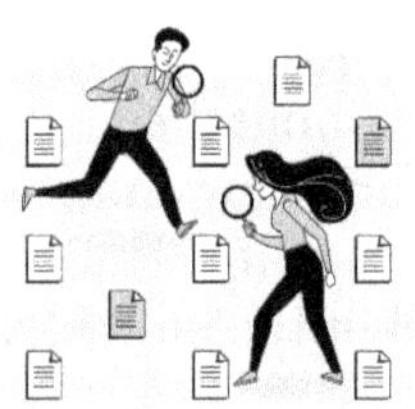

Additionally, many practice tests have a section explaining the answer choices. It can be tempting to read the explanation and think that you now have a good understanding of the concept. However, an explanation likely only covers part of the question's broader context. Even if the explanation makes perfect sense, **go back and investigate** every concept related to the question until you're positive you have a thorough understanding.

As you go along, keep in mind that the practice test is just that: practice. Memorizing these questions and answers will not be very helpful on the actual test because it is unlikely to have any of the same exact questions. If you only know the right answers to the sample questions, you won't be prepared for the real thing. **Study the concepts** until you understand them fully, and then you'll be able to answer any question that shows up on the test.

It's important to wait on the practice tests until you're ready. If you take a test on your first day of study, you may be overwhelmed by the amount of material covered and how much you need to learn. Work up to it gradually.

On test day, you'll need to be prepared for answering questions, managing your time, and using the test-taking strategies you've learned. It's a lot to balance, like a mental marathon that will have a big impact on your future. Like training for a marathon, you'll need to start slowly and work your way up. When test day arrives, you'll be ready.

Start with the strategies you've read in the first two Secret Keys—plan your course and study in the way that works best for you. If you have time, consider using multiple study resources to get different approaches to the same concepts. It can be helpful to see difficult concepts from more than one angle. Then find a good source for practice tests. Many times, the test website will suggest potential study resources or provide sample tests.

## Practice Test Strategy

If you're able to find at least three practice tests, we recommend this strategy:

### Untimed and Open-Book Practice

Take the first test with no time constraints and with your notes and study guide handy. Take your time and focus on applying the strategies you've learned.

### Timed and Open-Book Practice

Take the second practice test open-book as well, but set a timer and practice pacing yourself to finish in time.

### Timed and Closed-Book Practice

Take any other practice tests as if it were test day. Set a timer and put away your study materials. Sit at a table or desk in a quiet room, imagine yourself at the testing center, and answer questions as quickly and accurately as possible.

Keep repeating timed and closed-book tests on a regular basis until you run out of practice tests or it's time for the actual test. Your mind will be ready for the schedule and stress of test day, and you'll be able to focus on recalling the material you've learned.

# Secret Key #4 – Pace Yourself

Once you're fully prepared for the material on the test, your biggest challenge on test day will be managing your time. Just knowing that the clock is ticking can make you panic even if you have plenty of time left. Work on pacing yourself so you can build confidence against the time constraints of the exam. Pacing is a difficult skill to master, especially in a high-pressure environment, so **practice is vital**.

Set time expectations for your pace based on how much time is available. For example, if a section has 60 questions and the time limit is 30 minutes, you know you have to average 30 seconds or less per question in order to answer them all. Although 30 seconds is the hard limit, set 25 seconds per question as your goal, so you reserve extra time to spend on harder questions. When you budget extra time for the harder questions, you no longer have any reason to stress when those questions take longer to answer.

Don't let this time expectation distract you from working through the test at a calm, steady pace, but keep it in mind so you don't spend too much time on any one question. Recognize that taking extra time on one question you don't understand may keep you from answering two that you do understand later in the test. If your time limit for a question is up and you're still not sure of the answer, mark it and move on, and come back to it later if the time and the test format allow. If the testing format doesn't allow you to return to earlier questions, just make an educated guess; then put it out of your mind and move on.

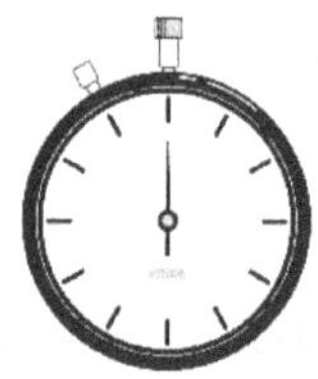

On the easier questions, be careful not to rush. It may seem wise to hurry through them so you have more time for the challenging ones, but it's not worth missing one if you know the concept and just didn't take the time to read the question fully. Work efficiently but make sure you understand the question and have looked at all of the answer choices, since more than one may seem right at first.

Even if you're paying attention to the time, you may find yourself a little behind at some point. You should speed up to get back on track, but do so wisely. Don't panic; just take a few seconds less on each question until you're caught up. Don't guess without thinking, but do look through the answer choices and eliminate any you know are wrong. If you can get down to two choices, it is often worthwhile to guess from those. Once you've chosen an answer, move on and don't dwell on any that you skipped or had to hurry through. If a question was taking too long, chances are it was one of the harder ones, so you weren't as likely to get it right anyway.

On the other hand, if you find yourself getting ahead of schedule, it may be beneficial to slow down a little. The more quickly you work, the more likely you are to make a careless mistake that will affect your score. You've budgeted time for each question, so don't be afraid to spend that time. Practice an efficient but careful pace to get the most out of the time you have.

# Secret Key #5 – Have a Plan for Guessing

When you're taking the test, you may find yourself stuck on a question. Some of the answer choices seem better than others, but you don't see the one answer choice that is obviously correct. What do you do?

The scenario described above is very common, yet most test takers have not effectively prepared for it. Developing and practicing a plan for guessing may be one of the single most effective uses of your time as you get ready for the exam.

In developing your plan for guessing, there are three questions to address:

- When should you start the guessing process?
- How should you narrow down the choices?
- Which answer should you choose?

## When to Start the Guessing Process

Unless your plan for guessing is to select C every time (which, despite its merits, is not what we recommend), you need to leave yourself enough time to apply your answer elimination strategies. Since you have a limited amount of time for each question, that means that if you're going to give yourself the best shot at guessing correctly, you have to decide quickly whether or not you will guess.

Of course, the best-case scenario is that you don't have to guess at all, so first, see if you can answer the question based on your knowledge of the subject and basic reasoning skills. Focus on the key words in the question and try to jog your memory of related topics. Give yourself a chance to bring the knowledge to mind, but once you realize that you don't have (or you can't access) the knowledge you need to answer the question, it's time to start the guessing process.

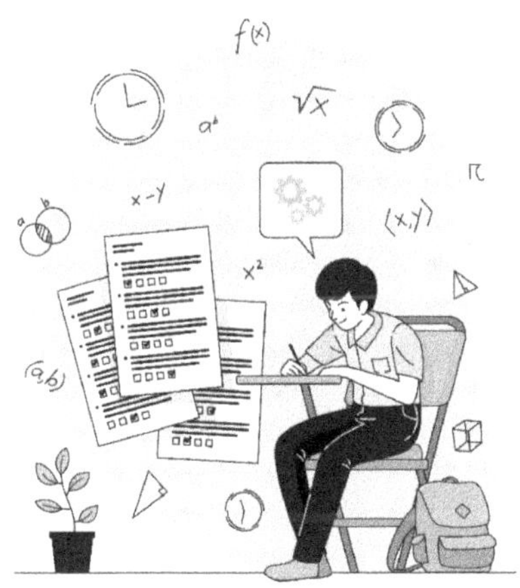

It's almost always better to start the guessing process too early than too late. It only takes a few seconds to remember something and answer the question from knowledge. Carefully eliminating wrong answer choices takes longer. Plus, going through the process of eliminating answer choices can actually help jog your memory.

**Summary**: Start the guessing process as soon as you decide that you can't answer the question based on your knowledge.

## How to Narrow Down the Choices

The next chapter in this book (**Test-Taking Strategies**) includes a wide range of strategies for how to approach questions and how to look for answer choices to eliminate. You will definitely want to read those carefully, practice them, and figure out which ones work best for you. Here though, we're going to address a mindset rather than a particular strategy.

Your odds of guessing an answer correctly depend on how many options you are choosing from.

| **Number of options left** | 5 | 4 | 3 | 2 | 1 |
|---|---|---|---|---|---|
| **Odds of guessing correctly** | 20% | 25% | 33% | 50% | 100% |

You can see from this chart just how valuable it is to be able to eliminate incorrect answers and make an educated guess, but there are two things that many test takers do that cause them to miss out on the benefits of guessing:

- Accidentally eliminating the correct answer
- Selecting an answer based on an impression

We'll look at the first one here, and the second one in the next section.

To avoid accidentally eliminating the correct answer, we recommend a thought exercise called **the $5 challenge**. In this challenge, you only eliminate an answer choice from contention if you are willing to bet $5 on it being wrong. Why $5? Five dollars is a small but not insignificant amount of money. It's an amount you could afford to lose but wouldn't want to throw away. And while losing $5 once might not hurt too much, doing it twenty times will set you back $100. In the same way, each small decision you make—eliminating a choice here, guessing on a question there—won't by itself impact your score very much, but when you put them all together, they can make a big difference. By holding each answer choice elimination decision to a higher standard, you can reduce the risk of accidentally eliminating the correct answer.

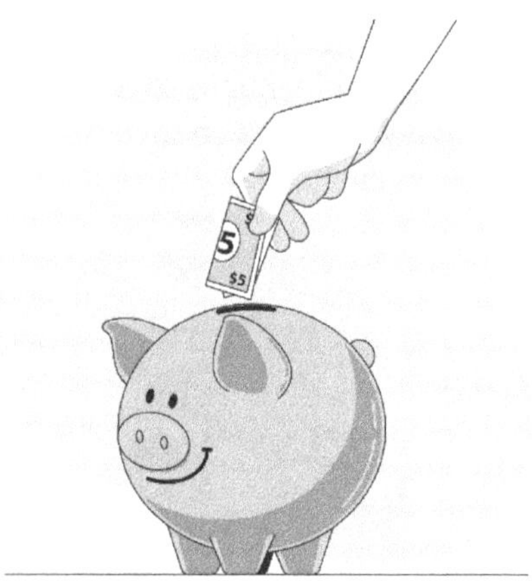

The $5 challenge can also be applied in a positive sense: If you are willing to bet $5 that an answer choice *is* correct, go ahead and mark it as correct.

**Summary**: Only eliminate an answer choice if you are willing to bet $5 that it is wrong.

# Which Answer to Choose

You're taking the test. You've run into a hard question and decided you'll have to guess. You've eliminated all the answer choices you're willing to bet $5 on. Now you have to pick an answer. Why do we even need to talk about this? Why can't you just pick whichever one you feel like when the time comes?

The answer to these questions is that if you don't come into the test with a plan, you'll rely on your impression to select an answer choice, and if you do that, you risk falling into a trap. The test writers know that everyone who takes their test will be guessing on some of the questions, so they intentionally write wrong answer choices to seem plausible. You still have to pick an answer though, and if the wrong answer choices are designed to look right, how can you ever be sure that you're not falling for their trap? The best solution we've found to this dilemma is to take the decision out of your hands entirely. Here is the process we recommend:

**Once you've eliminated any choices that you are confident (willing to bet $5) are wrong, select the first remaining choice as your answer.**

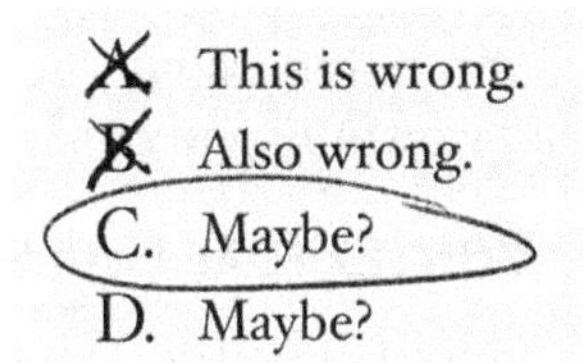


Whether you choose to select the first remaining choice, the second, or the last, the important thing is that you use some preselected standard. Using this approach guarantees that you will not be enticed into selecting an answer choice that looks right, because you are not basing your decision on how the answer choices look.

This is not meant to make you question your knowledge. Instead, it is to help you recognize the difference between your knowledge and your impressions. There's a huge difference between thinking an answer is right because of what you know, and thinking an answer is right because it looks or sounds like it should be right.

**Summary**: To ensure that your selection is appropriately random, make a predetermined selection from among all answer choices you have not eliminated.

# Test-Taking Strategies

This section contains a list of test-taking strategies that you may find helpful as you work through the test. By taking what you know and applying logical thought, you can maximize your chances of answering any question correctly!

It is very important to realize that every question is different and every person is different: no single strategy will work on every question, and no single strategy will work for every person. That's why we've included all of them here, so you can try them out and determine which ones work best for different types of questions and which ones work best for you.

## Question Strategies

### ✓ Read Carefully

Read the question and the answer choices carefully. Don't miss the question because you misread the terms. You have plenty of time to read each question thoroughly and make sure you understand what is being asked. Yet a happy medium must be attained, so don't waste too much time. You must read carefully and efficiently.

### ✓ Contextual Clues

Look for contextual clues. If the question includes a word you are not familiar with, look at the immediate context for some indication of what the word might mean. Contextual clues can often give you all the information you need to decipher the meaning of an unfamiliar word. Even if you can't determine the meaning, you may be able to narrow down the possibilities enough to make a solid guess at the answer to the question.

### ✓ Prefixes

If you're having trouble with a word in the question or answer choices, try dissecting it. Take advantage of every clue that the word might include. Prefixes can be a huge help. Usually, they allow you to determine a basic meaning. *Pre-* means before, *post-* means after, *pro-* is positive, *de-* is negative. From prefixes, you can get an idea of the general meaning of the word and try to put it into context.

### ✓ Hedge Words

Watch out for critical hedge words, such as *likely, may, can, often, almost, mostly, usually, generally, rarely*, and *sometimes*. Question writers insert these hedge phrases to cover every possibility. Often an answer choice will be wrong simply because it leaves no room for exception. Be on guard for answer choices that have definitive words such as *exactly* and *always*.

### ✓ Switchback Words

Stay alert for *switchbacks*. These are the words and phrases frequently used to alert you to shifts in thought. The most common switchback words are *but, although*, and *however*. Others include *nevertheless, on the other hand, even though, while, in spite of, despite*, and *regardless of*. Switchback words are important to catch because they can change the direction of the question or an answer choice.

### ⊘ Face Value

When in doubt, use common sense. Accept the situation in the problem at face value. Don't read too much into it. These problems will not require you to make wild assumptions. If you have to go beyond creativity and warp time or space in order to have an answer choice fit the question, then you should move on and consider the other answer choices. These are normal problems rooted in reality. The applicable relationship or explanation may not be readily apparent, but it is there for you to figure out. Use your common sense to interpret anything that isn't clear.

## Answer Choice Strategies

### ⊘ Answer Selection

The most thorough way to pick an answer choice is to identify and eliminate wrong answers until only one is left, then confirm it is the correct answer. Sometimes an answer choice may immediately seem right, but be careful. The test writers will usually put more than one reasonable answer choice on each question, so take a second to read all of them and make sure that the other choices are not equally obvious. As long as you have time left, it is better to read every answer choice than to pick the first one that looks right without checking the others.

### ⊘ Answer Choice Families

An answer choice family consists of two (in rare cases, three) answer choices that are very similar in construction and cannot all be true at the same time. If you see two answer choices that are direct opposites or parallels, one of them is usually the correct answer. For instance, if one answer choice says that quantity $x$ increases and another either says that quantity $x$ decreases (opposite) or says that quantity $y$ increases (parallel), then those answer choices would fall into the same family. An answer choice that doesn't match the construction of the answer choice family is more likely to be incorrect. Most questions will not have answer choice families, but when they do appear, you should be prepared to recognize them.

### ⊘ Eliminate Answers

Eliminate answer choices as soon as you realize they are wrong, but make sure you consider all possibilities. If you are eliminating answer choices and realize that the last one you are left with is also wrong, don't panic. Start over and consider each choice again. There may be something you missed the first time that you will realize on the second pass.

### ⊘ Avoid Fact Traps

Don't be distracted by an answer choice that is factually true but doesn't answer the question. You are looking for the choice that answers the question. Stay focused on what the question is asking for so you don't accidentally pick an answer that is true but incorrect. Always go back to the question and make sure the answer choice you've selected actually answers the question and is not merely a true statement.

### ⊘ Extreme Statements

In general, you should avoid answers that put forth extreme actions as standard practice or proclaim controversial ideas as established fact. An answer choice that states the "process should be used in certain situations, if…" is much more likely to be correct than one that states the "process should be discontinued completely." The first is a calm rational statement and doesn't even make a definitive, uncompromising stance, using a hedge word *if* to provide wiggle room, whereas the second choice is far more extreme.

### ⊘ Benchmark

As you read through the answer choices and you come across one that seems to answer the question well, mentally select that answer choice. This is not your final answer, but it's the one that will help you evaluate the other answer choices. The one that you selected is your benchmark or standard for judging each of the other answer choices. Every other answer choice must be compared to your benchmark. That choice is correct until proven otherwise by another answer choice beating it. If you find a better answer, then that one becomes your new benchmark. Once you've decided that no other choice answers the question as well as your benchmark, you have your final answer.

### ⊘ Predict the Answer

Before you even start looking at the answer choices, it is often best to try to predict the answer. When you come up with the answer on your own, it is easier to avoid distractions and traps because you will know exactly what to look for. The right answer choice is unlikely to be word-for-word what you came up with, but it should be a close match. Even if you are confident that you have the right answer, you should still take the time to read each option before moving on.

## General Strategies

### ⊘ Tough Questions

If you are stumped on a problem or it appears too hard or too difficult, don't waste time. Move on! Remember though, if you can quickly check for obviously incorrect answer choices, your chances of guessing correctly are greatly improved. Before you completely give up, at least try to knock out a couple of possible answers. Eliminate what you can and then guess at the remaining answer choices before moving on.

### ⊘ Check Your Work

Since you will probably not know every term listed and the answer to every question, it is important that you get credit for the ones that you do know. Don't miss any questions through careless mistakes. If at all possible, try to take a second to look back over your answer selection and make sure you've selected the correct answer choice and haven't made a costly careless mistake (such as marking an answer choice that you didn't mean to mark). This quick double check should more than pay for itself in caught mistakes for the time it costs.

### ⊘ Pace Yourself

It's easy to be overwhelmed when you're looking at a page full of questions; your mind is confused and full of random thoughts, and the clock is ticking down faster than you would like. Calm down and maintain the pace that you have set for yourself. Especially as you get down to the last few minutes of the test, don't let the small numbers on the clock make you panic. As long as you are on track by monitoring your pace, you are guaranteed to have time for each question.

### ⊘ Don't Rush

It is very easy to make errors when you are in a hurry. Maintaining a fast pace in answering questions is pointless if it makes you miss questions that you would have gotten right otherwise. Test writers like to include distracting information and wrong answers that seem right. Taking a little extra time to avoid careless mistakes can make all the difference in your test score. Find a pace that allows you to be confident in the answers that you select.

### ✓ Keep Moving

Panicking will not help you pass the test, so do your best to stay calm and keep moving. Taking deep breaths and going through the answer elimination steps you practiced can help to break through a stress barrier and keep your pace.

## Final Notes

The combination of a solid foundation of content knowledge and the confidence that comes from practicing your plan for applying that knowledge is the key to maximizing your performance on test day. As your foundation of content knowledge is built up and strengthened, you'll find that the strategies included in this chapter become more and more effective in helping you quickly sift through the distractions and traps of the test to isolate the correct answer.

Now that you're preparing to move forward into the test content chapters of this book, be sure to keep your goal in mind. As you read, think about how you will be able to apply this information on the test. If you've already seen sample questions for the test and you have an idea of the question format and style, try to come up with questions of your own that you can answer based on what you're reading. This will give you valuable practice applying your knowledge in the same ways you can expect to on test day.

**Good luck and good studying!**

# Assessment and Diagnosis

## Anatomy, Physiology, and Pathophysiology

### Aneurysms

An **aneurysm** is defined as a localized, blood-filled dilation of a blood vessel (artery or vein) caused by cardiac disease or weakening of the blood vessel wall. Aneurysms most commonly occur within the intracranial vessels but are also found along the thoracic aorta, abdominal aorta, and in vessels of the extremities.

Aneurysms typically occur in elderly patients but can present in patients of any age group. However, aneurysms are uncommon in individuals under 20 years of age. The risk of aneurysm increases with age and is most likely to occur in individuals between the ages of 50 and 80.

Aneurysms are more common in Caucasian patients than individuals of other ethnicities. Typically, men develop aneurysms more often than women. However, women with aneurysms have a significantly higher risk of rupture than men.

Approximately 15,000 individuals in the United States die each year from **ruptured aneurysms**. Ruptured aneurysms are the 10th leading cause of death in men over age 50 in the United States.

A **peripheral aneurysm** is more likely to affect individuals aged 60–80.

**Cerebral aneurysms** are more likely to occur in people aged 35–60. Approximately 0.2–3% of individuals in the United States with a brain aneurysm suffer from hemorrhage per year, with 10–15% of these individuals dying prior to obtaining care and over 50% dying within the first month post rupture. Approximately half of patients surviving a rupture suffer from permanent neurological damage.

**Abdominal aortic aneurysms** are four times more common in men than in women and are most prevalent in Caucasians aged 40–70. Less than 50% of individuals with a ruptured abdominal aortic aneurysm survive.

#### *Symptoms*

Typically, aneurysms are asymptomatic until they grow large enough to cause symptoms. **Associated symptoms** vary by location of the aneurysm. Aneurysms located closer to the surface of the body may present with swelling and pain; however, most aneurysms within the body are asymptomatic.

- Aneurysms in the **brain** can present with symptoms of localized severe headache, intense pressure, nausea and vomiting, neck pain, blurred or double vision, pain in or around the eye, dilated pupils, sensitivity to light, and loss of sensation.
- Aneurysms in the **abdomen** may present with a deep, dull, penetrating pain in the lower back or abdomen that lasts for hours to days.
- Signs and symptoms of a **peripheral** aneurysm may include leg or arm cramping, coldness, and numbness or tingling in the feet due to blocked blood flow to the peripheral arteries.

### *Risk Factors*

**Risk factors** that can potentially lead to aneurysm formation include the following:

- **Smoking** is a strong risk factor for the development of an aneurysm, with risk increasing according to the number of pack years.
- **Increased blood pressure** and **atherosclerosis** are also risk factors for aneurysms due to increased pressure within the blood vessels and damage to blood vessel walls.
- **Genetic disorders**, including Marfan syndrome, can lead to aneurysm formation, as the disease affects connective tissue throughout the body, including the tissues of the blood vessels.
- Another risk factor is a **family history** of aneurysms. Individuals with a family history of aneurysms typically develop aneurysms at an earlier age and should be monitored by a specialist.
- Additional risk factors include obesity, head or body trauma, alcohol consumption, use of oral contraceptives, tuberculosis, untreated syphilis, vasculitis, Caucasian ethnicity, and male gender.

### *Diagnosis*

**Physical examination** sometimes suggests aneurysms. For example, a pulsating abdominal mass suggests an aneurysm of the abdominal aorta. Medical imaging is used for definitive diagnosis, including chest x-ray, ultrasound, magnetic resonance imaging (MRI), angiography, and computer tomography (CT) scan. Aneurysms are often incidentally found while imaging a patient for other reasons.

Patients at high risk for aneurysms should be followed regularly by a cardiothoracic, vascular, or neurological surgeon. Current guideline recommendations suggest that men who are 65–75 years old and are ex-smokers should be checked for aneurysms routinely. Men aged 60 and older with a family history of aneurysms should also consider routine screening.

### *Clinical Manifestations of Ruptured Aneurysms*

Aneurysm rupture can lead to complications such as sudden death, stroke, and brain damage. **Signs and symptoms of aneurysm rupture** include hypotension, rapid heartbeat, lightheadedness, fainting, nausea, vomiting, sweating, shortness of breath, chest pain, lower back/abdominal pain, and dizziness. The risk of death is high with aneurysm rupture, except for rupture in the extremities. Also, the risk of rupture increases as the blood vessel dilation increases.

Another complication of aneurysms is the risk of blood clots. The occlusion of blood flow can lead to complications such as brain damage, lack of peripheral blood flow to end organ systems or extremities, and sudden death. Blood clots can also dislodge from the site of origin and cause the above complications.

### *Abdominal Aortic Aneurysms*

Most **aortic aneurysms** are asymptomatic, making early detection more difficult. If the patient presents with symptoms, the most common will be dull pain, deep within the abdominal cavity and radiating into the back. The pain may be alleviated or eased by change of position. The other noticeable symptom that might be detected by the patient or medical personnel is a palpable, abnormal pulsation within the abdominal cavity. Identification of the aneurysm is made with ultrasound or CT scan. Surgical repair is the primary route of treatment. When the aneurysm is small enough that it doesn't require surgery, treatment focuses on preventing growth or rupture through smoking cessation and controlling blood pressure and cholesterol levels, while monitoring the aneurysm size every 6–12 months.

## Atherosclerosis

**Atherosclerosis** is a disease caused by the formation of plaque in the walls of arteries. Plaque formation is caused by a chronic inflammatory response and endothelial dysfunction where lipids, cholesterol, calcium, and other substances build up in the arteries. There is an imbalance between deposition of plaque and removal by low-density lipoproteins in smooth muscle cells. Two types of plaque can form in the arteries, including stable plaques and unstable plaques:

- **Stable plaques** consist of a thick fibrous cap of smooth muscle cells that, upon stimulation, can lead to reduced blood flow to heart, lung, and other organ systems.
- **Unstable plaques** consist of a thin fibrous cap of smooth muscle cells that can rupture, leading to a heart attack and/or stroke.

The disease can affect arteries in the heart, brain, lungs, and extremities. Therefore, based on the origin of the condition, atherosclerosis can be referred to as coronary heart disease when present in coronary arteries, carotid artery disease when present in the carotid artery, and peripheral arterial disease when present in the arteries supplying the extremities.

### *Incidence, Prevalence, and Mortality*

In the United States, more than 11 million Americans have atherosclerosis. Atherosclerosis is the leading cause of coronary heart disease and stroke, with the disease responsible for more than half of annual deaths. Over 1 million individuals in the United States annually are diagnosed with coronary artery disease, and nearly 700,000 individuals suffer a stroke.

Atherosclerosis is a condition that develops over time, presenting symptoms in patients between the ages of 40 and 70 due to hardening of plaques, vascular remodeling, blood flow abnormalities, and diminished oxygen flow to end organ systems. Patients between the ages of 50 and 60 typically present with advanced complications of the condition as well as organ system dysfunction.

Individuals with an **increased risk** of atherosclerosis include men and patients with a family history of cardiovascular disease. The lower prevalence of atherosclerosis in women may be due to the protective effects of estrogen and progesterone. However, this hormonal protective effect has been shown to decrease after menopause, unless the individual is undergoing hormone replacement therapy.

### *Symptoms*

Typically, atherosclerosis is asymptomatic until plaques grow large enough to cause symptoms or rupture. The disease typically progresses slowly over time, and the symptoms vary by location of the condition. The most common site of atherosclerotic formation is the lower abdominal aorta. Other sites include coronary arteries, popliteal arteries, descending thoracic aorta, internal carotid arteries, and other vessels.

**Common symptoms** include chest pain, peripheral pain, weakness, numbness, shortness of breath, dizziness, intermittent claudication, and erectile dysfunction in men. Specifically, individuals presenting with obstruction to coronary arteries experience chest pain, weakness, and fatigue. Individuals who present with obstruction of carotid arteries may experience weakness, numbness, and dizziness. Obstruction of peripheral arteries to extremities may result in intermittent claudication.

### *Risk Factors and Complications*

Factors that can increase an individual's **risk** for atherosclerosis include elevated low-density lipoprotein (LDL) cholesterol, decreased high-density lipoprotein (HDL) cholesterol, elevated triglyceride levels, menopause, lack of physical activity, obesity, infection of the vascular smooth muscle cells, high blood pressure, history of smoking, and diabetes.

Smoking not only predisposes individuals to atherosclerosis, but it also increases the progression of the disease. The progression of atherosclerosis itself also further increases the extent and degree of the condition, as further accumulation of lipids, cholesterol, and other substances stimulates the endothelium to produce other substances that cause increased plaque buildup.

Atherosclerosis leads to altered vascular function including coronary heart disease, myocardial ischemia and myocardial infarction, cerebrovascular insufficiency, stroke, peripheral vascular disease, limb ischemia, renal disease, aortic aneurysm, and vasculitis. The final mechanism of the above complications usually occurs via plaque rupture or severe vessel narrowing and blood clotting.

### *Screening and Diagnosis*

**Physical examination** often hints at atherosclerosis, but further blood testing and medical imaging is needed for diagnosis. For example, a bruit heard over the carotid artery or abdomen is suggestive of atherosclerosis in the carotids or abdominal aorta. Hairless legs are suggestive of peripheral atherosclerosis. Initial blood tests showing elevated low-density lipoprotein (LDL) cholesterol, low high-density lipoprotein (HDL) cholesterol, and elevated triglycerides also suggest it. Diagnostic tools used to determine the presence of plaque formation include electrocardiogram, exercise stress test, echocardiogram, nuclear scan, coronary angiography, electron beam computed tomography, coronary computed tomography (CT) angiography, and magnetic resonance angiography.

**Screening** for atherosclerosis includes annual blood tests in patients over 20 years of age with a history of cardiovascular disease. Patients 20 years or older should have cholesterol levels checked every 5 years, including LDL cholesterol, HDL cholesterol, and triglycerides.

Assessment of other atherosclerosis risk factors should be done as well, including modifiable risk factors such as smoking, uncontrolled diabetes, and obesity as well as unmodifiable risk factors such as family history and aging. Individuals with multiple risk factors should be followed on a more regular basis than every 5 years.

## Buerger's Disease

**Buerger's disease**, also known as *Thromboangiitis obliterans*, is a rare condition resulting in impaired blood flow to extremities due to clot formation and inflammation in peripheral arteries and veins. The disease typically progresses from the hands and feet and extends to arms and legs.

The disease is more common in men than in women and typically occurs between 20 and 45 years of age. However, women over the age of 50 have more recently been diagnosed with the condition. The disease is most common in East Asia and the Middle East and is rare in the Americas.

Complications of the disease include ulcerations, infections, and gangrene, which result from tissue damage.

### *Risk Factors, Symptoms, and Complications*

The main **risk factor** for Buerger's disease is smoking. The onset of Buerger's disease is dependent on the degree and extent of cigarette smoking. Nearly all cases of Buerger's disease occur in patients who are current smokers or tobacco users, previous smokers or tobacco users, or were exposed to smoke for an extended period.

**Symptoms** of Buerger's disease include pain and weakness in extremities, swelling of the hands and feet, Raynaud's phenomenon, and open sores on digits.

**Complications** of Buerger's disease include gangrene in digits and infection of the hands and feet as well as amputation of digits/extremities. Symptoms associated with gangrene include black or blue digits, numbness or tingling in digits, and foul smell from the infected area.

### *Diagnosis and Screening*

**Physical examination**, specifically distal ischemia and ulcerations, suggests Buerger's disease, especially in a male smoker under 45 years old. A positive Allen test also suggests the disorder. Blood tests are useful to rule out other etiologies. However, there are currently no definitive tests available to diagnose the disease, and diagnosis is based on a process of elimination.

**Diagnostic screening tools** used to aid in the diagnosis of Buerger's disease include blood tests to rule out scleroderma, lupus, diabetes and other blood clotting conditions. The Allen test is used to assess blood flow to the hands and feet. Angiography, ultrasound, and echocardiography can be used to assess vascular flow.

The most commonly used **criteria for the diagnosis** of Buerger's disease include an age younger than 45, past or present tobacco use, presence of distal extremity ischemia (ischemic ulcers and gangrene), exclusion of autoimmune disorders, and consistent angiographic findings in extremities.

## Raynaud's Phenomenon

**Raynaud's phenomenon** is a condition where an individual's fingers and toes become discolored, pale, numb, and/or cold due to exposure to changes in temperature or emotional stress. Typical color changes are white, blue, and then red. The symptoms of Raynaud's syndrome occur due to the mechanism of action, where the small arteries carrying blood to the digits constrict and spasm. Thus, oxygen-rich blood is denied to the distal extremities, and this causes the corresponding symptoms.

Raynaud's phenomenon is used to describe two conditions: 1) Raynaud's disease, also known as primary Raynaud's phenomenon, and 2) Raynaud's syndrome, also known as secondary Raynaud's phenomenon, where the condition is secondary to another comorbid disease.

Recent data has shown that Raynaud's syndrome is more common in women than men. Symptoms of Raynaud's syndrome typically present within the 4th decade of life, whereas symptoms of Raynaud's disease occur earlier in life.

### *Primary and Secondary Raynaud's Phenomenon*

**Primary Raynaud's** or Raynaud's disease is typically an inherited condition, exacerbated by smoking, with a hormonal component.

However, **Raynaud's syndrome, or secondary Raynaud's**, is associated with numerous environmental factors and diseases. Those most often associated include scleroderma, lupus, rheumatoid arthritis, eating disorders, atherosclerosis, Buerger's disease, and drugs such as beta-blockers, cytotoxins, cyclosporin, ergotamine, or sulfasalazine. Additionally, occupational hazards including exposure to vibrating equipment, vinyl chloride, and cold as well as other comorbid conditions like hypothyroidism, cryoglobulinemia, cancer, and reflex sympathetic dystrophy have also been associated with secondary Raynaud's phenomenon.

### *Risk Factors*

The exact **cause** of Raynaud's disease and Raynaud's syndrome is unknown. In this phenomenon, blood vessels in the digits overreact to cold temperatures or stress.

**Risk factors of primary Raynaud's disease** include sex, age, residing in colder climates, and family history. Women tend to present with primary Raynaud's phenomenon more often than men. Also, individuals aged 15–25 present with primary Raynaud's disease more often than individuals in other age groups. Additionally, individuals who live in colder climates and have a family history of the phenomenon also present more frequently with primary Raynaud's disease.

The **risk factors for secondary Raynaud's syndrome** include patients with underlying comorbid conditions such as lupus and diabetes as well as individuals who operate machinery for their occupation.

### *Symptoms*

Patients with either primary or secondary Raynaud's phenomenon present with painful, pale, discolored, and/or cold digits. Patients may also experience numbness or tingling as well as dull sensory perception in response to cold or stress.

Primary Raynaud's phenomenon, or Raynaud's disease, is considered systemic, whereas secondary Raynaud's phenomenon typically only presents in the extremities. Patients with secondary Raynaud's phenomenon also experience symptoms of the comorbid condition when experiencing Raynaud's symptoms. The symptoms of the phenomenon depend on the extent and degree of vasospasm the individual is experiencing.

For the most part, Raynaud's phenomenon mainly affects the digits, but it can also cause symptoms in other areas of the body including the nose, nipples, lips, and ears. Also, the phenomenon may not always affect the same digits or areas of the body. The phenomenon can occur for short or long durations, ranging from minutes to several hours.

### *Diagnosis and Screening*

**Physical examination and diagnostic screening** are typically used to diagnose both Raynaud's disease and Raynaud's syndrome, as no single test is available to diagnose these disorders.

Although clinical practitioners can easily diagnose Raynaud's phenomenon by the signs and symptoms patients present with (cold extremities with color changes onset by cold or stress), it remains difficult to determine if the phenomenon is primary or secondary. In order to distinguish between Raynaud's disease and Raynaud's syndrome, a nail fold capillaroscopy is typically performed. Distorted or fewer capillaries than normal suggests secondary Raynaud's. Diagnostic measurement of hand temperature gradients, digital artery pressure measurements, Doppler ultrasound, blood counts, and measurement of urea and electrolyte levels are other tools used to distinguish between primary and secondary forms of the phenomenon. Additionally, blood tests to assess for secondary disorders like lupus or hypothyroidism are helpful.

#### *Complications and Prognosis*

**Raynaud's phenomenon** is typically not severe, but it can lead to digit deformity due to lack of proper oxygenation and blood flow to digits. Other complications include skin ulcers, infection, and gangrene. Patients with Raynaud's phenomenon should address any cuts or scrapes in the affected areas to prevent infection. A clinical practitioner should address any cuts or scrapes that do not heal properly or in a timely manner. In severe cases of Raynaud's phenomenon, patients may have to undergo surgery and/or have digits amputated.

In terms of prognosis, primary Raynaud's phenomenon is rarely life-threatening; rather, it is more often annoying and a cause of discomfort. Over time, with proper management and care, the phenomenon typically improves. However, secondary Raynaud's phenomenon may be a sign of a rheumatic condition and should be monitored closely by a specialist.

### Cardiomyopathy

**Cardiomyopathy** is defined as deterioration of myocardium function. The World Health Organization categorizes cardiomyopathy into two categories: extrinsic cardiomyopathy and intrinsic cardiomyopathy. Cardiomyopathies are considered extrinsic if their primary pathology is outside the myocardium. However, intrinsic cardiomyopathies are either secondary to genetic, infectious, or idiopathic.

Cardiomyopathy can also be classified as primary or secondary. **Primary** cardiomyopathy is idiopathic in nature, whereas **secondary** cardiomyopathies can be attributed to a specific cause such as high blood pressure, heart valve disease, or coronary heart disease.

#### *Causes*

Factors that increase **risk of cardiomyopathy** include ischemic damage to the heart musculature from a heart attack, hypertension, gene mutation, and/or viral infection. However, in some cases, the actual cause of cardiomyopathy remains unknown.

In terms of the specific **subtypes of cardiomyopathies**, dilated cardiomyopathy can be inherited but also can be caused by coronary heart disease, heart attacks, infections, alcohol consumption, pregnancy complications, toxins, certain drugs such as amphetamines, or other diseases such as diabetes or thyroid disease. Hypertrophic cardiomyopathy can also be inherited but can be caused by high blood pressure or natural aging. Restrictive cardiomyopathy can be caused by hemochromatosis, amyloidosis, sarcoidosis, and connective tissue disorders.

#### *Sub-Types*

More specific **subtypes of cardiomyopathies** include dilated cardiomyopathy, hypertrophic cardiomyopathy, restrictive cardiomyopathy, and arrhythmogenic right ventricular dysplasia:

- **Dilated cardiomyopathy** is the most common type of cardiomyopathy. It presents most often in individuals aged 20–60 years, with the condition more common in men than women.
- **Hypertrophic cardiomyopathy** can occur at any age and occurs due to abnormal thickening of cardiac muscle. Hypertrophic cardiomyopathy consists of two types of disease: obstructive and nonobstructive. Both types lead to thickening of cardiac muscle that, in turn, reduces the size of the left ventricle.
- **Restrictive cardiomyopathy** tends to affect elderly patients. It occurs because the ventricles become thick due to abnormal tissue growth that replaces cardiac tissue, reducing blood flow and proper cardiac muscle function.

- **Arrhythmogenic right ventricular dysplasia** is a rare cardiomyopathy that typically affects young adults. It is the leading cause of sudden death in young athletes. The disease presents due to formation of scar tissue in the right ventricle, which can lead to arrhythmias.

### *Diagnosis and Screening*

**Physical examination and diagnostic screening tools** are typically used to diagnose cardiomyopathies. However, cardiomyopathies are typically found when assessing other conditions or during routine examinations.

Hypertension is a **risk factor** for cardiomyopathy and can be diagnosed by measurement of blood pressure. **Symptoms** of high blood pressure include headaches, fatigue, dizziness, blurred vision, nausea and vomiting, facial flushing, or tinnitus.

Cardiomyopathy diagnostic tools include chest x-ray to determine if the heart is enlarged, echocardiogram to assess the size and motion of the heart, electrocardiogram to determine the presence of electrical disturbances, and blood tests to assess BNP levels. Thyroid levels and serum iron counts are also helpful. Clinical practitioners may also perform cardiac stress testing to assess cardiac muscle function as well as electrical activity when the heart is under physical stress. MRI and PET scans may also be used to evaluate cardiac structures, rhythm, and chemical activity in different areas of the heart. Other more invasive diagnostic techniques include cardiac angiography and biopsy.

### *Risk Factors*

Natural aging is an independent **risk factor** for cardiomyopathy. However, certain types of cardiomyopathies are more prevalent in certain age and ethnic groups. Men and individuals of African American descent are at increased risk for dilated cardiomyopathy as compared to women and individuals of Caucasian descent. Also, young adults are more prone to arrhythmogenic right ventricular dysplasia as compared to elderly individuals.

Other risk factors include family history of cardiomyopathy, congestive heart failure, and sudden cardiac death. The presence of other comorbid conditions includes coronary heart disease, diabetes, metabolic disorders, alcohol abuse, and high blood pressure.

### *Symptoms*

Typically, cardiomyopathies are asymptomatic until they inhibit blood flow or restrict cardiac muscle contraction. They also vary by type of cardiomyopathy. With progression of disease, symptoms include fatigue, weakness, shortness of breath with exertion, swelling of abdomen and extremities, dizziness, fainting, and palpitations. These symptoms tend to get worse as the degree and extent of disease progresses. However, the time to progression varies from patient to patient and ranges from sudden attack to a slow progression.

### *Complications and Prognosis*

The prognosis of **cardiomyopathy** varies by the type and extent of disease. Current treatments reduce symptoms and complications of the disease. However, in some patients the disease can progress rapidly and result in serious complications such as heart attack and death.

The complications of cardiomyopathy include congestive heart failure, arrhythmias, heart murmur, endocarditis, cardiac arrest, and sudden death. Blood clots may also occur, which can lead to heart attacks and strokes. Patients need to be aware of these complications and manage these risks effectively with self-care, proper pharmacologic regimens, and clinical follow-up on a regular basis.

## Congestive Heart Failure

**Congestive heart failure** is a condition in which the heart is unable to pump adequate oxygenated blood throughout the body.

Congestive heart failure is caused by diseases that weaken or stiffen cardiac muscle. It can also be caused by diseases that increase oxygen demand, which the heart is unable to support.

The **prevalence** of congestive heart failure is approximately 5 million individuals in the United States, with half a million cases diagnosed each year and approximately 300,000 deaths per year. An important prognostic factor associated with congestive heart failure is the development of arrhythmias. Mortality due to congestive heart failure can be attributed to arrhythmias in 50% of patients and progressive heart failure in another 50% of patients. Congestive heart failure is prevalent in individuals 65 years of age and older. It is also prevalent among African Americans, obese individuals, and individuals with type II diabetes. Congestive heart failure is more prevalent among men than women.

### *Diagnosis and Screening*

Physical examination and diagnostic screening tools are typically used in addition to symptoms to **screen for congestive heart failure**. However, congestive heart failure is typically found when assessing other conditions or during routine examinations.

During **physical examination**, practicing clinicians aim to uncover excess fluid in the lungs, heart, liver, or other end organ systems as well as to estimate the level of cardiac function.

Congestive heart failure **diagnostic tools** include chest x-ray to determine if the heart is enlarged, echocardiogram to assess the size and motion of the heart, electrocardiogram to determine the presence of electrical disturbances, and blood tests to assess BNP levels, thyroid levels, and iron counts. Clinical practitioners may also perform cardiac stress testing to assess cardiac muscle function as well as electrical activity when the heart is under physical stress. MRI and PET scans may also be used to evaluate cardiac structures, rhythm, and chemical activity in different areas of the heart. Occasionally, a biopsy of the myocardium is necessary.

### *Risk Factors*

Factors that can lead to congestive heart failure include heart muscle weakness, systolic dysfunction, heart valve disorders, viral infections, thyroid disorders, and arrhythmias. The most common causes of congestive heart failure include hypertension and coronary artery disease.

Other **risk factors** include a family history of congestive heart failure, presence of other comorbid conditions including previous heart attack, diabetes, metabolic disorders, and alcohol consumption.

Additional factors that can contribute to the progression of congestive heart failure include the use of pharmacologic agents such as NSAIDs, corticosteroids, calcium channel blockers, and diabetic agents.

### *Symptoms*

Congestive heart failure can be asymptomatic until later stages of the disease. However, some patients may present with fatigue and muscle weakness during earlier stages of the disease.

**Symptoms** vary among patients and are based on end organ system involvement. With progression of disease, symptoms may include fatigue, weakness, shortness of breath after exertion, swelling of abdomen and extremities, dizziness, fainting, arrhythmias, increased urination, decreased appetite, nausea, and palpitations. These symptoms tend to get worse as the degree and extent of disease progresses. However, the time to progression varies from patient to patient and ranges from sudden onset to a slow progression.

## Chronic Heart Failure

### *Priority Nursing Diagnoses and Best Practices*

Potential **nursing diagnoses for CHF** include decreased cardiac output, excess fluid volume, activity intolerance, deficient knowledge, risk for impaired gas exchange, and impaired skin integrity.

Medical treatment is a careful balancing act between medications, lifestyle adaptations, and surgical interventions.

Medication choices might include angiotensin-converting enzyme (ACE) inhibitors to lower blood pressure and improve blood flow. Other options might include angiotensin II receptor blockers and beta-blockers. Diuretics may be used to try and maintain proper fluid balances and improve lung perfusion. If diuretics are used, carefully monitor the patient's electrolytes as well as blood pressure.

Other areas to monitor include oxygen saturation levels and activity tolerance. Education efforts and long-term planning might include energy conservation, diet, and cardiac rehabilitation to increase activity tolerance levels.

Surgical procedures might include coronary bypass to relieve severely blocked arteries, heart valve surgery, pacemaker placement, implantable cardioverter-defibrillators (ICD), or ventricular assist devices (pumps).

### *Physical Signs and Symptoms*

Key identifiers for many cardiovascular disorders are the presence of cyanosis (peripheral and central) and pallor. This, combined with shortness of breath related to position (supine) and exertion, fatigue, fluid retention and swelling, changes in heart rate, weight gain, and wheezing and/or productive cough (white or pink fluid) all suggest the presence of congestive heart failure (CHF).

Treatment priorities include oxygenation and fluid reduction with diuretics. Other priorities, depending on individual patient needs, might include anxiety reduction and blood pressure reduction.

### *Complications and Prognosis*

**Complications of congestive heart failure** include end organ system dysfunction such as renal failure, pulmonary edema, liver dysfunction due to fluid buildup, and insufficient absorption of nutrients and pharmacologic agents by the small intestines.

Congestive heart failure is typically a progressive disease. The prognosis of the disease varies by the degree and extent of progression. Current treatments reduce symptoms and complications of the disease. However, in some patients the disease can progress rapidly, while in others the disease can become chronically maintained.

Factors that determine prognosis include underlying comorbid conditions, symptoms, response to pharmacologic management, and degree and severity of the end organ system involvement.

## Cor Pulmonale

By definition, **cor pulmonale** is failure of the right heart not caused by and unrelated to left heart failure. Cor pulmonale is a disease that affects the structure and function of the right ventricle due to respiratory system abnormalities such as prolonged pulmonary hypertension. Pathophysiologic mechanisms that can lead to cor pulmonale include pulmonary vasoconstriction, compromise of vascular bed due to lung disease such as emphysema and interstitial lung disease, increased blood viscosity due to diseases like sickle cell anemia, and primary pulmonary hypertension. The disease can present as a chronically evolving condition but can also occur acutely due to pulmonary embolism or acute respiratory distress syndrome. In the United States, the prevalence of cor pulmonale associated with adult-onset cardiac disease is approximately 6–7%. Nearly half of these cases are due to underlying chronic bronchitis, chronic obstructive pulmonary disease, or emphysema. Acute pulmonary embolism is the most common cause of death in patients with cor pulmonale. Of the 50,000 patients that die of acute pulmonary embolism in the United States, nearly half are associated with cor pulmonale. Of those patients with chronically evolving disease due to chronic obstructive pulmonary disease, 30% have a chance of surviving for 5 years.

### *Diagnosis and Screening*

**Physical examination and diagnostic screening** tools are typically used to diagnose cor pulmonale. Patients typically present with a bluish hue to their skin as well as distension of the neck veins caused by elevated right side heart pressures. Other indicators of the disease include abnormal fluid collection in the abdomen, liver enlargement, increased chest diameter, prominent A or V waves, cyanosis, ankle and foot swelling, and abnormal heart sounds.

Diagnostic tools used to diagnose the disease include echocardiogram, chest x-ray, CT scan, pulmonary angiography, magnetic resonance imaging, ECG-gated CT scanning, pulmonary function tests, ventilation/perfusion lung scans, arterial blood gas measurements, antibody testing, and brain natriuretic peptide measurements. Additionally, more invasive diagnostic approaches include Swan-Ganz catheterization and lung biopsy.

### *Causes*

Cor pulmonale is **caused** by any condition that leads to prolonged pulmonary hypertension and can occur secondary to an array of cardiopulmonary diseases. Chronic pulmonary diseases that can put patients at a predisposition for cor pulmonale include COPD, obstructive sleep apnea, central sleep apnea, cystic fibrosis, primary pulmonary hypertension, pneumoconiosis, kyphoscoliosis, interstitial lung disease, chronic thromboembolic pulmonary disease, pulmonary vascular disease, and pulmonary hypertension.

- **Acute causes** of cor pulmonale include massive pulmonary embolization and exacerbation of chronic cor pulmonale.
- **Chronic causes** of cor pulmonale include COPD, loss of lung tissue due to trauma or surgery, Pierre Robin sequence, and end stage pneumoconiosis.

Cor pulmonale is caused by several mechanisms, including pulmonary vasoconstriction, anatomic changes in vascularization, increased blood viscosity, and idiopathic or primary pulmonary hypertension.

### *Symptoms*

The **symptoms** associated with cor pulmonale are typically nonspecific and can be associated with a variety of cardiopulmonary diseases. The symptoms of the disease also depend on whether the disease presents chronically or acutely due to pulmonary embolism or acute respiratory distress syndrome.

The symptoms of cor pulmonale include shortness of breath, coughing, wheezing, swelling of feet and ankles, fluid retention, exercise intolerance, tachypnea, hemoptysis, labored respiratory efforts with retractions of chest wall, hoarseness, and chest pain or discomfort. Additionally, neurological symptoms may occur due to decreased cardiac output and hypoxemia.

### *Complications and Prognosis*

The **prognosis of cor pulmonale** depends on the underlying cause of disease. The more severe the underlying cause, the greater the risk for complications, and the lower the chance of survival. The administration of supplemental oxygen is typically effective in increasing survival and improving quality of life.

**Complications** of cor pulmonale include severe fluid retention, life-threatening shortness of breath, shock, and/or death. Other complications include syncope, hypoxia, pedal edema, and/or hepatic congestion. Additionally, complications associated with underlying disease leading to cor pulmonale may arise.

## Type I, Type II, and Gestational Diabetes

**Diabetes mellitus** is a condition resulting in a high blood glucose level. The condition is caused by metabolic dysfunction due to either low levels of insulin or abnormal resistance to insulin combined with inadequate levels of insulin secretion.

- **Type I diabetes** is also known as juvenile diabetes or insulin dependent diabetes. It is a chronic metabolic disorder that results in high blood glucose levels due to low levels of insulin. In type I diabetes, the pancreas does not produce enough insulin, resulting in high blood glucose levels.
- **Type II diabetes** is also known as adult onset or noninsulin dependent diabetes. It is a chronic metabolic disorder that results in high blood glucose levels due to insulin resistance and/or low secretion of insulin. In type II diabetes, the body is resistant to insulin, which in turn results in high blood glucose levels. Early in the disease, insulin levels may actually be greater than normal, but eventually the beta cells in the pancreas "burn out" and insulin levels are lower than normal.
- **Gestational diabetes** is not a chronic condition and typically occurs during pregnancy and resolves upon birth. The condition results in high blood glucose levels due to low insulin secretion and responsiveness.

### *Incidence and Prevalence*

**Type I diabetes** occurs in approximately 10% of all cases of diabetes mellitus. The condition can affect both adults and children but is referred to as juvenile diabetes because it typically affects adolescents. The incidence of type I diabetes is approximately 15 cases per 100,000 individuals annually.

**Type II diabetes** is the most common type of diabetes mellitus, comprising approximately 90% of all cases of diabetes mellitus. Additionally, more than half of patients diagnosed with type II diabetes are obese. It is also more common in patients over 40 years of age but can occur in young adults and adolescents. It is also more prevalent in Hispanics, Native Americans, African Americans, and Asians/Pacific Islanders than in Caucasians.

**Gestational diabetes** occurs in approximately 2–5% of all pregnancies and is treatable with careful supervision throughout pregnancy. Of those women affected with gestational diabetes, approximately 20–50% develop type II diabetes.

### *Diagnosis and Screening*

The **diagnosis** of both type I and type II diabetes is suggested by physical examination, patient symptoms, and diagnostic tools. Type I diabetes diagnosis is suggested by thc sudden onset of symptoms. A fasting glucose greater than 126 mg/dL or random glucose greater than 200 mg/dL on two different occasions is diabetes. Age, family history, comorbidities, and demographics help suggest type I, II, or gestational diabetes. Additionally, C-peptide levels serve as a marker for insulin production. Elevated C-peptide suggests type II, and low C-peptide suggests type I.

The diagnosis of type II diabetes is typically made during ordinary health examinations, but diagnosis can be made by detection of hyperglycemia during other examinations or based on the presence of secondary symptoms such as fatigue or vision changes. In many cases, type II diabetes is not diagnosed until the patient experiences complications caused by the condition, including heart attack, neuropathy, vision problems, and/or foot ulcers. Diabetes screening tools include random blood glucose testing, fasting blood glucose testing, and more formal blood glucose tolerance testing. Other lab studies include urine glucose and ketones as well as renal function tests. Blood tests include glycated hemoglobin, islet cell antibodies, thyroid function tests, antithyroid antibodies, lipid levels, and antigliadin antibodies.

### *Causes and Risk Factors*

Individuals with type I diabetes typically have a genetic predisposition for the condition. Therefore, individuals with a parent or sibling with the disease have a higher risk for developing the condition. The causes and risk factors for type I diabetes are poorly understood, aside from some individuals having a predisposition for the disease.

It remains unclear why individuals develop type II diabetes, but the disease is associated with certain predisposing risk factors. Risk factors that increase the risk for developing type II diabetes include obesity, physical inactivity, family history, increasing age, prediabetes, and gestational diabetes. Also, individuals of African American, Hispanic, Native American, and Asian American descent are at higher risk for developing type II diabetes.

Medical conditions associated with a higher risk for developing type II diabetes include high blood pressure, elevated cholesterol levels, coronary artery disease, polycystic ovary syndrome, chronic pancreatitis, liver dysfunction, hemochromatosis, and cystic fibrosis.

### *Symptoms*

The **symptoms of type I diabetes** include increased thirst, frequent urination, extreme hunger, weight loss, fatigue, and blurred vision. Patients diagnosed with type I diabetes may also present with diabetic ketoacidosis, which may include altered mental status, coma, hyperventilation, and abdominal pain. The symptoms associated with type I diabetes tend to develop rapidly over a short period.

The **symptoms of type II diabetes** also include increased thirst, frequent urination, extreme hunger, weight loss, fatigue, and blurred vision. The condition also includes slow healing sores or frequent infections. Also, patients diagnosed with type II diabetes may present in a hyperosmolar nonketotic state. The symptoms associated with type II diabetes develop over time and may be mistaken for other conditions or go unrecognized.

### *PROGNOSIS AND COMPLICATIONS*

**Acute complications associated with type I and type II diabetes** include diabetic ketoacidosis (type I), nonketotic hyperosmolar coma (type II), hyperglycemia, and hypoglycemia. Acute complications need to be addressed immediately; otherwise, individuals are at risk for seizures and/or coma.

Other **long-term complications** include vascular disease, coronary artery disease, stroke, peripheral vascular disease, diabetic myonecrosis, diabetic retinopathy, diabetic neuropathy, osteoporosis, Alzheimer's disease, infections, foot ulcers, and diabetic nephropathy. In an effort to avoid these complications, patients need to comply with blood sugar management and control other environmental risk factors.

In an effort to prevent long-term complications, diabetic patients should undergo yearly physicals and eye examinations, get necessary immunizations, maintain teeth and feet, avoid stress, maintain proper cholesterol and blood pressure levels, and avoid smoking and/or tobacco use.

The **prognosis** of diabetes depends on the individual patient and the presence of other comorbid conditions. It also depends on an individual's compliance to lifestyle modifications and pharmacologic management.

## METABOLIC SYNDROME

**Metabolic syndrome** is defined as a group of risk factors that put individuals at risk for developing cardiovascular disease or other comorbid conditions such as diabetes. The risk of developing metabolic syndrome is closely linked to obesity, lack of physical activity, genetic factors, and poor diet.

Metabolic syndrome is also known as syndrome X, insulin resistance syndrome, dysmetabolic syndrome, hypertriglyceridemic waist, and obesity syndrome.

The **five risk factors** associated with metabolic syndrome include a large waistline, higher than normal triglyceride levels, lower than normal high-density lipoprotein cholesterol, hypertension, and hyperglycemia. An increased number of risk factors raises an individual's risk of developing complications such as cardiovascular disease, diabetes, and/or stroke.

### *NCEP/ATP III AND WHO GUIDELINE DEFINITIONS*

The **NCEP/ATP III (National Cholesterol Education Program/Adult Treatment Panel)** defines metabolic syndrome as an individual with three or more of the following risk factors: waist circumference equal to or greater than 102 cm in men and 88 cm in women, triglyceride levels greater than 150 mg/dL, high-density lipid cholesterol less than 40 mg/dL in men and less than 50 mg/dL in women, blood pressure greater than or equal to 130/85 mmHg, and fasting plasma glucose greater than 100 mg/dL.

The **World Health Organization (WHO)** defines metabolic syndrome as an individual with diabetes, impaired glucose tolerance (IGT), impaired fasting glucose (IFG) or insulin resistance, plus two or more of the following risk factors: body mass index greater than 30 kg/m$^2$ and/or waist-to-hip ratio greater than 0.9 in men and greater than 0.85 in women, triglyceride levels greater than 150 mg/dL and/or high-density lipid cholesterol less than 35 mg/dL in men and less than 39 mg/dL in women, blood pressure greater than or equal to 140/90 mmHg, and urinary albumin excretion greater than or equal to 20 μg/min or urinary albumin: creatinine ratio greater than or equal to 30 mg/g.

### Incidence and Prevalence

Approximately 47 million individuals have been diagnosed with metabolic syndrome in the United States. The **incidence** continues to increase annually, which can be attributed to increasing obesity rates within the United States.

The **prevalence** of metabolic syndrome in individuals greater than 20 years of age is more than 20%, increasing to over 40% in individuals greater than 60 years of age. Gender and ethnic descent affect the prevalence of metabolic syndrome. Mexican Americans have the highest rate of metabolic syndrome in the United States, followed by Caucasian Americans and African Americans.

### Causes and Risk Factors

The exact mechanisms that induce metabolic syndrome in some individuals remain unclear. The pathophysiology is very complex and poorly understood. However, several **risk factors** put some individuals at an increased risk of developing the condition. Risk factors associated with metabolic syndrome include obesity, lack of physical activity, dyslipidemia, history of familial diabetes, polycystic ovarian syndrome, insulin resistance, stress, aging, genetic factors, and hormonal changes.

While genetic factors and aging cannot be addressed, individuals can prevent obesity by maintaining proper weight with diet and exercise as well as managing other comorbid conditions.

Patients diagnosed with metabolic syndrome also typically form blood clots and present with constant low-grade inflammation throughout the body. Additional conditions that have been associated with metabolic syndrome include fatty liver, polycystic ovary syndrome, gallstones, and sleep apnea.

### Symptoms

The **symptoms** of metabolic syndrome present as a combination of other conditions. Therefore, the symptoms of metabolic syndrome are based on underlying conditions that define the condition, such as hypertension, diabetes, or high cholesterol.

Other comorbid conditions associated with metabolic syndrome include elevated uric acid levels, fatty liver disease, polycystic ovary syndrome, hemochromatosis, and acanthosis nigricans.

### Screening and Diagnosis

**Physical examination** and diagnostic tools are used to diagnose metabolic syndrome. Patients are diagnosed with metabolic syndrome if they have three or more of the following risk factors: abdominal obesity, higher than normal triglyceride levels, lower than normal high-density lipid cholesterol levels, hypertension, and hyperglycemia. Patients with one or more of the above symptoms should seek medical attention to prevent other complications or comorbid conditions.

Patients with type II diabetes should be screened for metabolic syndrome, as more than 80% of type II diabetes patients have comorbid metabolic syndrome and are at a higher risk for cardiovascular disease.

### Complications

The main **complication of metabolic syndrome** is cardiovascular disease such as coronary artery disease, congestive heart failure, heart attack, stroke, and sudden death. Another complication in patients diagnosed with metabolic syndrome, who have not already been diagnosed with diabetes, is the development of type II diabetes. Most patients diagnosed with metabolic syndrome have abdominal obesity, which puts them at a high predisposition for developing type II diabetes.

Patients diagnosed with metabolic syndrome who have comorbid type II diabetes are at a much higher risk for the development of cardiovascular disease.

Patients diagnosed with metabolic syndrome are also at an increased risk for blood clotting abnormalities and peripheral vascular disease.

## Endothelial Dysfunction

**Endothelial dysfunction** is defined as abnormal functioning of the cells forming the endothelium, the innermost lining of blood vessels. It is characterized by reduced vasodilation, increased proinflammatory response, and prothrombotic properties.

Patients with endothelial dysfunction typically **present** with an inability of arteries and veins to dilate properly or fully. Biochemical dysfunction of the endothelium leads to problems with coagulation, platelet adhesion, immune function, and electrolyte balance.

Individuals diagnosed with endothelial dysfunction are at a higher risk for developing cardiovascular disease as well as having a heart attack or stroke due to the presence of atherosclerosis. They are also at risk for developing the following comorbid complications, if not already present: congestive heart failure, chronic renal failure, peripheral artery disease, and diabetes. The prognosis of endothelial dysfunction is dependent on the degree and extent of the disease as well as the presence of other comorbid conditions.

### *Diagnosis, Screening, and Symptoms*

**Physical examination and comorbid conditions** suggest the condition, and diagnostic tools can be used to diagnose endothelial dysfunction. Patients with elevated risk for the disease, including those with diabetes and other cardiovascular risk factors, should be screened for the condition.

**Diagnostic screening** for endothelial dysfunction can be determined using the following methods: iontophoresis of acetylcholine, intra-arterial administration of vasoactive agents, localized heating of the skin, and temporary arterial occlusion via inflating a blood pressure cuff to high pressures. Another more invasive approach is intracoronary catheterization, but it is not often performed due to increased risk of complications.

## Hypertension

**Hypertension** is defined as high blood pressure chronically elevated at greater than or equal to 140/90 mmHg. Hypertension can be classified as primary hypertension or as a result of a comorbid condition and referred to as secondary hypertension. Secondary hypertension can be attributed to kidney disease, metabolic disorders, or cancer. Primary hypertension occurs in 90–95% of individuals diagnosed with high blood pressure, as compared to secondary hypertension, which occurs in 2–10%.

The **incidence and prevalence** of hypertension increase with natural aging. In the United States, more than 40 million individuals have been estimated to have hypertension. In the United States, the prevalence of hypertension tends to be higher in blacks and Hispanics as compared to Caucasians. Women under the age of 50 tend to have a lower risk of hypertension than men. However, women over the age of 50 have a higher risk of hypertension than men.

### *Diagnosis, Screening, and Symptoms*

Hypertension is typically **diagnosed** during routine physical examinations or when addressing other conditions or concerns. The only test used for diagnosis of hypertension is blood pressure measurement. However, blood pressure measurements need to be taken on a regular basis when persistent high blood pressure is a concern. Also, proper measurement is necessary for accurate diagnosis. If other cardiovascular complications are suspected, other testing including echocardiogram, urinalysis, CBC, serum electrolytes, serum creatine, serum glucose, and x-rays may be performed.

Most patients present with no **symptoms**, but some patients experience headaches, fatigue, dizziness, confusion, chest pain, irregular heartbeat, nosebleed, blurred vision, facial flushing, or tinnitus. Hypertension is sometimes misdiagnosed as stress and/or anxiety. Although stress and anxiety can contribute to elevated blood pressure, they cannot cause persistent hypertension.

### *Causes and Risk Factors*

**Primary hypertension** can be attributed to a variety of causes, including emotional stress, licorice toxicity, salt sensitivity, high renin levels, insulin resistance, sleep apnea, genetic factors, natural aging, and other factors. Individuals with a family member with primary hypertension are at an increased risk of developing the condition. Also, being of African American descent increases risk of hypertension compared to Caucasians.

**Secondary hypertension** can be attributed to renal disease, adrenal disease, Cushing syndrome, spinal misalignment, adrenal gland tumor, alcohol poisoning, anxiety, stress, pain, arteriosclerosis, obesity, pregnancy, hyperthyroidism, hypothyroidism, retroperitoneal fibrosis, oral contraceptives, antihypertensive medication withdrawal, and drugs such as NSAIDS.

### *Nursing Diagnoses and Best Practices*

Potential **nursing diagnoses for hypertension** might include decreased cardiac output, pain (headache), activity intolerance, ineffective coping, and knowledge deficits. Nursing care priorities should first focus on blood pressure (and related pain) control with medication. Initial treatment choices would include a combination of a thiazide diuretic and ACE inhibitor, beta-blocker, or calcium-channel blocker.

Further interventions should focus on careful monitoring to reduce risk of HTN-related cardiovascular emergencies; educational interventions to promote lifestyle changes including smoking cessation, diet, and exercise; and being a patient advocate to support patient decisions regarding care.

### *Complications and Prognosis*

Persistent hypertension is a risk factor for developing **complications** such as stroke, heart attack, congestive heart failure, aneurysm, aortic dissection, arteriosclerosis, vision loss, and chronic renal failure. Other complications include intracerebral hemorrhage, lacunar infarcts, congestive heart failure, angina, encephalopathy, myocardial infarction, cardiomyopathy, retinopathy, and nephropathy.

The **prognosis** of hypertension is associated with the blood pressure level and the presence of other comorbid conditions and complications. Untreated hypertension increases the risk of cardiovascular complications, end organ system failure, and mortality. Untreated mild to moderate hypertension, after 8–10 years post onset, has been shown to be associated with atherosclerotic disease in 30% of individuals and end organ system damage in 50% of individuals.

## Dyslipidemia

**Dyslipidemia** is a disorder of lipoprotein metabolism, including hyperlipidemia and hypolipidemia. Dyslipidemia can be classified as primary dyslipidemia or as a result of a comorbid condition and referred to as secondary dyslipidemia. The condition is typically characterized by elevations in total cholesterol, low-density lipoprotein cholesterol, triglyceride levels, and a decrease in high-density cholesterol levels.

Primary dyslipidemia is more prevalent among adolescents and children than in adults. Secondary dyslipidemia is the main type of dyslipidemia in adults. African Americans and Hispanic Americans are at greater risk for the development of dyslipidemia and cardiovascular complications as compared to Caucasian Americans.

### *Causes and Risk Factors*

The **causes** of dyslipidemia include genetic as well as environmental contributions.

In secondary dyslipidemia, increases in low-density lipoprotein levels can be caused by diabetes, hypothyroidism, nephrotic syndrome, obstructive liver disease, anabolic steroids, progestins, beta-adrenergic blockers, and thiazides. Increases in triglyceride levels can be caused by diabetes, hypothyroidism, obesity, renal insufficiency, beta-adrenergic blockers, bile acid binding resins, estrogens, and ticlopidine. Decreases in high-density lipoprotein levels can be caused by cigarette smoking, diabetes, hypertriglyceridemia, menopause, obesity, puberty, uremia, anabolic steroids, beta-adrenergic blockers, and progestins.

The **risk factors** associated with dyslipidemia that can lead to coronary heart disease include natural aging, male gender, family history of cardiovascular disease, cigarette smoking or tobacco use, hypertension, and diabetes.

### *Diagnostic and Screening Tools and Symptoms*

The **goal of dyslipidemia treatment** is to control lipid levels, decreasing low-density lipoprotein levels and triglyceride levels and increasing high-density lipoprotein levels, as well as to prevent the onset of cardiovascular diseases such as coronary artery disease, peripheral artery disease, heart attack, and stroke. Treatment algorithms involve lifestyle modifications and pharmacologic management.

Individuals prescribed lifestyle modifications and pharmacologic drugs should be monitored by a clinical practitioner on a regular basis. Also, lipid levels should be checked on a periodic basis after starting treatment in case the dose needs to be titrated.

### *Presentation of a Patient*

Individuals are typically diagnosed with dyslipidemia during routine physical examinations or when seeking medical attention for other complaints. Xanthelasma, or yellow streaks on the eyelids, and xanthomas, yellow nodules on tendons, can be suggestive. Diagnostic testing involves measurement of fasting serum lipid levels, including low-density lipoprotein levels, high-density lipoprotein levels, and triglyceride levels. Diagnostic tests for secondary causes of dyslipidemia should be performed, including fasting serum glucose level, liver enzymes, creatinine levels, thyroid-stimulating hormone, and urinalysis.

Dyslipidemia does not typically present with any specific symptoms unless associated with comorbid cardiovascular disease, including coronary artery disease or peripheral artery disease. Increased low-density lipoprotein levels may cause symptoms including vision problems and joint problems. Individuals with elevated triglyceride levels may present with vision and joint problems as well.

## Myocardial Infarction

**Myocardial infarction** is defined as the lack of blood flow to the heart caused by plaque rupture or blockage. Myocardial infarction is also known as heart attack or acute myocardial infarction.

In the United States, myocardial infarction and other cardiac ischemic conditions are the leading cause of mortality. Coronary heart disease is responsible for 1 in 5 deaths in the United States. Currently, the prevalence of coronary artery disease is over 7 million cases in men and over 6 million cases in women. More than 1 million individuals suffer an acute myocardial infarction per year, with nearly 40% dying because of the incident. Men are at a higher risk of myocardial infarction than women, especially with increasing age.

### *Diagnosis and Screening*

Physical examination, patient history, and diagnostic tools are used for **diagnosis** of myocardial infarction. Diagnostic tools include echocardiogram, electrocardiogram, chest x-ray, nuclear ventriculography, magnetic resonance imaging (MRI), and blood tests to detect elevation in cardiac markers. More invasive diagnostic tools used for diagnosis of myocardial infarction and atherosclerosis include angiography and angioplasty.

The **World Health Organization criteria** used to diagnose myocardial infarction include clinical history of ischemic type chest pain lasting more than 20 minutes, changes in electrocardiogram tracing, and rise and fall of serum cardiac markers such as creatinine kinase-MB fraction and troponin I. Individuals that present with two or more of these criteria are typically diagnosed with having experienced a myocardial infarction.

### *Causes and Risk Factors*

**Risk factors** that can lead to myocardial infarction include a family history of vascular disease such as atherosclerosis, coronary artery disease and/or angina, previous heart attack or stroke, previous episodes of syncope or arrhythmias, natural aging, smoking or tobacco use, lack of physical activity, excessive alcohol consumption, abuse of drugs, elevated triglyceride levels, elevated low-density lipoprotein levels, decreased high-density lipoprotein levels, diabetes, hypertension, acute infections, obesity, chronic renal failure, stress, and anxiety.

Other contributing factors include socioeconomic factors, such as lack of education and lower income, that prevent individuals from seeking preventative care and/or routine management.

### *Symptoms*

**Symptoms** associated with myocardial infarction include chest pain, pain radiating from the left side of the neck or arm, feeling of fullness or pressure in the chest, prolonged pain in upper abdomen, syncope, lightheadedness, dizziness, shortness of breath, nausea, vomiting, palpitations, sweating, weakness, fatigue, and anxiety. Some patients present with no symptoms, which is referred to as a silent heart attack. Also, men present with different symptoms than women in most cases. Women tend to present with shortness of breath, fatigue, and weakness.

The onset of symptoms typically occurs over a short period of time, worsening without intervention. However, nearly half of patients do not experience any symptoms such as chest pain or shortness of breath.

### *Complications and Prognosis*

**Complications associated with myocardial infarction** can be acute or develop post-acute attack. Complications include recurrent myocardial infarction, congestive heart failure, valve problems, myocardial rupture, myocardial damage, life-threatening arrhythmia, pericarditis, and cardiogenic shock.

The **prognosis** of an individual who experiences a myocardial infarction depends on the degree and extent of the attack. It also depends on the presence of underlying comorbid conditions. Prognosis further depends on patient compliance with lifestyle modifications and pharmacologic management post-acute attack. Increased prognosis is associated with early reperfusion, preserved left ventricular function, and compliance with short-term and long-term pharmacologic agents.

## STROKE

**Stroke** is defined as an acute condition where blood flow, and thus oxygen, to the brain is hindered or significantly reduced. There are two types of stroke: ischemic stroke and hemorrhagic stroke. Ischemic stroke is defined as a condition where blood flow to the brain is blocked because of blood clot formation or embolism. Approximately 80–85% of strokes are ischemic strokes, while 15–20% are hemorrhagic strokes. Another type of stroke is a transient ischemic attack, where blood flow to the brain is temporarily hindered.

In the United States, approximately 400,000 individuals are diagnosed with stroke per year, which is expected to increase on a yearly basis because of the aging of the US population.

In the United States, stroke is the third leading cause of death annually, following cancer and cardiovascular diseases. It is also the leading the cause of adult disability in the United States.

### *ISCHEMIC AND HEMORRHAGIC STROKES*

**Ischemic strokes** include thrombotic strokes, which occur when a blood clot forms in arteries supplying the brain, and embolic strokes, which occur when a blood clot (or other embolus, like a cholesterol plaque) formed in the cardiovascular system dislodges and blocks more distal arteries.

**Hemorrhagic strokes** occur when a blood vessel ruptures and leaks into the brain. Hemorrhagic strokes include intracerebral hemorrhages, which occur when a blood vessel in the brain ruptures, hindering blood flow and damaging tissue, and subarachnoid hemorrhages, which occur when a blood vessel lining the brain membrane bursts and leaks into the subarachnoid space.

### *DIAGNOSIS AND SCREENING*

Early recognition of **signs and symptoms** of stroke is very important for prevention of complications and death. Physical examination, patient feedback, and diagnostic tools are used to diagnose an acute stroke.

**Screening tools** used to diagnose a stroke include carotid ultrasonography, arteriography, computerized tomography, magnetic resonance imaging, and echocardiography. Practicing clinicians may also perform blood work to assess other comorbid conditions that may have contributed to the stroke including lipids, glucose, and homocysteine levels.

More invasive approaches such as angiography may be performed to assess the degree and extent of cardiovascular disease.

### *CAUSES AND RISK FACTORS*

Patients at **highest risk** for an acute stroke are those individuals who have experienced a transient ischemic attack or experienced a previous stroke. Other risk factors include family history, natural aging, African American descent, hypertension, high cholesterol, cigarette smoking, diabetes, cardiovascular disease, alcoholism, illicit drug use, stress, anxiety, and elevated homocysteine levels.

Drugs may also increase an individual's risk of stroke, including birth control pills and hormone replacement therapy. Furthermore, men are at a higher risk for stroke than women. The elderly are especially at an increased risk, with nearly 75% of strokes occurring in individuals 65 years of age or older.

#### *Symptoms*

Patients experiencing an acute stroke typically present with sudden numbness or weakness of the arms, legs, and/or face, which occurs on one side of the individual's body. They also may experience confusion, slurred speech, difficulty speaking, vision loss, double vision, difficulty walking, dizziness, loss of balance, loss of coordination, pain, memory loss, problems with spatial orientation, perception loss, and severe headache of sudden onset.

Most patients who present with symptoms of stroke do not present with warning symptoms aside from the acute attack. However, in some cases, individuals may experience a transient ischemic attack with similar symptoms of an acute attack prior to experiencing an acute stroke.

#### *Complications and Prognosis*

**Complications associated with stroke** depend on the extent and degree of damage to the brain and associated tissues. They also depend on the location of the brain affected by the stroke. Complications include numbness and weakness on one side of the body, confusion, slurred speech, difficulty speaking, vision loss, double vision, difficulty walking, dizziness, loss of balance and coordination, pain, memory loss, problems with spatial orientation and swallowing, loss of bladder or bowel function, and perception loss.

Complications of stroke may be improved with physical therapy and/or rehabilitation. Practitioners involved in rehabilitation include psychiatrists, physical therapists, occupational therapists, recreational therapists, and/or speech therapists. Family or loved ones should keep in close touch with a patient who has had a stroke. They should also keep conversations at an adult level using a normal tone of voice and speaking at a comfortable pace.

Approximately 75% of individuals who have experienced a stroke are unable to maintain employment. Also, 30–50% of individuals who experience a stroke suffer depression.

### Peripheral Arterial Disease

**Peripheral arterial disease** is a condition in which blood flow is reduced to limbs and extremities. The prevalence of peripheral arterial disease increases with age, with individuals over the age of 55 having a prevalence of 10–25%. In the United States, approximately 10–20% of individuals 65 years or older are affected by peripheral arterial disease.

Most patients diagnosed with peripheral arterial disease are asymptomatic, with approximately 70–80% presenting with no symptoms upon diagnosis. However, the incidence of symptomatic peripheral arterial disease increases with age. Furthermore, the prevalence of symptomatic peripheral arterial disease varies based on the disease definition and the age of the patient population being evaluated.

#### *Causes and Risk Factors*

Atherosclerosis is the main **cause** of peripheral arterial disease. However, blood clots, injury to limbs, unusual anatomy of ligaments or muscles, or infection may lead to peripheral arterial disease. Other diseases that can lead to the onset of peripheral vascular disease include aortic aneurysms, Buerger's disease, pulmonary embolism, phlebitis, varicose veins, and Raynaud's syndrome.

Factors that increase an individual's **risk** for peripheral arterial disease include smoking, age over 50 years, diabetes, obesity, high blood pressure, high cholesterol or family history of cardiovascular diseases, and atherosclerosis. Male individuals of African American descent as well as overweight individuals and those with a family history of cardiovascular disease are at a particularly high risk of peripheral vascular disease.

Other risk factors under clinical investigation include inflammatory mediators such as C-reactive protein, homocysteine, and fibrinogen.

### *Symptoms*

More than half of individuals diagnosed with peripheral arterial disease do not present with **symptoms**. However, symptoms associated with peripheral arterial disease include leg numbness or weakness, cold legs and feet, sores or wounds on digits or extremities that will not heal, blue or pale hue to legs, feet, hands and/or arms, hair loss on feet and legs, and changes in composition of nails.

Approximately one-third to one-half of individuals diagnosed with peripheral arterial disease present with intermittent claudication. Intermittent claudication is defined as muscle pain or cramping in appendages triggered by walking and physical activity. Individuals may also experience ischemic rest pain.

### *Diagnosis and Screening*

Early **diagnosis** of peripheral arterial disease is necessary for prevention of complications such as cardiovascular disease, heart attack, stroke, and sudden death. Physical examination and diagnostic screening tools are used to determine if a patient has peripheral arterial disease.

Upon **physical examination**, practicing clinicians use a stethoscope to determine the presence of bruits. They also look for evidence of poor wound healing, sores, color changes, temperature changes, and decreased blood pressure in limbs. Diagnostic screening tools include the ankle-brachial index and angiography. Additional tests include angiography, electrocardiogram, magnetic resonance angiography, blood tests, and ultrasound.

### *Complications and Prognosis*

The main **complications of peripheral arterial disease** include limb ischemia, limb loss, pain, wound infection, poor wound healing, and decreased limb function.

Individuals diagnosed with peripheral arterial disease are at a greater risk of cardiovascular disease, heart attack, stroke, and/or transient ischemic attack than the general population.

Patients with diabetes and peripheral arterial disease are at a higher risk for developing critical limb ischemia, sometimes requiring amputation of affected limbs.

### *Risk Factors and Treatment Recommendations*

Patients with the greatest risk for PAD include individuals with diabetes, abnormal extremity pulses, known cardiac disease, high cholesterol, high blood levels of homocysteine, high blood pressure, impaired wound healing on extremities, age over 70, or a history of smoking. The presence of PAD in turn increases the patient's risk for myocardial infarction and stroke.

Treatment includes smoking cessation and other risk management. Further interventions might include physical or exercise rehabilitation, medication (including thrombolytics, vasodilators, and medications to treat related risk factors), and surgical interventions including stents or amputation in extreme cases.

## Inflammation

**Inflammation** is defined as a complex response of vascular tissues to irritants, pathogens, and/or damaged cells. It is a protective mechanism to remove harmful substances from the body and initiate the healing signal transduction cascade.

Inflammation can be classified as either acute or chronic:

- **Acute inflammation** is defined as the initial response by the body to irritants, pathogens, and/or damaged cells, recruiting neutrophils, monocytes, and macrophages from blood to affected tissue.
- **Chronic inflammation** is a prolonged inflammation process that recruits other cells such as monocytes, macrophages, lymphocytes, plasma cells, and fibroblasts involved in the pathogen removal and healing process.

### *Acute vs. Chronic Inflammation*

**Acute inflammation** is caused by pathogens, irritants and/or damaged cells. The major cells involved in the acute inflammation process include neutrophils, monocytes, and macrophages. The primary mediators include vasoactive amines and eicosanoids. The onset of action of acute inflammation is immediate and lasts for approximately a few days. The initiation of acute inflammation leads to healing, abscess formation, and chronic inflammation stimulation.

**Chronic inflammation** is triggered by acute inflammation due to the presence of pathogens, irritants, and/or damaged cells and the body's reaction to these initial triggers. The presence of neutrophils, monocytes, and pathogens as well as other signaling transduction mechanisms triggers chronic inflammation. The major cells involved in the chronic inflammation process include monocytes, macrophages, lymphocytes, plasma cells, and fibroblasts. The primary mediators include cytokines, growth factors, reactive oxygen species, and hydrolytic enzymes. The onset of action of chronic inflammation is delayed and lasts for approximately several months or years. The initiation of chronic inflammation leads to tissue destruction and fibrosis.

### *Diagnosis and Screening*

Inflammatory diseases are **diagnosed** after careful physical examination and use of diagnostic tools. Practicing clinicians will complete a physical examination and take an individual's medical history as well as a family history of inflammatory disorders. They will examine painful joints, muscles, and other organ systems. They will also examine and discuss the presence of other comorbid conditions.

**Diagnostic screening tools** used include x-rays, magnetic resonance imaging, and CT scans, as well as other imagining techniques to assess impact on end organ systems including the cardiovascular system, respiratory system, renal system, and gastrointestinal system.

### *Symptoms*

The **symptoms** of acute inflammation include swelling of joints and muscles, joint and muscle stiffness, redness, pain, heat, and loss of function. Chronic inflammation is sometimes characterized by the same symptoms as acute inflammation. However, fever, chills, fatigue, low energy, headaches, appetite loss, and muscle stiffness may characterize chronic inflammation.

Involvement of internal end organ systems may present with symptoms specific to that organ system. Involvement of the cardiovascular system may lead to chest pain, palpitations, hypertension, and/or high cholesterol. Involvement of the respiratory system may lead to asthma and/or allergic reactions. Involvement of the renal system may lead to kidney failure and/or infections. Involvement of the large intestines may lead to ulcerative colitis, Crohn's disease, diverticulitis, and/or inflammatory bowel disease.

### *Causes and Risk Factors*

The **causes of acute inflammation** include the presence of irritants, pathogens and/or damaged cells within the body. Acute inflammation is characterized by vascular changes, including vasodilation, increased permeability, and/or reduced blood flow. The signaling cascades involved in acute inflammation include the complement system, such as C3, C5a, membrane attack complex, and thrombin; the kinin system, such as bradykinin; the coagulation system, such as thrombin; and the fibrinolysis system, such as plasmin.

The **cause of chronic inflammation** is persistent acute inflammation due to bacterial infection, chemical exposure (including silica exposure), and/or autoimmune reactions, as in rheumatoid arthritis, lupus, or psoriasis.

### *Complications*

Examples of acute inflammation include acute appendicitis, acute dermatitis, acute infective meningitis, and acute tonsillitis.

**Complications of chronic inflammation** can lead to prolonged activation of the inflammatory cascade and inflammatory disorders caused by the presence of viral or bacterial infections or signaling malfunctions. Chronic inflammation can lead to development of inflammatory disorders such as asthma; autoimmune disease such as lupus, psoriasis, and rheumatoid arthritis; bursitis; gout; prolonged inflammation; chronic prostatitis; glomerulonephritis; hypersensitivities such as allergies; myopathies; leukocyte defects; inflammatory bowel disease such as Crohn's disease and ulcerative colitis; pelvic inflammatory disease; reperfusion injury; transplant rejection; obesity; and vasculitis.

## Pericarditis

**Pericarditis** is defined as inflammation of the pericardium, which is the thin membrane surrounding the heart muscle. Excess fluid can accumulate between the two layers of the membrane, impacting the proper function of the heart. There are two types of pericarditis: acute pericarditis and chronic pericarditis. Acute pericarditis is more prevalent than chronic pericarditis.

The condition is more **prevalent** among men than women and most often occurs between the ages of 20–50. Acute pericarditis episodes can last from 1 to 3 weeks, but additional episodes can occur in the future. Approximately 20% of individuals with pericarditis may have a reoccurrence within one month of the first episode.

Pericarditis occurs in approximately 15% of individuals who have experienced an acute myocardial infarction/heart attack. Approximately 25–85% of cases present with no clear reason and are idiopathic in nature.

### *Screening and Diagnosis*

Physical examination, medical history, and diagnostic tools are used to **diagnose** pericarditis. Practicing clinicians will evaluate the patient by listening to the individual's heart with a stethoscope and looking for other comorbid conditions. Indicators of pericarditis upon physical examination include abnormal heart sounds such as muffling and friction rub, crackles in lungs, and decreased breath sounds.

Diagnostic screening tools used to diagnose pericarditis include electrocardiogram, echocardiogram, chest x-ray, computerized tomography, and magnetic resonance imaging. Blood work may also be performed to rule out heart attack or congestive heart failure. Blood levels include complete blood count, C-reactive protein, and evaluation of erythrocyte sedimentation rate.

Physical and diagnostic findings include friction rub, diffuse ST-elevation, and PR depression on electrocardiogram, enlarged heart, fluid surrounding pericardium, cardiac tamponade, and/or congestive heart failure on echocardiogram.

### *Causes and Risk Factors*

The **cause** of pericarditis remains unclear. However, pericarditis can develop post heart attack or surgery. Other causes of pericarditis include systemic inflammatory disorders such as lupus and rheumatoid arthritis, trauma due to car accident, slip and fall or other traumatic events, comorbid conditions such as renal disease, bacterial infections such as tuberculosis, viral infections such as coxsackie virus or echo virus, fungal infections, myocardial infarction, uremia, aortic dissection, HIV/AIDS, malignancy metastasis, Dressler syndrome, hypothyroidism, renal disease, and radiation and pharmacologic agents such as tetracyclines, isoniazid, cyclosporine, and hydralazine.

In adolescents, pericarditis is most commonly caused by adenovirus or Coxsackie virus.

### *Symptoms*

The most common **symptoms** associated with pericarditis include sharp chest pain behind the breast bone or left side of the chest wall cavity, dull/sharp chest pain radiating to the back that is relieved by sitting up or forward and worsened by lying down, pressure or ache in the chest wall, shortness of breath, difficulty breathing when lying down, anxiety, low grade fever, weakness, fatigue, ill feeling, dry cough, and abdominal or extremity swelling.

The symptoms of pericarditis are very similar to other cardiovascular diseases such as heart attack and congestive heart failure and respiratory conditions such as asthma, emphysema, pulmonary embolism, and chronic obstructive pulmonary disease.

### *Complications and Prognosis*

The **complications of pericarditis** include pericardial effusion, arrhythmias, constrictive pericarditis, and cardiac tamponade. Early diagnosis of pericarditis can reduce the risk of developing these complications.

- **Constrictive pericarditis** is a permanent thickening of the pericardium, which hinders proper function of the heart muscle. Complications of constrictive pericarditis include swelling of the abdomen and legs as well as shortness of breath.
- **Cardiac tamponade** is accumulation of fluid in the pericardium, leading to improper functioning of the heart. The excess fluid does not allow the heart to pump blood effectively and can lead to sudden death if not properly treated.

Pericarditis can range from mild to very severe cases, and prognosis depends on the extent and degree of disease. Most cases resolve within two weeks to three months.

## VASCULITIS

**Vasculitis** is a condition that involves inflammation of blood vessels such as arteries, veins, and capillaries. Vasculitis causes thickening, weakening, narrowing, and scarring of the blood vessels, leading to abnormal blood flow, cardiovascular complications, and organ system damage. Vasculitis can be classified as primary vasculitis, having no known cause, and secondary vasculitis, caused by another comorbid condition or pharmacologic approaches.

The **incidence** of vasculitis in the general population is rare, even though there are various types of the condition and it can affect a variety of end organ systems. Women, children, current or ex-smokers, and individuals with chronic hepatitis B or hepatitis C are at increased risk for certain types of vasculitis. The course of disease is difficult to predict and can go into remission, recur, or remain chronic.

### *DIAGNOSIS AND SCREENING*

Physical examination, medical history, and diagnostic screening tools are used to **diagnose** vasculitis. However, the symptoms and physical findings of vasculitis resemble those of other conditions and can be difficult to diagnose.

Blood tests used for diagnosis of vasculitis and to rule out other conditions include erythrocyte sedimentation rate, C-reactive protein, anti-nuclear antibodies, complement levels, antineutrophil cytoplasmic antibody, and complete blood count such as red blood cells and platelets. A urinalysis may also be performed to detect any abnormalities, such as increased protein in urine or presence of red blood cells.

### *CAUSES AND RISK FACTORS*

Various diseases and conditions can be classified as vasculitis or can lead to the condition. Some conditions that are commonly associated with vasculitis include Behcet's syndrome, Buerger's syndrome, Churg-Strauss syndrome, cryoglobulinemia, giant cell arthritis, Henoch-Schönlein purpura, hypersensitivities, Kawasaki disease, microscopic polyangiitis, polyarteritis nodosa, polymyalgia rheumatica, rheumatoid conditions, lupus, Sjögren's syndrome, Takayasu's arteritis, and Wegener's granulomatosis. Pharmacologic approaches that can lead to vasculitis include antibiotics and diuretics.

Vasculitis can affect men, women, and children. Its cause remains unclear, but certain risk factors have been associated with the condition. Individuals most affected by vasculitis include current or ex-smokers, children, young women, middle-aged adults, and individuals with chronic hepatitis B and/or hepatitis C.

### *SYMPTOMS*

The **symptoms** of vasculitis vary depending on which blood vessels and end organ systems are affected by the condition. The symptoms are also dependent on the extent and degree of vasculitis. Patients may experience few symptoms or have more extensive symptoms depending on the organ systems that are involved.

The most common symptoms among individuals diagnosed with vasculitis include weight loss, fever, general aches and pains, skin changes such as purple or red spots, shortness of breath, ulcers, abdominal pain, bloody stool, sinus infections, chronic middle ear infections, ulcers in nostrils, blurring or vision loss, headaches, confusion, changes in behavior, strokes, muscle and joint pain, loss of appetite, numbness, tingling, and weakness.

### *Complications and Prognosis*

**Complications of vasculitis** are dependent on the degree and extent of disease as well as the blood vessel systems and end organ systems involved. Most cases of vasculitis are minor and resolve on their own without medical intervention. However, some cases are severe and involve major end organ systems and result in serious complications. Serious complications include end organ system damage, cardiovascular disease, heart attack, stroke, and death.

Other complications include renal insufficiency, digital gangrene, pulmonary hemorrhage, central nervous system infarction, arterial or venous thrombosis, and subglottic stenosis.

The **prognosis** of individuals diagnosed with vasculitis depends on the type, extent, and degree of vasculitis as well as end organ involvement.

## Endocarditis

**Endocarditis** is defined as inflammation of the endocardium, which is the inner lining of the heart chambers and valves. Endocarditis can lead to cardiovascular disease, improper functioning of heart valves and chambers, and sudden death. The disease can be classified as infective or noninfective, but noninfective endocarditis is very rare and uncommon in clinical practice. Endocarditis is most common in individuals with damaged hearts either from heart attack or disease.

In the United States, the incidence of endocarditis is 1.4–4.2 cases per 100,000 individuals per year. Men are more prone to endocarditis than women. More than half of the cases of endocarditis occur in individuals ages 50 years or older.

### *Causes and Risk Factors*

The main **cause** of endocarditis is bacterial infection that resides in the endocardium. Bacteria entering the blood stream and attaching to the walls of the endocardium typically cause endocarditis. Other causes of endocarditis include common activities such as teeth brushing or chewing food; infection; other medical conditions such as skin sores, gum disease, inflammatory bowel disease and sexually transmitted disease; insertion of contaminated catheters or needles; and/or certain dental or respiratory tract procedures.

Individuals most at **risk** for developing endocarditis include those who have had a heart attack or have damaged heart valves or underlying heart abnormalities. Others at risk include those with artificial heart valves, congenital heart defect, and prior history of endocarditis. Also, individuals who have healthy hearts but use illicit drugs with needles or are hospitalized with IV tubes may be at risk for endocarditis.

### *Diagnosis and Screening*

The **diagnosis** of endocarditis involves physical examination, medical history, and diagnostic screening tools. Upon physical examination, clinical practitioners will use a stethoscope to determine the presence of heart murmur or other arrhythmia problems. They will also look for enlarged end organ systems such as the spleen. Other diagnostic testing involves blood tests such as complete blood count, culture and erythrocyte sedimentation rate, serology, chest x-ray, echocardiogram, electrocardiogram, and transesophageal echocardiogram. More invasive approaches such as cardiac catheterization may be performed to determine the extent of heart valve damage.

Practicing clinicians look for signs of endocarditis in individuals with high-risk conditions such as congenital heart disease, intravenous drug use, recent dental work, and/or rheumatic fever.

### Symptoms

Endocarditis can be acute or may develop over an extended period. The **signs and symptoms** of endocarditis are dependent on the underlying cause of the disease. The most common symptoms include fever; chills; heart murmur; fatigue; aching joints and muscles; swelling of feet, legs or abdomen; night sweats; shortness of breath; paleness; persistent cough; unexplained weight loss; blood in urine; nail abnormalities; weakness; and tenderness of spleen.

Other signs include red and tender spots under the skin of the fingers as well as purple or red spots on other areas of the skin, such as the whites of the eyes or inside the mouth (known as petechiae).

### Complications and Prognosis

**Complications associated with endocarditis** are dependent on the extent and degree of disease. In more severe cases, where debris and bacteria reside in the endocardium, individuals may experience heart attack, stroke, other end organ system damage, and sudden death. Other complications include arrhythmias, blood clots, brain abscess, brain or nervous system damage, congestive heart failure, glomerulonephritis, jaundice, cardiac valvular insufficiency, aneurysm, cardiac abscesses, and severe heart failure.

Untreated endocarditis can be very serious and permanently damage the inner lining of the heart chambers and valves, leading to congestive heart failure due to an inability of the heart to pump effectively.

The prognosis in individuals who receive early intervention is better than for those who receive delayed treatment. However, complications such as heart attack and stroke can lead to sudden death.

## Renal Artery Occlusion

**Renal artery occlusion** is a condition that involves narrowing or blockage of one or both of the renal arteries. Alternative names used for renal artery occlusion include acute renal arterial thrombosis, renal artery embolism, acute renal artery occlusion, and renal artery stenosis.

Renal artery occlusion is the primary cause of hypertension in approximately 1–10% of the 50 million individuals diagnosed with hypertension in the United States. Renal artery occlusion is more prevalent among elderly individuals with atherosclerosis. The disease is more common in Caucasian Americans than African Americans.

### Causes and Risk Factors

Renal artery occlusion can be **caused** by a variety of other comorbid conditions including atheroembolic renal disease; atherosclerosis; fibromuscular dysplasia of the renal wall; trauma to abdomen, back, or side; emboli residing in renal arteries; and scar formation in the renal artery.

Other **risk factors** include hypertension, aging, renal insufficiency, extrarenal atherosclerosis, diabetes, presence of other comorbid conditions such as cardiovascular disease or renal disease, and smoking. Elderly Caucasian individuals with atherosclerosis are at highest risk for the development of renal artery occlusion.

### Diagnosis and Screening

Physical examination, medical history, and diagnostic tools are used to **diagnose** renal artery occlusion. The disease typically presents with few or no symptoms and is usually diagnosed upon routine physical examination or when being examined for other cardiovascular or renal conditions.

Practicing clinicians will use a stethoscope to listen for bruits of the kidney and check blood pressure to see if the patient presents with high blood pressure. Other diagnostic tools used to diagnose renal artery occlusion include magnetic resonance imaging, computerized tomography, kidney ultrasound, radionucleotide conventional arteriography, contrast nephrotoxicity, renogram, renal perfusion scintiscan, urine concentration testing, urine specific gravity, and renal arteriography.

Blood work includes complete blood counts, serum creatinine levels, and serologic levels such as antinuclear antibodies, C3, C4, and antinuclear cytoplasmic antibodies.

### *Symptoms*

Most individuals with renal artery occlusion typically present with no **symptoms**. The reason that patients present with few or no symptoms is that the second kidney takes over for the lack of functioning by the impaired kidney.

**Diagnosis** is typically made upon routine physical examination or when being examined for other cardiovascular or renal conditions. Some signs associated with renal artery occlusion include high blood pressure, history of high blood pressure, and/or bruits of the kidneys.

### *Complications and Prognosis*

**Complications associated with renal artery occlusion** include hypertension, chronic renal failure, and malignant hypertension. Hypertension associated with renal artery occlusion may be difficult to control and require intervention with multiple pharmacologic approaches, including angiotensin-converting enzyme inhibitors such as captopril and enalapril and angiotensin II receptor antagonists such as losartan.

Untreated renal artery occlusion can result in chronic renal failure and potentially death. Although balloon angioplasty and stenting may improve blood flow from arteries of kidneys, blockage may reoccur. Early diagnosis and careful monitoring can prevent progression of the disease and improve outcomes.

## Renal Vein Thrombosis

**Renal vein thrombosis** is a condition in which the veins leaving the kidney become occluded by a thrombus. The condition leads to a reduction in blood drainage by the kidney, which can cause further complications.

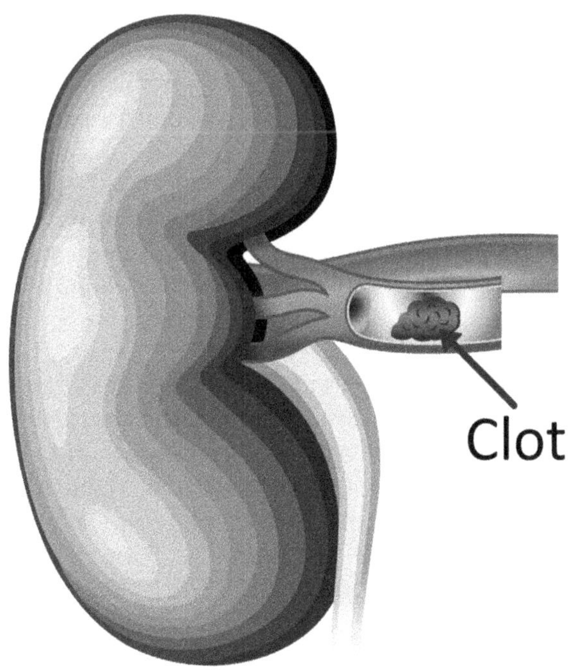


Renal vein thrombosis is a rare condition that typically presents with other conditions including nephrotic syndrome, kidney cancer, and/or other blood clotting disorders. Renal vein thrombosis occurs more often in adults than in infants, toddlers, or adolescents. However, it is typically more serious in infants, toddlers, or adolescents.

In the United States, the **prevalence** of renal vein thrombosis remains unknown. It is most commonly associated with nephrotic syndrome, but prevalence rates among these patients vary greatly, ranging from 5% to 60% on average.

### *Diagnosis and Screening*

**Diagnosis** of renal vein thrombosis is made by physical examination as well as the use of diagnostic imaging tools. Abdominal CT angiography scan is typically used to confirm the diagnosis of renal vein thrombosis, as physical examination does not always reveal renal vein thrombosis. Other diagnostic tools used for screening of renal vein thrombosis include abdominal MRI scan, x-ray, Doppler ultrasound, or abdominal ultrasound, which may reveal the occluded vein. Urinalysis may also be performed to detect increased protein levels and/or red blood cells. Blood tests may also indicate evidence of renal failure. Blood tests may involve lipid level testing, albumin levels, and serum complement levels.

Renal biopsy may also be performed in patients who present with nephrotic syndrome.

### *Causes and Risk Factors*

**Renal vein thrombosis** is an uncommon and rare condition but can occur after trauma to the abdomen and/or back as well as due to scar formation, stricture, and/or tumor. It is also, more commonly, associated with nephrotic syndrome.

In infants, toddlers, and adolescents, renal vein thrombosis can occur due to severe dehydration, which is considered to be a much more serious condition than when it occurs in adults. Other possible causes of renal vein thrombosis include blood clotting disorders such as hypercoagulability disorder; protein C or S deficiency; antiphospholipid antibody syndrome; pregnancy; post renal transplant; Behçet's syndrome; extrinsic compression such as lymph nodes, tumor, retroperitoneal fibrosis, or aortic aneurysm; sickle cell anemia; diabetes that affects the kidney; oral contraceptive use; illicit drug abuse; steroid use; or thrombophlebitis migrans.

### *Symptoms*

The **symptoms** of renal vein thrombosis are minimal unless the vein becomes occluded suddenly. Patients who present with symptoms of renal vein thrombosis typically present with blood in urine or decreased urine volume upon excretion. Other signs of renal vein thrombosis include protein and/or red blood cells upon urinalysis.

Pulmonary embolism (from embolization of the thrombus) may be a sign that a patient has renal vein thrombosis. With pulmonary embolism, patients present with shortness of breath and chest pain made worse by breathing. Infants, toddlers, and adolescents typically present with lower back/abdominal pain, decreased urine excretion, fever, and blood in the urine.

### *Complications and Prognosis*

**Renal vein thrombosis** typically improves over time, with limited permanent damage to kidneys and other end organ systems. However, complications that can arise from renal vein thrombosis include acute renal failure if occurring due to dehydration in an infant or adolescent; embolization of blood clot to lungs, heart, brain, or other organ systems; and formation of new blood clots.

The **prognosis** of renal vein thrombosis depends on the degree and extent of the condition and the impact on other organ systems such as the lungs and/or brain. It also depends largely on the extent of renal system damage. The effects on kidney function depend on whether one or both kidneys are affected, whether blood flow can be restored, and on the health of the kidney prior to the presence of renal vein thrombosis. Death is typically rare but can occur due to an underlying comorbid condition.

## Atheroembolic Renal Disease

**Atheroembolic renal disease** is a condition that involves lipid build-up and clot formation within the small arteries that serve the capillaries of the kidneys. The condition is also known as renal atheroembolism, cholesterol embolization syndrome, or atherosclerotic disease. It is a condition that slowly progresses over time and can lead to severe complications such as heart attack, stroke, and brain damage. It is most commonly associated with atherosclerotic disease.

Approximately 25% of patients with renal failure due to atheroembolic renal disease recover renal function.

### *Diagnosis and Screening*

Physical examination and diagnostic testing are used to **diagnose** atheroembolic renal disease. Practicing clinicians will look for signs of swelling of the ankles, wrists, and other parts of the body (signs of kidney failure), particles in blood vessels of the retina, abnormal blood flow from the heart, increased blood pressure, and skin ulcers on lower feet.

Diagnostic imaging tests used include abdominal CT scan, abdominal MRI, abdominal x-ray, and kidney or abdominal ultrasound. Blood work performed may include chem.-7, chem.-20, complete blood count, serum complement levels, and serum lipid levels. More invasive diagnostic tools include kidney biopsy and renal arteriography. Urinalysis may also be performed to look for increases in protein excretion and/or red blood cells.

### *Causes and Risk Factors*

Atheroembolic renal disease is strongly associated with atherosclerotic disease, which is a very common disorder among patients with cardiovascular disease. The **risk factors** for atheroembolic renal disease are the same as for atherosclerotic disease.

Factors that can increase an individual's risk for atherosclerosis include high low-density lipoprotein cholesterol, low high-density lipoprotein, evaluated triglyceride levels, menopause, lack of physical activity, obesity, infection of the vascular smooth muscle cells, high blood pressure, history of smoking, and diabetes.

Smoking not only predisposes individuals for atherosclerosis, but it also increases the progression of the disease. The progression of atherosclerosis itself also further increases the extent and degree of the condition, as further accumulation of lipids, cholesterol, and other substances stimulates the endothelium to produce substances that cause increased plaque buildup.

### *Symptoms*

The **symptoms** of atheroembolic renal disease include foot pain and/or ulcers, discoloration of feet such as blue or purple feet or toes, claudication, pain in the abdomen, nausea, vomiting, pancreatitis, hepatitis, strokes, blindness, flank pain, blood in urine, decrease or no urine excretion, and uncontrolled high blood pressure.

In some patients, renal failure may also occur, which would present with nausea, vomiting, bad taste in mouth, chest pain, high blood pressure, high cholesterol, weight loss, decreased or no urine excretion, swelling, decreased sensation, skin pigmentation changes, dry and itchy skin, drowsiness, fatigue, confusion, and/or lethargy.

### *Complications*

The **complications of atheroembolic renal disease** are similar to those of atherosclerotic disease. Complications associated with atheroembolic disease include acute renal failure, chronic renal failure, high blood pressure, embolization of blood clots, and formation of blood clots in other organ systems such as the heart, intestines, lungs, and legs.

Complications associated with atherosclerosis include risk of blood clotting, in which a plaque increases in size to reduce blood flow, and risk of rupture, which can lead to heart attack and/or stroke. If blood flow is reduced to the peripheral vasculature, then patients may have walking and dexterity complications, erectile dysfunction, and abdominal aortic aneurysms.

Atherosclerosis leads to altered vascular function, including coronary heart disease, myocardial ischemia and myocardial infarction, cerebrovascular insufficiency, stroke, aortic aneurysm, and vasculitis. The prognosis of atheroembolic renal disease depends on the degree and extent of disease as well as presence of other comorbid conditions. The disease typically progresses over time, and outcomes are generally poor.

Lifestyle modifications may slow the progression of the disease, but progression typically occurs.

## Marfan Syndrome

**Marfan syndrome** is a connective tissue disorder affecting the skeleton, lungs, eyes, heart, and major blood vessels. It is a genetic disorder that causes a reduction in fibrillin, leading to a decrease in the elasticity and a weakening of connective tissue.

Marfan syndrome affects men and women equally, as well as individuals of all races and ethnic groups. In the United States, approximately 60,000 individuals have been diagnosed with Marfan syndrome. Most individuals with Marfan syndrome have a family history of disease. However, approximately 15–30% of individuals diagnosed with the disease have new genetic mutations.

### *Diagnosis and Screening*

Physical examination and medical history are key in **diagnosing** Marfan syndrome. There are no key diagnostic tools solely used to confirm Marfan syndrome. However, patients with Marfan syndrome are typically tall and thin with tapering fingers and have a narrow face, loose joints, long arms and legs, curvature of the spine, chest wall abnormalities, and eye problems.

Therefore, diagnosis is made by a combination of clinical practitioners including cardiologists, ophthalmologists, orthopedic surgeons, and/or medical geneticists. Diagnostic tools used to diagnose Marfan syndrome include echocardiogram, chest x-ray, MRI, and genetic testing. The Ghent criterion is typically used to make a diagnosis of Marfan syndrome.

### *Ghent Criteria for Diagnosis*

Practicing clinicians use the **Ghent criteria** to diagnose patients with Marfan syndrome correctly since the symptoms of the condition resemble those of other connective tissue disorders. The criteria are divided into two categories: major and minor. In patients with a family history of Marfan syndrome, they must have one major criterion in one organ system and involvement of another organ system to be diagnosed with the condition. If patients do not have a family history of the condition, then these individuals need to have two major criteria affecting different organs and the involvement of another organ system.

The major criteria for Marfan syndrome include an enlarged aorta, with or without aortic dissection; aortic dissection affecting ascending aorta; dislocation of the lens of an eye; dural ectasia; at least four skeletal problems such as chest deformities, long and thin arms and legs, flat footedness, and scoliosis; family history; and/or having an abnormal gene for Marfan syndrome.

Minor criteria that occur are symptoms and signs that occur in both patients with the disease as well as in the general population.

### Causes and Risk Factors

Marfan syndrome is a genetic disorder that results from a defect in the gene that enables the production of fibrillin. In this syndrome, the defect leads to lower production of fibrillin, which leads to weakened connective tissue in the skeletal system, aorta, and ligaments. The greatest **risk factor** for the condition is a parent with the disease.

Marfan syndrome is an autosomal dominant condition, which means that only one parent needs to have the gene for the condition to pass it on to offspring. Offspring have a 50% chance of inheriting the disease from one parent diagnosed with the condition.

### Symptoms

Some patients with Marfan syndrome present with few or no **symptoms**. Also, patients typically present with varying symptoms depending on the organ system affected. Symptoms can vary from very mild in some patients to severe in others. The degree and extent of symptoms also varies from patient to patient, which makes diagnosis difficult. However, most patients have common traits and characteristics such as being tall, being thin with tapering fingers, chest wall abnormalities, high arched palate, long arms and legs, narrow face, loose joints, curvature of the spine, crowded teeth, flat feet, weakened part of aorta, heart murmur, nearsightedness, glaucoma, cataracts, detached retina, stretch marks, hernia, painful abdomen, weakened legs, collapsed lung, stiff air sacs, and snoring.

### Complications and Prognosis

**Complications of Marfan syndrome** include aortic dissection due to weakening of the aorta, heart valve disease that can lead to enlargement of the heart, mitral valve prolapse, mitral valve regurgitation, endocarditis, optical complications, lung complications such as breathing difficulties, abnormal heart sounds, and aortic aneurysm. Aortic aneurysm accounts for the most deaths associated with Marfan syndrome.

Vision complications associated with Marfan syndrome include shifting or dislocation, extreme nearsightedness, glaucoma, cataract and/or detachment or tear in the retina. Skeletal complications include scoliosis, spondylolisthesis, and foot pain. Other complications include stretch marks and dural ectasia.

Pregnant women with Marfan syndrome are at greater risk for aortic dissection or rupture due to increased stress to the aortic walls.

## Atrial Septal Defect

**Atrial septal defect** is a congenital birth defect involving an abnormality of the atrial chambers of the heart, which causes them not to close appropriately. Smaller defects may close on their own during infancy, toddler years, or early childhood. However, larger defects may cause problems later in life, damaging the heart, lungs, or other organ systems.

The disease is relatively uncommon and typically difficult to diagnose due to lack of symptoms. The risk of congenital heart disease in the general population is less than 1%. In children of parents with congenital heart disease, the risk of atrial septal defects increases to between 2 and 20%. The condition occurs equally in men and women, as well as across racial and ethnic groups.

### *Diagnosis and Screening*

**Physical examination and diagnostic tools** are used to diagnose atrial septal defect, but diagnosis is difficult in patients who present with few or no symptoms. Practicing clinicians typically use a stethoscope to determine the presence of abnormal heart sounds. Murmur is a quiet ejection sound heard at the left upper sternal border, often with a split-second heart sound. Murmur is not usually heard until after 1 year of age. Other diagnostic tools used to determine atrial septal defect include chest x-ray, echocardiography, Doppler ultrasound, transesophageal echocardiography, magnetic resonance imaging, pulse oximetry, and electrocardiogram. A more invasive approach such as cardiac catheterization may also be used.

Patients experiencing poor appetite; failure to gain weight; bluish discoloration of skin; shortness of breath; easy tiring; swelling of legs, feet, or abdomen; and heart palpitations should seek medical attention.

### *Causes and Risk Factors*

Atrial septal defect is a genetic condition that is congenital. It occurs during fetal circulation, leading to the formation of a shunt, which can be either left-to-right or right-to-left, depending on the nature of the condition. It can occur in combination with other genetic conditions such as Down syndrome. It can occur due to genetic inheritance or mutations during pregnancy or birth.

The following conditions during pregnancy may increase the **risk** of an offspring having a congenital heart defect such as atrial septal defects: rubella infection, poorly controlled diabetes, and illicit drug and/or alcohol abuse.

### *Symptoms*

Individuals may present with few or no symptoms, making diagnosis rather difficult. However, **symptoms** may begin to present in infancy through childhood, yet some individuals may not present with symptoms until later in life due to the presence of other comorbid conditions or progression of the defect. Individuals with small or minor defects may present with no symptoms or present with symptoms later in life.

Symptoms associated with atrial septal defect include frequent respiratory infections in children; difficulty breathing; shortness of breath with activity; fatigue; swelling of legs, feet, or abdomen; and heart palpitations in adults.

### *Consequences and Prognosis*

The **prognosis** for patients with small atrial septal defect is very good, with most living a normal life without symptoms. However, patients with larger defects may have complications later in life, including disabilities due to shunting of blood between atria and increased blood flow in pulmonary circulation.

**Complications associated with atrial septal defects** include pulmonary hypertension, arrhythmias such as atrial fibrillation, Eisenmenger syndrome, right-sided heart failure, shortened life expectancy, stroke, and heart failure. Patients with larger defects have a higher risk of high blood pressure leading to lung problems and congestive heart failure. If surgery is not performed, patients with these comorbid conditions are at a higher risk for death. Eisenmenger syndrome occurs when pulmonary resistance increases because of prolonged high blood flow from the shunt. Eventually, the shunt reverses and causes cyanosis.

Surgical mortality rate is less than 0.1%. In younger adolescents, surgical closure is effective in preventing complications, with excellent prognosis.

**Review Video: What is the Pulmonary Circuit**
Visit mometrix.com/academy and enter code: 955608

## Pulmonary Embolism

**Pulmonary embolism** is a condition that involves the blockage of arteries that supply the lungs. Typically, pulmonary embolism occurs due to the traveling of a blood clot to the lungs from another organ system.

In the United States, the incidence of pulmonary embolism is 0.9 cases per 100,000 individuals per year. The mortality rate associated with untreated pulmonary embolism in the United States averages between 18 and 30%. The mortality rate upon early diagnosis is approximately 8%.

Pregnant women in their third trimester as well as women undergoing treatment with hormone replacement therapy or oral contraceptives are at high **risk** of pulmonary embolism. The **prevalence** of pulmonary embolism increases with age.

### *Diagnosis and Screening*

Physical examination, medical history, and diagnostic tools are used to **diagnose** pulmonary embolism. However, the condition is difficult to diagnose because patients may present with varying symptoms and have other comorbid conditions such as respiratory or heart disease.

Diagnostic tools used to diagnose pulmonary embolism include chest x-ray, ventilation-perfusion scan, spiral computerized tomography scan, magnetic resonance imaging, ultrasound, and pulmonary angiogram. Blood tests may also be used to detect blood clots including D-dimer blood tests. Other blood tests used to aid in the diagnosis of pulmonary embolism include complete blood count, lipid levels, and metabolic levels. More invasive approaches include venography. Of all these methods, most modern hospitals use computed tomography (CT) scans with intravenous (IV) contrast.

### *Causes and Risk Factors*

**Risk factors** for pulmonary embolism or clot formation include genetic predisposition, history of cardiovascular disease, and/or family history of clot formation. Other factors that may lead to pulmonary embolism and clot formation include surgery such as hip and knee surgery, long periods of inactivity such as prolonged bedrest or long plane or car trips, increased levels of clotting factors in the blood as associated with certain types of cancer, previous cardiovascular conditions such as heart attack or stroke, and injury to veins. The most common risk factor is the presence of deep venous thrombosis.

Additional factors that put one at high risk for pulmonary embolism include obesity, comorbid cardiovascular diseases such as high cholesterol and hypertension, pacemakers or venous catheters, pregnancy, childbirth, hormone replacement therapy, and smoking.

### *Symptoms*

The **symptoms** of pulmonary embolism vary depending on how much lung is involved, the size of the clot, the patient's comorbid conditions, and general health. However, many patients with pulmonary embolism are asymptotic and diagnosed during routine physical examination or when being evaluated for other conditions.

Symptoms associated with pulmonary embolism include shortness of breath; chest pain that can radiate to an individual's arm, shoulder, neck, or jaw; chest wall tenderness; back pain; upper abdominal pain; painful respiration; cardiac arrhythmia; persistent cough with blood-streaked sputum; tachycardia; wheezing; leg swelling; clamminess; discoloration of skin including bluish-colored skin; excessive sweating; anxiety; weak pulse; lightheadedness; fainting; and/or fever.

### *Complications and Prognosis*

**Complications associated with pulmonary embolism** depend on the extent and degree of disease. The most common complications associated with the condition include pulmonary hypertension, cor pulmonale, heart failure, heart attack, and stroke.

Pulmonary embolism can lead to death if left untreated. Approximately 33% of undiagnosed or untreated individuals die of the condition due to complications. Also, reoccurrence of the condition increases with initial diagnosis of the disease. Early treatment of pulmonary embolism decreases the risk of serious side effects, and proactive continued monitoring of the condition prevents the reoccurrence of pulmonary embolism.

Patients who develop pulmonary embolism from deep venous thrombosis may develop permanent leg swelling, discomfort, discoloration, chronic nonhealing ulcerations, and atrophic skin changes.

## Deep Venous Thrombosis

**Deep venous thrombosis** is a condition that involves the formation of blood clots in the veins deep within the body, which can dislodge and embolize into other organ systems such as the lungs, heart, and brain. The condition mainly affects the lower legs and thighs. Deep venous thrombosis is also known as blood clots in the legs, venous thrombosis, and venous thrombus.

In the United States, the **incidence** of deep venous thrombosis is approximately 4.2 cases per 100,000 individuals per year. The incidence of deep venous thrombosis increases with age, with those over the age of 60 at higher risk.

### *Diagnosis and Screening*

Physical examination, medical history, and diagnostic testing are used to **diagnose** deep venous thrombosis. Upon physical examination, practicing clinicians may recommend a patient for further diagnostic testing when deep venous thrombosis is suspected.

Diagnostic testing tools include venography, Doppler ultrasound of leg in question, nuclear medicine imaging studies, magnetic resonance imaging, impedance plethysmography of leg, and D-dimer blood test. Other blood tests to evaluate the presence of blood clots include antithrombin III, protein C, protein S, factor V Leiden, prothrombin 2020a mutation, disseminated intravascular coagulation (DIC) test, and lupus anticoagulant and anticardiolipin antibodies.

### *Causes and Risk Factors*

**Risk factors** for deep venous thrombosis include prolonged sitting such as long car trips, plane trips, or prolonged bedrest as well as recent surgery, fractures, childbirth, and use of oral contraceptives and hormone replacement therapy. Malignancy and smoking are also important risk factors.

Individuals at higher risk for deep venous thrombosis include those with a history of deep venous thrombosis, inherited blood disorders, injury to deep vein from surgery or other trauma, slowed blood flow due to lack of physical activity, pregnancy, recent or ongoing cancer treatment, central venous catheter, obesity, and age over 60.

Deep venous thrombosis can be **caused** by damage to the vein's inner lining due to physical, chemical, or biochemical factors such as surgery, injury, inflammation, or immune response. Other causes include hindered blood flow and more viscous blood.

#### *Symptoms*

The **symptoms** of deep venous thrombosis include pain in one leg, tenderness in one leg, swelling of one leg, increased heat or warmth in one leg, and discoloration of skin color in one leg.

Individuals with deep venous thrombosis may also present with pulmonary embolism. Symptoms of pulmonary embolism include unexplained shortness of breath, pain with deep breathing, coughing up blood, and tachycardia.

A majority of patients diagnosed with deep venous thrombosis may also present with tendonitis, arterial insufficiency, arthritis, asymmetric peripheral edema, cellulitis, hematoma, lymphedema, soft tissue injury, neurogenic pain, and postphlebitic syndrome.

#### *Complications and Prognosis*

The **complications of deep venous thrombosis** include pulmonary embolism and postphlebitic syndrome. Blood clots in the thigh have a higher rate of leading to pulmonary embolism than deep venous thrombosis of the lower leg.

The **prognosis** of deep venous thrombosis is good with early intervention. However, untreated deep venous thrombosis can lead to serious complications such as pulmonary embolism, stroke, heart attack, and sudden death. Also, maintaining regular checkups, being compliant with pharmacologic agents, using graduated compression stockings, and increasing physical activity all decrease complications of deep venous thrombosis.

### Venous Insufficiency

**Venous insufficiency** is a condition that involves abnormal blood flow through the veins, which can lead to complications such as heart failure and sudden death. Typically, the condition occurs when veins in the legs do not properly send blood back to the heart. Venous insufficiency can be associated with deep venous thrombosis, varicose veins, and static dermatitis and ulcers.

The **risk** of venous insufficiency increases with age, with women over the age of 50 at highest risk for developing the condition. In the United States, the prevalence of venous insufficiency ranges from 7% to 60% on average.

#### *Diagnosis and Screening*

Physical examination, medical history, and diagnostic tools are used to **diagnose** venous insufficiency. Newer guidelines recommend the use of standard diagnostic tools. Practicing clinicians may use a clinical scoring system that rates signs and symptoms of venous insufficiency. The scoring system ranks five symptoms including pain, cramps, heaviness, pruritus, and paresthesia and six signs including edema, hyperpigmentation, induration, venous ectasia, redness, pain, and calf compression on a scale of 0–3, with 3 being most severe. Scores of 5–14 on two visits greater than six months apart indicate mild to moderate disease, and scores greater than 15 indicate severe disease.

### *Causes and Risk Factors*

Patients diagnosed with venous insufficiency are also at **risk** for skin color changes around the ankles, redness of legs and ankles, thickening of skin on legs and ankles, and ulcers on the legs and ankles.

The most common risk factor for venous insufficiency is deep venous thrombosis. Other risk factors include natural aging, pregnancy, limited physical activity, smoking, sitting for long periods of time, obesity, phlebitis, family history, medical history of cardiovascular disease, and presence of other comorbid conditions. Blood pressure that is higher than normal in the leg can also lead to venous insufficiency.

### *Symptoms*

The **symptoms** of venous insufficiency can vary based on the extent and degree of disease. However, some patients present with few or no symptoms. Also, symptoms may mimic other conditions and should be evaluated by a clinical practitioner to eliminate the presence of other comorbid conditions.

Common symptoms include throbbing, cramping, burning sensations, fatigue, ulcerations that do not heal, varicose veins, fluid retention, and skin changes and discoloration in the legs. Other symptoms include pain that improves when raising the legs but gets worse when standing as well as dullness, aching, heaviness, and/or cramping in the legs. Varicose veins are complications that can lead to death if they rupture and bleed.

### *Complications and Prognosis*

**Complications of venous insufficiency** include chronic pain, dermatitis, chronic non-healing ulcers, hemorrhage, recurrent cellulitis, deep and superficial thrombophlebitis, pulmonary embolism, heart attack, stroke, and even sudden death. Complications associated with nontreatment of venous insufficiency include recruitment of veins, deep venous thrombosis, pulmonary embolism, venous ulceration, and secondary lymphedema.

Potential complications associated with surgical ablation include infection, peripheral nerve damage, and arterial injury. Adverse events associated with radiofrequency ablation and endovenous laser therapy include skin burns, injury to adjacent tissues, and injury to deep veins. Additionally, side effects associated with sclerotherapy include allergic reaction, cutaneous necrosis, and loss of limb.

The **prognosis** of venous insufficiency depends on the extent and degree of the condition, presence of other comorbid conditions, and the patient's age and overall general health.

## Valvular Disease

**Valvular disease** is a condition that affects one of the four main cardiac valves including the aortic, tricuspid, mitral, and pulmonic valves.

**Valvular stenosis** is a condition that involves narrowing, stiffening, thickening, and/or blockage of one or more of the heart valves. Depending on the valve site, the condition can be referred to as aortic stenosis, tricuspid stenosis, mitral stenosis, and/or pulmonic stenosis.

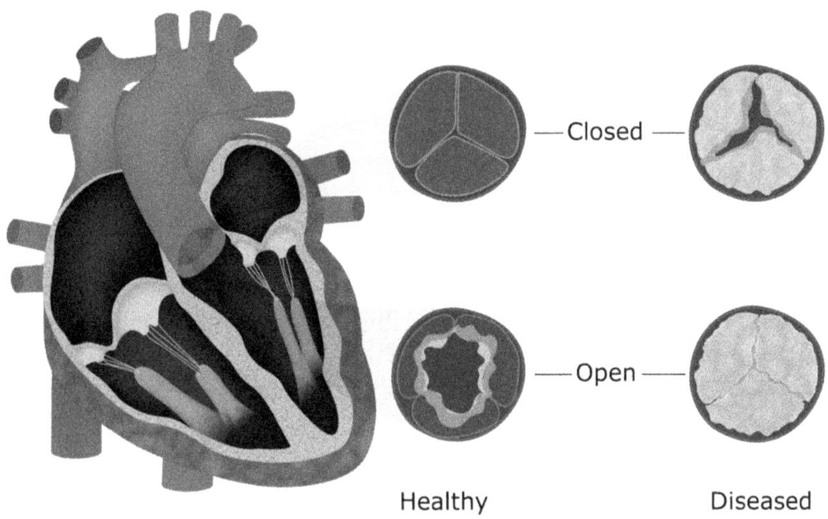


**Valvular regurgitation** is a condition that occurs when blood leaks back through the valve in the wrong direction due to improper closing of one or more of the cardiac valves. Depending on the valve site, the condition can be referred to as aortic regurgitation, tricuspid regurgitation, mitral regurgitation, and/or pulmonic regurgitation.

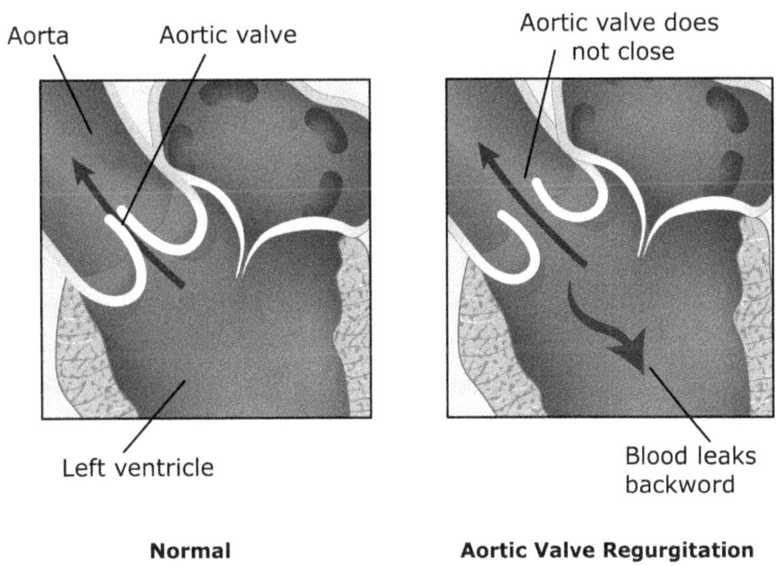

**Atresia** is a condition where one or more of the cardiac valves fail to develop properly, and there is a small or no opening between the respective chambers. Depending on the valve site, the condition can be referred to as aortic atresia, tricuspid atresia, pulmonic atresia, and/or mitral atresia. Aortic atresia is often associated with a patent ductus arteriosus and, sometimes, coarctation of the aorta.

**Mitral valve prolapse** is a very common condition characterized by excessive retrograde movement of one or both mitral valve leaflets. It is often associated with regurgitation through the mitral valve due to anatomical defects in the valve flaps. It occurs in 1–2% of the population in the United States, affecting men and women equally. In most cases, the condition is considered benign with few or no symptoms. However, in some cases, it can lead to more serious complications and various symptoms. Rarely, it is secondary to rheumatic carditis, Marfan syndrome, or ruptured chorda tendinea.

### *Incidence and Prevalence*

**Valvular disease** accounts for approximately 20,000 deaths in the United States annually. It is also considered a contributing factor to increased mortality in over 40,000 individuals annually. The majority of patients with valvular disease leading to death have aortic valve dysfunction, accounting for over 60% of cases, with over 10% having a contribution from mitral valve dysfunction. Deaths due to tricuspid and pulmonic valve dysfunctions are uncommon. Pregnant women with valvular disease are at higher risk for complications to the mother and fetus. Women aged 75 years or older are at an increased risk for developing atherosclerosis and potentially valvular disease than men of the same age group.

### *Diagnosis and Screening*

The **diagnosis** of valvular disease can be difficult, especially when patients present with few or no symptoms. Most patients are diagnosed during routine physical examination or when examining the patient for other conditions.

Physical examination, medical history, and diagnostic tools are used to diagnose valvular disease. Practicing clinicians examine the patient for abnormal heart sounds such as murmur, evidence of heart enlargement, and fluid buildup in the lungs.

Diagnostic tools used to screen for valvular disease include electrocardiogram, echocardiography, magnetic resonance imaging, and chest x-ray. Other diagnostic tests to rule out any other comorbid cardiovascular conditions include cardiac catheterization and cardiac stress testing.

### *Causes and Risk Factors*

The **causes** of valvular disease can be a combination of genetic and environmental factors. The most common causes of valvular disease are congenital defects such as Marfan syndrome and infections such as rheumatic fever.

Diseases or other disorders that can lead to valvular disease include damage and scar tissue due to heart attack, endocarditis, other infections, high blood pressure, heart failure, and/or atherosclerosis. Other conditions that have been associated with valvular disease include systemic lupus erythematosus, cardiomyopathy, syphilis, hypertension, aneurysms, connective tissue disorders, carcinoid syndrome, metabolic disorders, diet medications, and radiation therapy.

Individuals at highest **risk** for developing valvular disease include those with comorbid cardiovascular diseases such as congestive heart failure, those older than 65 years of age, and those with endocarditis and/or rheumatic fever.

### Symptoms

The severity of **symptoms** associated with valvular disease depends on the extent and degree of the disease and the particular valves affected. However, patients with mild disease may present with few or no symptoms, while patients with more severe disease may have symptoms that are more extensive.

Gradual progression of valvular disease typically presents with fewer symptoms than sudden onset of valvular disease. Symptoms that can be associated with valvular disease include chest pain; palpitations; loss of breath; fatigue; fainting; swelling of ankles, feet, or abdomen; weakness; dizziness; and rapid weight gain.

### Complications and Prognosis

Most patients diagnosed with **valvular disease** can live their normal lifespan without any interruption of quality of life or impact from symptoms. However, in some patients diagnosed with the condition, the disease progresses over time, leading to complications such as congestive heart failure, stroke, blood clot formation, myocardial infarction, and sudden death.

The **prognosis** of individuals diagnosed with valvular disease depends on the extent and degree of the condition, age of the patient, and presence of other comorbid conditions. Pharmacologic management and lifestyle changes may improve a patient's prognosis and prevent the onset of more serious complications such as congestive heart failure, stroke, blood clot formation, myocardial infarction, and sudden death.

## Cardiac Vasospasm

**Vasospasm** is a condition that occurs when blood vessels spasm, leading to vasoconstriction. The condition can cause ischemia, blood clot formation, hemorrhage, stroke, aneurysm, heart attack, and sudden death. The genetic and/or environmental factors that contribute to vasospasm remain vague, and a combination of factors is usually the cause of vasospasm. Some patients present with few or no symptoms, while others present with more symptoms.

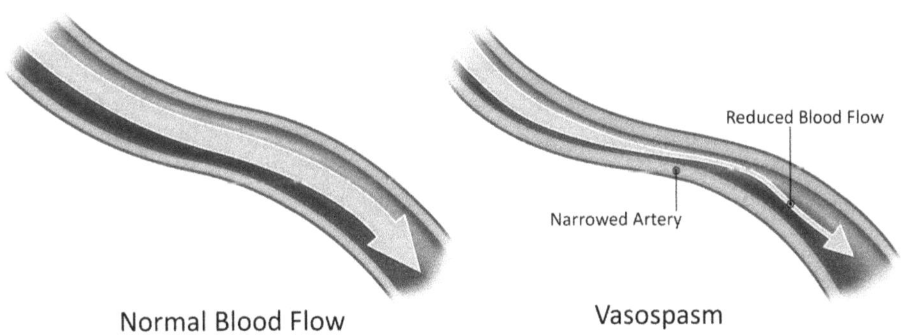


Cardiac vasospasm can be treated with lifestyle modifications, pharmacologic management and, in more severe cases, surgery. Pharmacologic approaches include nitrates such as nitroglycerin, isosorbide dinitrate and isosorbide mononitrate, and calcium channel blockers such as nifedipine, amlodipine, verapamil, and diltiazem.

### Complications and Prevention

**Complications associated with cardiac vasospasm** include myocardial infarction, arrhythmias, tachycardia, ventricular fibrillation, heart failure, stroke, and sudden death. Complications depend on the degree and extent of cardiac vasospasm, age of the patient, and presence of other comorbid conditions.

General preventive measures that individuals can take to reduce the risk of cardiac vasospasm and disease complications include avoiding the triggers of vasospasm such as cocaine or stress. Decreasing risk factors for heart disease in general is also beneficial.

## Angina Pectoris

**Angina pectoris** is a condition defined by chest pain and/or discomfort due to myocardial ischemia. The condition is reversible and dissipates over a short period. It can be associated with pain that radiates to the shoulders, neck, or jaw.

In the United States, the **prevalence** of angina pectoris is over 6 million individuals. The condition is more prevalent among women than men, with more than 4 million women being affected and over 2 million men affected. Individuals over the age of 50 are at an increased risk for angina pectoris, especially those individuals with other cardiovascular comorbid conditions.

### *Causes and Risk Factors*

**Angina pectoris** is typically caused by the presence of atherosclerotic disease or blood clot formation in the coronaries. Other conditions contributing to angina pectoris include valvular disease, coronary artery spasm or abnormalities, and other cardiovascular conditions. Angina pectoris is typically precipitated by cold, stress, exertion, or large meals.

**Non-modifiable risk factors** for angina pectoris include a medical history of cardiovascular disease, family history of heart disease, increasing age, female gender, and African American or Hispanic American descent.

**Modifiable risk factors** include cigarette smoking, hypertension, elevated low-density lipoprotein levels, elevated triglycerides, low serum high-density lipoprotein, diabetes, previous stroke, alcohol or illicit drug abuse, obesity, and/or physical inactivity.

### *Diagnosis and Screening*

Physical examination, medical history, and diagnostic tools are used to **screen** for angina pectoris. Practicing clinicians examine the patient for abnormal heart sounds, evidence of heart enlargement, presence of other cardiovascular comorbid conditions, and/or fluid build-up in the lungs. Individuals suspected of angina pectoris or other comorbid conditions may be observed over a few days in a hospital setting to determine the reason for their chest pain and/or discomfort, specifically to rule out myocardial infarction.

Diagnostic tools used to **diagnose** angina pectoris include response to nitroglycerin and echocardiography. Other diagnostic tools used in the screening for angina pectoris to exclude other comorbid conditions include echocardiography, electrocardiogram, magnetic resonance imaging, ultrasound, and chest x-ray. Other more invasive diagnostic approaches include cardiac catheterization and cardiac stress testing.

### *Symptoms*

Patients diagnosed with angina pectoris typically present with chest pain, vomiting, nausea, fatigue, and other cardiovascular **symptoms**. The pain often radiates across the precordium, to the jaw, and to the shoulders. The degree and extent of symptoms depend on the condition, underlying cause of the condition, age of the patient, and/or presence of other comorbid conditions.

Chronic stable angina pectoris typically presents with increased symptoms upon physical exertion and/or fatigue. Individuals with unstable angina pectoris typically present with similar symptoms, but the symptoms are typically more severe, frequent, and /or prolonged.

Physical findings upon diagnosis include S4 heart sounds, cardiac murmur, dysrhythmia, tachycardia, hypertension, and/or hypotension.

### Complications and Prognosis

In most cases, **angina pectoris** is typically a symptom and dissipates as the underlying condition is treated. It is not a typically a serious condition, and most patients will not experience any complications such as myocardial infarction, heart failure, or stroke due to angina pectoris.

Treating underlying causes of angina pectoris decreases the risk of developing complications or other comorbid conditions. However, in more severe cases in individuals with comorbid cardiovascular conditions, patients may experience myocardial infarction and/or arrhythmias. Elderly patients who are in poor health with other comorbid conditions are more likely to experience more serious complications compared to younger patients who are in good health.

Angina pectoris, especially unstable angina and cases not responding to nitrates, should always be taken seriously.

### Comparison to Myocardial Infarction

**Angina pectoris** often serves as a warning sign for myocardial infarction. Angina is chest pain occurring from reduced blood flow to the myocardium. This pain is described as squeezing, burning, or pressure and is focused on the chest cavity. It is intermittent, often correlating with increased activity and dissipating with rest and/or the use of nitroglycerine.

**Myocardial infarction** occurs when the lack of oxygen perfusion to the heart causes myocardial tissue death. This pain is more extreme, often referred to as crushing, and extends beyond the chest to radiate out toward the back, shoulder, neck, and jaw. Rest and nitroglycerin will have no effect on this type of pain. Initial treatments will include oxygen and morphine sulfate for pain control.

Angina may be diagnosed with an exercise stress test. In the face of an MI, an electrocardiogram will show ST changes, and laboratory results will show elevated troponin and creatinine levels.

## Arrhythmias

**Arrhythmia** is defined as a condition that involves dysregulation of cardiac electrical activity. Arrhythmia can cause a slowing or speeding up of the heart rate, or irregular heartbeat. Tachycardia is a condition that occurs when an arrhythmia is faster than normal, whereas bradycardia is a condition that occurs when an arrhythmia beats slower than normal.

There are many **types of arrhythmias** including premature beats, supraventricular arrhythmias, ventricular arrhythmias, and bradyarrhythmias. Premature beats can originate in both the atria and the ventricles. Supraventricular arrhythmias originate in the atria and include atrial fibrillation, atrial flutter, and Wolf-Parkinson-White syndrome. Arrhythmias that originate in the ventricles include ventricular tachycardia, ventricular fibrillation, and long QT syndrome. Bradycardias occur when the heart rate is below 60 bpm and can be categorized as sick sinus or conduction block.

### *Factors and Causes*

Both genetic and environmental factors can contribute to the development of arrhythmias. However, sometimes the **cause** of an arrhythmia may remain unknown. Factors that increase an individual's risk for developing arrhythmias include age; family history; medical history of cardiovascular conditions such as congestive heart failure, rheumatic heart disease, coronary artery disease, or previous heart surgery; thyroid dysfunction, including hyperthyroidism and hypothyroidism; drugs containing pseudoephedrine or other stimulants; alcohol or illicit drug abuse; high blood pressure; obesity; diabetes; stress; excessive exercise; obstructive sleep apnea; electrolyte imbalance; and/or stimulant use such as caffeine or tobacco.

### *Diagnosis and Screening*

**Diagnosis** of arrhythmias can be difficult if patients present with few or no symptoms. Physical examination, medical history, and diagnostic tools are used to screen for atrial fibrillation. Upon physical examination, practicing clinicians will look for a rapid or irregular heart rate, varying heart rate, and/or hypotension.

Diagnostic screening tools used to confirm diagnosis of an arrhythmia primarily include electrocardiogram, Holter monitor, and event recorders. Of note, echocardiography, chest x-ray, magnetic resonance imaging, and thyroid function tests will help elucidate the underlying cause. Also, blood work may be completed to assess other contributing factors including thyroid function tests, electrolyte levels, and metabolic function tests. More invasive diagnostic tools used include stress test, tilt table test, and/or electrophysiologic testing.

### *Symptoms*

Some patients who are diagnosed with an arrhythmia present with few or no **symptoms**. However, many patients present with symptoms upon diagnosis. Yet, these symptoms vary from patient to patient and in terms of severity. Cardiovascular comorbid conditions may also impact the symptoms that patients diagnosed with arrhythmias present with.

Symptoms commonly associated with different types of arrhythmias include cardiac palpitations, slow heartbeat/heart rate, irregular heartbeat, skipped heartbeats, feeling of pauses between heartbeats, anxiety, weakness, dizziness, lightheadedness, fainting, sweating, shortness of breath, chest pain, inability to perform activities of daily living, confusion, fatigue, physical activity intolerance, and hypotension.

## Atrial Arrhythmias

**Atrial arrhythmias** are the most common type of cardiac arrhythmia. These include:

- **Premature atrial contractions (PAC):** Normal rhythm, irregular rate with irregular P waves. Patient may complain of a "fluttering" sensation or exhibit low blood pressure.

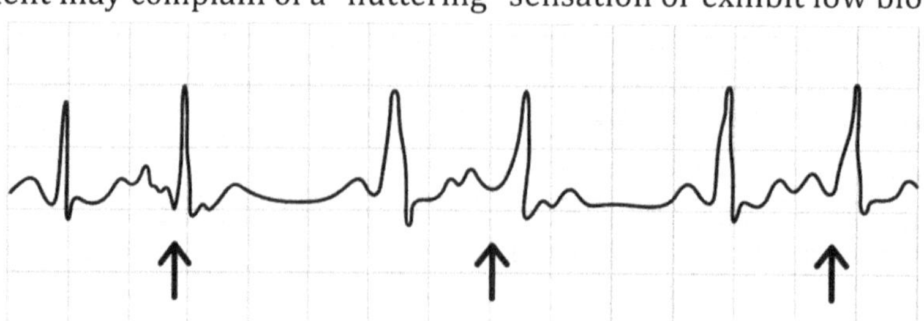

- **Atrial flutter:** A form of supraventricular tachycardia. Atrial rate of 250–400 bpm. Saw-toothed appearance on ECG. Critical nature increases with higher ventricular rates. Pulse may be normal but patient exhibits signs of decreased cardiac output.

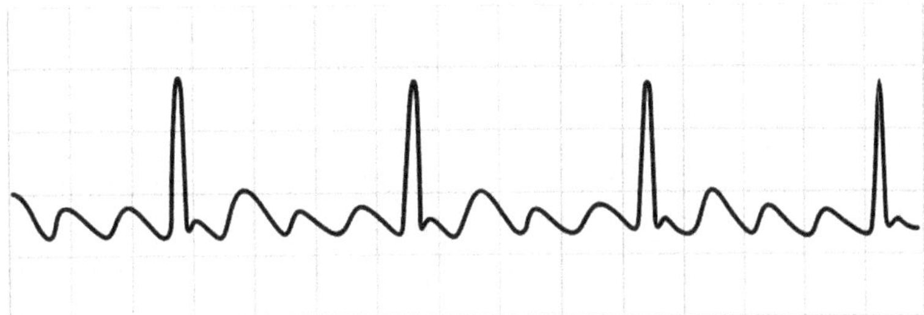

- **Atrial fibrillation (A-fib):** Chaotic electrical impulses of the atrium with a rate of 400–600 bpm and irregular ventricular rate. Cannot identify or measure P wave, PR interval, T wave, or QT interval. High risk for shock, heart failure, or embolism. Pulses may not match audible heart rate. Patient exhibits low blood pressure and change of consciousness.

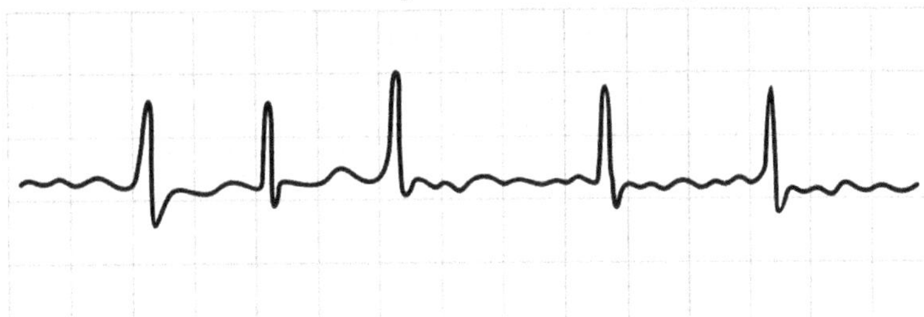

- **Atrial tachycardia:** A form of supraventricular tachycardia. Exhibits a regular atrial and ventricular rate of 150–250 bpm. Patient shows decreased cardiac output and is at risk for angina, heart failure, or myocardial infarction. Common cause is digoxin toxicity.

### *Nursing Diagnoses and Treatments*

Arrhythmias include any malfunction of the normal beating of the heart. This can include beating too fast, too slow, or irregularly. An arrhythmia may be constantly present when not controlled or may appear sporadically due to known or unknown causes.

**Nursing diagnoses** might include decreased cardiac output, deficient knowledge, and in the case of digitalis, toxicity poisoning. Treatment for an arrhythmia may only occur in the symptomatic patient; this treatment might include cardiac monitoring, medication, cardioversion, or use of a pacemaker.

### *Complications and Prognosis*

**Complications of arrhythmias** include stroke, congestive heart failure, and thromboembolism. Severe complications including myocardial infarction, thromboembolism, and stroke occur more often in undiagnosed individuals and those noncompliant with treatment.

Treating the underlying causes of arrhythmias and the arrhythmia itself decreases the risk of developing complications. However, in more severe cases, especially in individuals with comorbid cardiovascular conditions, patients may experience myocardial infarction and/or arrhythmias. Elderly patients who are in poor health with other comorbid conditions are more likely to experience more serious complications compared to younger patients who are in good health.

## ATRIAL FIBRILLATION

**Atrial fibrillation** is a dysfunctional cardiac arrhythmia. The condition is caused by absent P waves, irregular R-R intervals, and F waves of variable shape and amplitude. Atrial fibrillation can occur as an acute condition or a chronic condition. Chronic atrial fibrillation is better tolerated than acute atrial fibrillation.

The **incidence** of atrial fibrillation increases with age and is the most common dysrhythmia. The condition occurs in approximately 20–30% of individuals undergoing coronary artery bypass surgery. In the general population, atrial fibrillation occurs in just under 10% of individuals over the age of 70. In the United States, the prevalence of atrial fibrillation is approximately 2 million individuals.

### *DIAGNOSIS AND SCREENING*

**Symptoms** of atrial fibrillation vary, and therefore, patients may not present with symptoms upon diagnosis. Physical examination, medical history, and diagnostic tools are used to screen for atrial fibrillation. Upon physical examination, practicing clinicians will look for rapid or irregular heart rate, varying intensity and frequency of S1, and hypotension. Diagnostic screening tools used to confirm diagnosis of atrial fibrillation and likely etiologies include echocardiogram, electrocardiogram, Holter monitor, event recorder, chest x-ray, magnetic resonance imaging, and thyroid function tests.

Also, blood work may be completed to access other contributing factors, including thyroid function tests, electrolyte levels, and metabolic function tests.

### *CAUSES AND RISK FACTORS*

The key **risk factors** for atrial fibrillation include increasing age, heart disease, other chronic diseases such as thyroid dysfunction or lung disease, alcohol abuse, and/or family history.

Other risk factors associated with atrial fibrillation include pulmonary disease, valvular disease, congenital heart disease, coronary artery bypass surgery, congestive heart failure, atherosclerosis, myocardial infarction, rheumatic heart disease, and thyrotoxicosis.

Other possible **causes** of atrial fibrillation include high blood pressure, congenital heart defects, hyperthyroidism, metabolic imbalance, exposure to stimulants such as caffeine, illicit drugs, alcohol or tobacco, sick sinus syndrome, emphysema, lung disease, previous heart surgery, viral infections, stress due to pneumonia or other illnesses, and/or sleep apnea.

### *SYMPTOMS*

Many individuals with atrial fibrillation do not have any **symptoms** of disease but are diagnosed during routine physical examination or when being assessed for another ailment or condition. However, some patients present with more extensive symptoms. Symptoms may also vary from patient to patient. In addition, the severity of symptoms and impact on quality-of-life parameters may vary from patient to patient.

Symptoms associated with atrial fibrillation include fatigue, dizziness, weakness, physical activity intolerance, hypotension, inability to perform daily living activities, cardiac palpitations, shortness of breath, fainting, confusion, chest pain, and lightheadedness.

### *Complications and Prognosis*

**Chronic atrial fibrillation** leads to **complications** that include clot formation, thromboembolism, heart failure, and potential for heart attack and stroke. Acute atrial fibrillation can lead to more serious complications, as the body is unable to handle the severity of the condition.

Nearly half of patients experiencing atrial fibrillation treated with pharmacologic agents including dysrhythmia agents do not experience a reoccurrence at 12 months. However, individuals with underlying comorbid conditions should have those conditions addressed to prevent reoccurrence of atrial fibrillation as well as other comorbid cardiovascular complications. Severe complications, including myocardial infarction, thromboembolism, and stroke, occur more often in undiagnosed individuals and those who are noncompliant with treatment.

## Atrial Flutter

**Atrial flutter** is a condition that is similar to atrial fibrillation. However, the condition presents with a more organized and less chaotic abnormal heartbeat compared with atrial fibrillation. However, atrial flutter may develop into atrial fibrillation, and the reverse is also possible.

In atrial flutter, the atrial rhythm is regular, and the ventricular rhythm may be regular or irregular. In atrial fibrillation, the atrial rhythm is irregular, so the ventricular rhythm is also irregular.

The symptoms, diagnosis, risk factors, and complications of atrial flutter are similar to those of atrial fibrillation. However, atrial flutter is as not as life threatening as atrial fibrillation. Also, patients diagnosed with atrial flutter respond better to catheter ablation than patients diagnosed with atrial fibrillation. Both conditions are more common in elderly patients.

### *Diagnosis and Screening*

The **diagnosis** of atrial flutter can be difficult if patients present with few or no symptoms. Physical examination, medical history, and diagnostic tools are used to screen for atrial fibrillation. Upon physical examination, practicing clinicians will look for rapid or irregular heart rate and/or hypotension.

Diagnostic screening tools used to confirm diagnosis and cause of atrial flutter include echocardiogram, electrocardiogram, Holter monitor, event recorder, chest x-ray, magnetic resonance imaging, and thyroid function tests. Also, blood work may be completed to assess other contributing factors including thyroid function tests, electrolyte levels, and metabolic function tests. More invasive diagnostic tools used include stress test, tilt table test, and/or electrophysiologic testing.

### *Causes and Risk Factors*

The **causes and risk factors** for atrial flutter are similar to those of atrial fibrillation. Both genetic and environmental factors can lead to the onset of atrial flutter.

The most common **causes** include rheumatic heart disease, high blood pressure, coronary artery disease, alcohol or illicit drug abuse, hyperthyroidism, hypothyroidism, pulmonary disease, valvular disease, congenital heart disease, coronary artery bypass surgery, congestive heart failure, atherosclerosis, myocardial infarction, rheumatic heart disease, metabolic imbalance, exposure to stimulants such as caffeine or tobacco, sick sinus syndrome, emphysema, lung disease, previous heart surgery, viral infections, stress due to pneumonia or other illnesses, and/or sleep apnea.

### *Symptoms*

Some patients diagnosed with an atrial flutter present with few or no **symptoms**. However, many patients present with a variety of symptoms upon diagnosis. These symptoms vary from patient to patient and in terms of severity. Cardiovascular comorbid conditions may also affect the symptoms that are presented in patients diagnosed with atrial flutter.

Symptoms commonly associated with atrial flutter include cardiac palpitations, irregular heartbeat, anxiety, weakness, dizziness, lightheadedness, fainting, sweating, shortness of breath, chest pain, inability to perform activities of daily living, confusion, fatigue, physical activity intolerance, and hypotension.

### *Complications and Prognosis*

Typically, **atrial flutter** is not considered as life threatening as atrial fibrillation. However, complications associated with atrial flutter include stroke, embolization, rate-related complications, clot formation, sudden cardiac death, congestive heart failure, severe bradycardia, and myocardial rate-related ischemia.

The risk of developing stroke with atrial fibrillation and atrial flutter is approximately 4%. In more severe cases of atrial flutter, especially those with comorbid cardiovascular conditions, patients may experience myocardial infarction or stroke. Elderly patients who are in poor health with other comorbid conditions are more likely to experience more serious complications compared to younger patients who are in good health.

## Wolff-Parkinson-White Syndrome

**Wolff-Parkinson-White syndrome** develops because of the formation of extra electrical circuits within the heart. The condition leads to a rapid heart rate and abnormal electrocardiogram.

In the United States, Wolff-Parkinson-White syndrome occurs in less than 0.2% of the general population. Most patients diagnosed with the syndrome have no evidence of other cardiovascular comorbid conditions. Wolff-Parkinson-White syndrome is the most common cause of tachycardia in young children, toddlers, and infants. The syndrome is more common in men than women, with 60–70% of cases in men. However, the syndrome can occur in individuals of all ages and ethnic/racial descents. The highest incidence occurs in individuals between the ages of 30 and 40.

### *Diagnosis, Screening, Causes, and Risk Factors*

Physical examination, medical history, and diagnostic tools are used to **screen** for Wolff-Parkinson-White syndrome. Upon physical examination, practicing clinicians will look for rapid or irregular heart rate, varying heart rate, and/or hypotension. The Wolff-Parkinson-White syndrome (a preexcitation syndrome) is characterized by a short PR interval and a delta wave, which appears as a slurred upstroke into the QRS complex, so the PR interval is missing. The QRS complex is prolonged because of the delta wave. The rhythm is very irregular and the rate is often 250-300 bpm. The delta wave is produced because of premature depolarization of part of the ventricles.

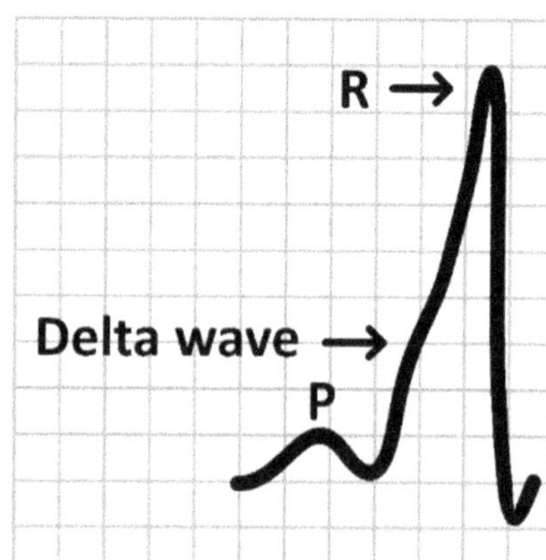


Diagnostic screening tools used to confirm **diagnosis** of Wolff-Parkinson-White syndrome include electrocardiogram, Holter monitor, event recorders, and electrophysiologic testing and mapping.

Wolff-Parkinson-White syndrome is a syndrome, and by definition, an identifiable external **cause** is not known. It is caused by an accessory pathway in the cardiac conduction system that causes arrhythmias in some individuals. The condition is congenital, and thus there are no risk factors.

### *Symptoms*

The **symptoms** of Wolff-Parkinson-White syndrome include rapid heart rate and abnormal electrocardiogram. Patients diagnosed with the condition may have a few episodes of increased heart rate, while others may present with more consistent episodes of increased heart rate, as many as a few times per week. Symptoms may also vary from patient to patient and may vary in terms of severity. Cardiovascular comorbid conditions may further affect the symptoms that present in patients who are diagnosed with the syndrome.

The most common symptoms associated with the syndrome include cardiac palpitations, lightheadedness, fainting, confusion, dizziness, shortness of breath, chest pain, chest tightness, fluttering in the chest, anxiety, sweating, inability to perform activities of daily living, fatigue, physical activity intolerance, and hypotension. Wolff-Parkinson-White is one of the most common causes of tachycardia in infants and children.

### *Complications and Prognosis*

**Complications of Wolff-Parkinson-White syndrome** include hypotension, congestive heart failure, and other comorbid cardiovascular conditions.

The **prognosis** of patients diagnosed with Wolff-Parkinson-White syndrome varies depending on the degree and extent of disease. However, most patients respond well to lifestyle modifications and pharmacologic management. Also, more invasive approaches such as radiofrequency catheter ablation cure the condition by ablating the extra pathway, which has demonstrated good outcomes. Elderly patients who are in poor health and have other comorbid conditions are more likely to experience more serious complications compared to younger patients who are in good health.

## Ventricular Fibrillation

**Ventricular fibrillation** is a very serious condition caused by uncoordinated contractions of cardiac muscle in the ventricles of the heart. In this condition, the contractions of the atria and ventricles are uncoordinated. If not addressed promptly, the condition can lead to heart failure and sudden death.

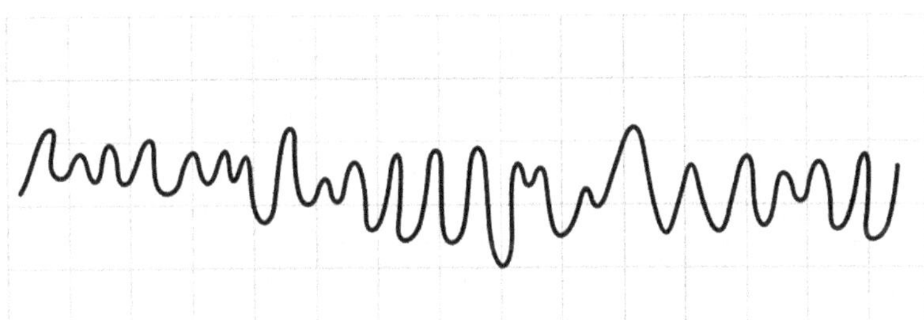

In the United States, approximately 300,000 individuals are diagnosed with ventricular fibrillation. The condition is more common in men than women. Individuals of African American descent are also at higher risk for ventricular fibrillation. The condition rarely occurs in infants under the age of 6 months or in adults age 45–75 years old.

### Diagnosis and Screening

Ventricular fibrillation is an emergency condition that requires immediate attention to prevent serious complications such as congestive heart failure and sudden death. Physical examination, medical history, and diagnostic tools are used to **screen** for ventricular fibrillation. Upon physical examination, practicing clinicians will look for rapid or irregular heart rate, hypertension, or hypotension. The patient may also present with a very low or no heart rate, and a cardiac monitor will demonstrate a disorganized heart rate.

Diagnostic screening tests used to confirm **diagnosis** of ventricular fibrillation include electrocardiogram, cardiac monitor, Holter monitor, and event recorder.

### Causes and Risk Factors

The main **cause** of ventricular fibrillation is myocardial infarction, but the condition can result from other cardiovascular comorbid conditions and/or when the heart does not get enough oxygen. Other conditions that can lead to ventricular fibrillation include congenital heart disease, coronary artery disease, shock, electrical shock, drowning, very low levels of potassium, electrocution accidents, injury to heart, cardiomyopathies, congestive heart failure, heart surgery, administration of drugs that affect electrical currents such as sodium blockers, and/or ischemia.

Additional **risk factors** include family history of cardiovascular disease, medical history of cardiovascular conditions, hypertension, high cholesterol, diabetes, smoking, and/or alcohol or illicit drug abuse.

### Symptoms

The **symptoms** associated with ventricular fibrillation can resemble those of other cardiovascular conditions and can vary from patient to patient. Individuals with an acute ventricular fibrillation episode typically present by fainting or suddenly collapsing and/or becoming unconscious. They also typically present with a very rapid or undetectable heart rate.

Symptoms that typically occur before an individual having an acute ventricular fibrillation episode faints or becomes unconscious include chest pain, seizures, dizziness, nausea, vomiting, rapid heartbeat, shortness of breath, confusion, and weakness.

### Consequences and Prognosis

**Ventricular fibrillation** is a very serious condition with severe complications, including congestive heart failure and sudden cardiac death. The degree and extent of complications depends on when a patient receives treatment for the condition or whether the patient recognizes the symptoms and seeks treatment.

Other complications in patients who survive an acute ventricular fibrillation episode include coma, reduced mental perception, neurological problems, congestive heart failure, central nervous system (CNS) ischemic injury, myocardial injury, post defibrillation arrhythmias, aspiration pneumonia, defibrillation injury, injuries from cardiopulmonary resuscitation, skin burns, stroke, and other cardiovascular conditions.

The **prognosis** for patients who experience an acute ventricular fibrillation episode depends on the length of time the patient was in fibrillation. However, for those patients who survive an acute ventricular fibrillation episode, the survival rate averages around 2–25% post hospital stay. Patients who seek treatment sooner rather than later tend to have better outcomes long term. Elderly patients who are in poor health and have other comorbid conditions are more likely to experience more serious complications compared to younger patients who are in good health.

## VENTRICULAR TACHYCARDIA

**Ventricular tachycardia** is a condition that is initiated in the ventricle and results in a very rapid or irregular heartbeat. The condition is triggered by three or more consecutive premature ventricular heartbeats. Ventricular tachycardia can result in heartbeats ranging from 160 to 240 bpm. The condition can be classified as nonsustained or sustained.

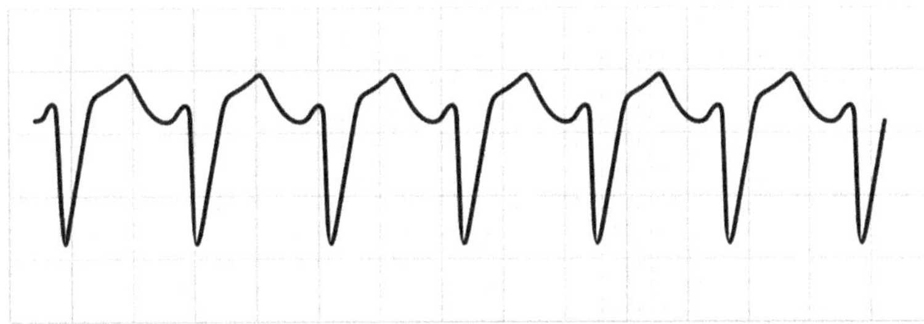

In the United States, ventricular tachycardia occurs in approximately 2 out of 10,000 individuals. The **incidence** of ventricular tachycardia in the United States remains unknown due to overlap with ventricular fibrillation. Ventricular tachycardia is more **prevalent** among men than women but varies with the risk factors for atherosclerosis. The incidence of ventricular tachycardia increases with natural aging and with prevalence of coronary artery disease.

### *DIAGNOSIS AND SCREENING*

Physical examination, medical history, and diagnostic tools are used to **diagnose** ventricular tachycardia. Upon physical examination, practicing clinicians will look for rapid or irregular heart rate and changes in blood pressure. The patient may also present with a very low or no heart rate and normal or low blood pressure. Individuals with ventricular tachycardia may present with fainting or in an unconscious state.

Diagnostic tools used to screen for ventricular tachycardia and assess for causes include electrocardiogram, echocardiogram, Holter monitor, intracardiac electrophysiology studies, event recorder, chest x-ray, magnetic resonance imaging, and thyroid function tests. Also, blood work may be completed to access other contributing factors including thyroid function tests, electrolyte levels, and metabolic function tests.

### *CAUSES AND RISK FACTORS*

The most common **cause** of ventricular tachycardia is the presence of coronary artery disease. Ventricular tachycardia can result from the presence of other comorbid cardiovascular conditions or in the absence of any other cardiac diseases. It can also occur as a result of myocardial infarction, congestive heart failure, cardiomyopathy, cardiac valvular disease, myocarditis, ischemia, electrolyte abnormalities, high potassium levels, high magnesium levels, adrenergic stimulation, and post cardiovascular surgery.

Additional **risk factors** include family history of cardiovascular disease, medical history of cardiovascular conditions, hypertension, high cholesterol, diabetes, smoking, and/or alcohol or illicit drug abuse.

### *SYMPTOMS*

The **symptoms** of ventricular tachycardia can vary depending on the degree and extent of disease. Some patients present with severe symptoms that require emergency treatment. However, other patients may present with few or no symptoms, which may or may not require medical intervention. In addition, symptoms may start and stop suddenly. Ventricular tachycardia is most commonly associated with coronary artery disease and can present with a nonsustained or sustained rapid heart rate.

The most common symptoms individuals with ventricular tachycardia present with include heart palpitations, rapid heartbeat, lightheadedness, dizziness, confusion, weakness, fatigue, fainting, shortness of breath, and chest discomfort.

#### Complications and Prognosis

**Complications associated with ventricular tachycardia** can be benign or very serious, including congestive heart failure and cardiac sudden death. The prognosis of patients with ventricular tachycardia depends on the degree and extent of the condition. Patients who seek treatment sooner rather than later tend to have better outcomes long term. Elderly patients who are in poor health and have other comorbid conditions are more likely to experience more serious complications compared to younger patients who are in good health.

The **mortality rate** of ventricular tachycardia in patients with cardiomyopathy and nonsustained disease averages 30% in two years. In patients with idiopathic disease, prognosis is excellent. However, patients with long QT syndrome, right ventricular dysplasia, and hypertrophic cardiomyopathy are at an increased risk of sudden cardiac death.

## PSVT

Paroxysmal Supraventricular Tachycardia (**PSVT**) refers to occasional, intermittent rapid heart rate that lasts from a few minutes to several hours. This most often occurs in younger patients and can be brought on by alcohol, caffeine, smoking, illicit drug use, or digitalis toxicity. Intervention of any kind might not be needed unless the patient is presenting symptoms such as anxiety, dizziness, shortness of breath, an uncomfortable feeling of chest tightness, racing heart, or fainting. Emergency treatment options might include the Valsalva maneuver (instructing the patient to bear down as if having a bowel movement), splashing the face with ice water, IV adenosine, or cardioversion. Long-term stability may be maintained by oral medications such as propafenone, flecainide, moricizine, sotalol, and amiodarone; the use of a pacemaker; or, more often, radiofrequency catheter ablation.

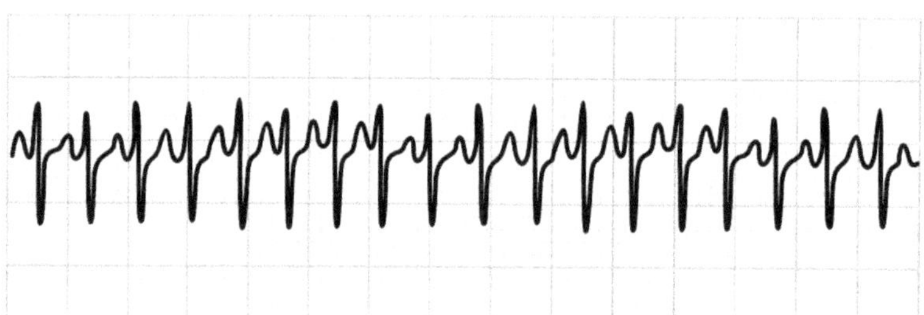

### Intermittent Claudication

**Intermittent claudication** is a condition that arises from peripheral arterial disease. Approximately one-third to one-half of individuals diagnosed with peripheral arterial disease present with intermittent claudication. The condition occurs after physical exertion and consists of pain during physical activity, which resolves once the activity is stopped. The pain most commonly occurs in the calves, thighs, and/or buttocks.

The condition is defined as muscle pain or cramping in appendages triggered by walking and physical activity. Individuals may also experience ischemic rest pain. The condition results from inadequate oxygen supply to the legs because of impeded blood flow.

### *Incidence and Prevalence*

Intermittent claudication occurs more commonly in men than women. It also occurs more often in individuals with a history of smoking, cardiovascular comorbid conditions, diabetes, and high blood pressure.

The estimated **prevalence** of intermittent claudication is approximately 4.5 million individuals. It has been estimated that 60–70% of individuals with intermittent claudication have persistent symptoms, 20–25% of symptoms get worse, and 10% require surgical intervention. The rate of amputation is approximately 1–2% per year.

### *Diagnostic Screening*

The **symptoms** of individuals with intermittent claudication may vary. Therefore, practicing clinicians should assess the patient's medical history and presence of comorbid conditions and examine the patient. Physical examination, medical history, and diagnostic screening tools are used to determine if a patient has intermittent claudication.

Upon physical examination, practicing clinicians use a stethoscope to determine the presence of bruits. They also look for evidence of poor wound healing, sores, color changes, muscle pain or cramping upon physical activity, temperature changes, and decreased blood pressure in limbs. Diagnostic screening tools include the ankle-brachial index and angiography. Additional tests include electrocardiogram, magnetic resonance angiography, blood tests, and ultrasound.

### *Causes and Risk Factors*

Intermittent claudication is most commonly associated with peripheral arterial disease. Both genetic and environmental factors can contribute to the onset of intermittent claudication.

The **risk factors** and causes for intermittent claudication are very similar to peripheral arterial disease, as the former is a symptom of the latter. Conditions that can lead to intermittent claudication include blood clots, injury to limbs, and unusual anatomy of ligaments or muscles or infection. Other diseases that can lead to onset of peripheral vascular disease include aortic aneurysms, Buerger's disease, pulmonary embolism, phlebitis, varicose veins, and Raynaud's syndrome.

Factors that increase an individual's risk for peripheral arterial disease and intermittent claudication include smoking, being 50 years of age or older, diabetes, obesity, high blood pressure, high cholesterol, or family history of cardiovascular diseases and/or arthrosclerosis. Male individuals of African American descent as well as overweight individuals and those with a family history of cardiovascular disease are at a higher risk of peripheral vascular disease and intermittent claudication.

### *Symptoms*

The main **symptoms** of intermittent claudication include pain in a functional muscle group located in the legs such as calf, buttock, and thigh; pain after strenuous activity such as brisk walking or physical activity; and reduction of pain once physical activity is stopped.

The symptoms of intermittent claudication are associated with other symptoms of peripheral arterial disease, including leg numbness or weakness; cold legs and feet; sores or wounds that will not heal on digits or extremities; blue or pale hue to legs, feet, hands, and/or arms; hair loss on feet and legs; and changes in composition of nails.

### COMPLICATIONS AND PROGNOSIS

The **prognosis** of individuals diagnosed with **intermittent claudication** is good because the condition typically stabilizes or improves over time. The condition tends to improve over a few months when new, smaller blood vessels form to make up for the blockage or lack of blood flow to larger blood vessels in the legs.

Typically, approximately one-third of patients with intermittent claudication tend to improve over time, while one-third remain stable, and another one-third deteriorate, mainly due to continued smoking. Graduated increased physical activity can improve the condition over time, as regular walks have demonstrated improvement in the condition.

Early intervention with physical activity provides better outcomes and improvements in the condition. Patients who seek treatment sooner rather than later tend to have better outcomes long term. Elderly patients who are in poor health and have other comorbid conditions are more likely to experience more serious complications compared to younger patients who are in good health.

## HYPOTENSION

**Hypotension** is defined as low blood pressure, particularly pressure lower than 90/60 mmHg. However, what practicing clinicians consider low blood pressure varies from patient to patient because some individuals have naturally low blood pressure with no symptoms. Also, patients with comorbid conditions like hepatic disease (cirrhosis) may have lower than normal blood pressure at baseline.

Drops in blood pressure of more than 20 mmHg from a patient's normal blood pressure are more of a concern, as this can cause symptoms of dizziness, fainting, and decreased mental capacity. This can also be an indicator of a more serious underlying condition such as uncontrolled bleeding, severe infections, and/or allergic reactions.

### ORTHOSTATIC HYPOTENSION

**Orthostatic hypotension** or postural hypotension is defined as low blood pressure upon standing. In this condition, an individual's blood pressure drops when going from a sitting to standing position, leading to dizziness, lightheadedness, blurred vision, and fainting or syncope. The causes of orthostatic hypotension include dehydration, prolonged bedrest, pregnancy, diabetes, heart problems, burns, excessive heat exposure, large varicose veins, and certain neurological disorders. Drugs that can lead to orthostatic hypotension include diuretics, beta-blockers, calcium channel blockers, angiotensin-converting enzyme inhibitors, and antidepressants.

This condition is more common in older individuals, with 20% of cases occurring in individuals aged 65 or older.

### POSTPRANDIAL HYPOTENSION

**Postprandial hypotension** is a condition that involves a sudden drop in blood pressure after eating. It typically affects elderly individuals with other cardiovascular comorbid conditions or neurological disorders. Symptoms of the condition include dizziness, fatigue, syncope or fainting, mental confusion, and/or lightheadedness. Postprandial hypotension is more common among individuals with high blood pressure or autonomic nervous system disorders. Lifestyle modifications such as eating smaller, more frequent meals that are low in carbohydrates may reduce symptoms. Also, lowering the dose of blood pressure medications may decrease the onset of postprandial hypotension.

### *Shy-Drager Syndrome*

**Shy-Drager syndrome**, also known as multiple system atrophy with orthostatic hypotension, is a rare disease that causes progressive damage to the autonomic nervous system. Deterioration of the autonomic nervous system leads to improper functioning of blood pressure, heart rate, breathing, and digestion. The main characteristic of Shy-Drager syndrome is severe hypotension when standing and severe hypertension when lying down. Other symptoms of the disease include muscle tremors, slowed movement, problems with coordination and speech, and incontinence. The disease is progressive with few treatment approaches and usually leads to death within 7–10 years from time of diagnosis.

### *Neurally Mediated Hypotension*

**Neurally mediated hypotension** is a condition that causes a drop in blood pressure after standing for long periods. The symptoms associated with neurally mediated hypotension include dizziness, lightheadedness, heart palpitations, sweating, nausea, confusion, and fainting or syncope. The condition tends to affect younger adults and is caused by a malfunction between the brain and cardiovascular system, which causes blood to pool in the legs and feet, leading to sudden blood pressure drops. Lifestyle modifications that may improve symptoms include the vagal maneuver, increased sodium intake, and use of graduated compression stockings. Pharmacologic agents such as beta-blockers, alpha-adrenergic inhibitors, and agents that maintain salt in the kidneys can improve symptoms.

### *Causes and Risk Factors*

The **causes and risk factors** associated with hypotension vary from individual to individual. Athletes and individuals who exercise regularly tend to have lower blood pressure than unfit and/or obese individuals. The main risk factors and causes of hypotension, as outlined by the American Heart Association, include pregnancy; certain pharmacologic agents such as diuretics, beta-blockers, Parkinson disease drugs, tricyclic antidepressants, sildenafil (particularly in combination with nitroglycerine), narcotics, and alcohol; cardiac conditions such as bradycardia, cardiac valvular disease, myocardial infarction and congestive heart failure; endocrine problems such as hypothyroidism, hyperthyroidism, Addison's disease, hypoglycemia and diabetes; blood loss such as from major surgery or severe injury; severe infection; allergic reaction; nutritional deficiencies such as a lack of vitamins B-12 and folate; natural aging; and dehydration.

### *Diagnosis and Screening*

Physical examination, medical history, and diagnostic tools are used to **diagnose** hypotension and determine which type of hypotension a patient presents with. The goal is to determine the underlying cause of hypotension in order to treat the symptoms of hypotension or treat the underlying cause to improve an individual's blood pressure.

Diagnostic tools used to assess hypotension include blood tests such as red blood cell counts and blood glucose levels, electrocardiogram, echocardiogram, stress test, Valsalva maneuver, and/or tilt-table test.

### *Symptoms*

The **symptoms** of hypotension vary from patient to patient and depend on the extent and degree of the condition. It also depends on the patient's overall health and presence of other comorbid conditions. Also, some individuals experience more severe symptoms than others, even if their blood pressure is relatively normal. However, patients with relatively low blood pressure may experience few or no symptoms.

Symptoms associated with hypotension include dizziness; lightheadedness; fainting or syncope; lack of concentration or decrease in mental capacity; weakness; fatigue; blurred vision; nausea; cold, clammy, and/or pale skin; rapid or shallow breathing; depression; and/or thirst.

### *Complications and Prognosis*

**Complications associated with hypotension** or low blood pressure include dizziness, fainting, confusion and, in more serious cases, severe heart, endocrine, and/or neurological disorders. Shock is a complication of very severe hypotension, where the brain and other organ systems are deprived of oxygen and vital nutrients.

Most healthy individuals with hypotension can maintain their condition with lifestyle modifications. However, in more severe cases, practicing clinicians will prescribe pharmacologic agents and treat the underlying cause of the condition. Individuals with hypotension, including neurally mediated hypotension or orthostatic hypotension, need to be careful to avoid fainting and dizziness, which can be dangerous. In very severe cases of hypotension, shock is a life-threatening condition that is fatal if not treated immediately.

## Compartment Syndrome

**Compartment syndrome** is a condition that involves the compression of nerves and blood vessels within an enclosed space, which leads to decreased blood flow as well as muscle and nerve damage. Compartment syndrome can be acute or chronic, depending on the underlying cause. Chronic compartment syndrome can be caused by repetitive activities that lead to swelling, such as running or excessive physical activity.

The **incidence** of compartment syndrome in the United States is relatively low, averaging up to 12%. The mortality rate depends on the time of diagnosis and treatment of the condition. The condition is more common in men than women.

### *Diagnosis and Screening*

**Diagnosis** of compartment syndrome involves physical examination, medical history, and diagnostic screening tools. A practicing clinician will examine a patient for any swollen toes, legs, or feet. They will also move or squeeze muscle groups potentially affected to see if the patient expresses severe pain.

The diagnosis is made by directly measuring the pressure in the compartment with a needle and pressure meter, which is called the compartment pressure measurement. If the compartment pressure is greater than 45 mmHg or the diastolic blood pressure is within 30 mmHg, then a diagnosis of compartment syndrome is made. Other diagnostic screening tools used include blood tests such as complete metabolic profile, complete blood count, creatine phosphokinase and urine myoglobin, serum myoglobin, toxicity screen, and prothrombin and activated partial thromboplastin time. Urinalysis may also be performed along with the use of imaging tools such as radiography and ultrasonogram.

If chronic compartment syndrome is suspected, then direct blood pressure measurement needs to be determined post physical exertional activity.

### *Causes and Risk Factors*

**Risk factors** and causes of compartment syndrome include swelling due to high-energy trauma from a car accident or surgery, tight bandages, or casts with significant swelling. In addition, a variety of physical injuries can lead to compartment syndrome. Compartment syndrome can be caused by increased pressure, swelling, and/or decreased compartment size. Increased swelling or fluid buildup can be caused by intensive muscle use, daily physical exertion, burns, intraarterial injection, envenomation, decreased serum osmolarity, infiltrated infusion, and hemorrhage. Decreased compartment size can be caused by military anti-shock trousers, burns, tight bandages, and/or casts. The abdomen can also be a site of compartment syndrome if excessive swelling occurs.

### *Symptoms*

The **main symptom** associated with compartment syndrome is severe pain that does not respond to elevation or pain medication. However, in more severe cases, patients may present with decreased sensation, weakness, and paleness of the skin. The degree and extent of symptoms depend on the severity of compartment syndrome and whether or not it is a chronically occurring condition.

Typically, patients diagnosed with compartment syndrome present with severe pain when a muscle running through a compartment is passively moved or squeezed, such as a toe, foot, or leg. The skin covering the affected compartment will be shiny and swollen.

### *Complications and Prognosis*

Prompt diagnosis and treatment of **compartment syndrome** results in good outcomes, with recovery of affected nerves and blood vessels of the muscle. However, the prognosis of compartment syndrome is determined by the underlying injury leading to the condition. Delayed diagnosis and treatment can result in permanent nerve damage and loss of muscle function. Other complications include impaired function due to muscle damage, infection, cosmetic deformity, and death and limb amputation.

Increased education in patients at high risk for compartment syndrome improves prognosis and prevents serious complications due to early diagnosis and treatment.

## Pulmonary Edema

**Pulmonary edema** is a condition that involves increased blood pressure in the blood vessels of the lungs forcing fluid into the air sacs, which prevents the absorption of oxygen. The elevated pulmonary capillary pressures lead to increased fluid in the interstitial compartment and alveoli. Decreased cardiac output, inadequate tissue perfusion, and acute pulmonary congestion are characteristic of the condition.

**Acute pulmonary edema** is a serious condition that requires prompt medical attention. However, if treated aggressively and immediately, prognosis is generally good. Delayed intervention can lead to severe complications, including death. In the acute care setting, the mortality rate associated with pulmonary edema is as high as 15–20%, on average.

### *Diagnosis and Screening*

Physical examination, medical history, and diagnostic screening tools are used to **diagnose** pulmonary edema. Acute pulmonary edema requires prompt medical attention for prevention of severe complications. Patients with pulmonary edema typically present with rapid breathing, increased heart rate, crackles in lungs, and pale or blue skin.

Diagnostic tools used for screening of pulmonary edema include blood tests such as arterial blood gas concentrations, chest x-ray, electrocardiogram, echocardiogram, and transesophageal echocardiography. A more invasive diagnostic approach used to diagnose pulmonary edema when diagnosis is unclear is pulmonary artery catheterization.

### Causes and Risk Factors

The **causes and risk factors** for pulmonary edema are generally environmental and can be exacerbated by the presence of other comorbid conditions. The causes and risk factors for pulmonary edema include coronary artery disease, congestive heart failure, myocardial infarction, cardiomyopathy, cardiac valve dysfunction, and high blood pressure.

Noncardiac causes and risk factors for pulmonary edema include lung infections; exposure to certain toxins such as chlorine, ammonia, and nitrogen dioxide; kidney disease; smoke inhalation; adverse drug reaction to drugs, such as illicit drugs and chemotherapy drugs; acute respiratory syndrome; and high altitudes.

### Symptoms

The **symptoms** of pulmonary edema can vary from patient to patient. The symptoms are also dependent on the degree and extent of the condition as well as a patient's overall general health and presence of other comorbid conditions. However, the most common symptoms associated with pulmonary edema include extreme shortness of breath or difficulty breathing, a feeling of suffocating or drowning, wheezing or gasping for breath, anxiety, restlessness, a sense of apprehension, a cough that produces frothy sputum that may be tinged with blood, excessive sweating, grunting or gurgling sounds when breathing, restlessness, anxiety, nasal flaring, inability to speak, decreased awareness, pale skin, and chest pain.

Symptoms that may develop more gradually include difficulty breathing while lying down, awakening at night out of breath, increased shortness of breath, and significant weight gain.

### Complications and Prognosis

**Complications associated with pulmonary edema** include leg swelling, abdominal swelling, and pleural effusion. If treated promptly, individuals diagnosed with pulmonary edema have a good prognosis. However, individuals who are not promptly diagnosed or treated may have more serious complications or death.

Early intervention provides better outcomes and improvements in the condition. Patients who seek treatment sooner rather than later tend to have better outcomes long term. Elderly patients who are in poor health and have other comorbid conditions are more likely to experience more serious complications compared to younger patients who are in good health.

## First-Degree Atrioventricular Block

**First-degree atrioventricular block** is defined as a delay in conduction of impulses from the sinoatrial (SA) node to the atrioventricular (AV) node. The condition is typically asymptomatic and undiagnosed. It can occur in individuals of all ages. The disease is typically benign and not associated with an increase in morbidity and mortality.

In the United States, the **prevalence** of first-degree atrioventricular block varies up to 1.6%. There is a higher prevalence in younger adult athletes. The condition is more prevalent in African Americans than Caucasian Americans. The condition also increases with natural aging and is more prevalent among elderly patients with other cardiovascular comorbid conditions.

### Diagnosis and Screening

Physical examination, patient history, and diagnostic screening tools are used to **diagnose** first-degree atrioventricular block. The condition is often hard to diagnose, as patients typically present with few or no symptoms. Many individuals go undiagnosed due to lack of symptoms. Additionally, some individuals have prolonged PR interval due to a normal variant that is typically asymptomatic.

The condition is often diagnosed during routine electrocardiogram screening and is found incidentally. Diagnosis is made by a PR interval greater than 200 msec.

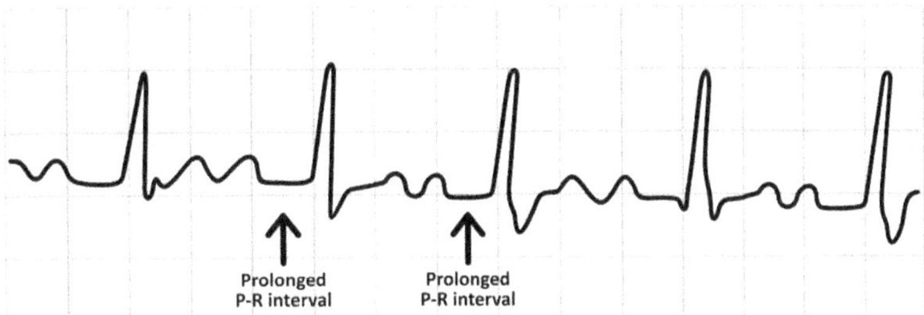


### Causes and Risk Factors

Other **comorbid conditions** that can lead to first-degree atrioventricular block include cardiac ischemia, myocardial infarction, congestive heart failure, coronary artery disease, scarring of atrial tissue in internodal pathways, infiltration by amyloid, sarcoid, Lyme carditis, endocarditis, degenerative diseases, rheumatic cardiac disease, electrolyte imbalances, atrial stretch, increased vagal tone, and inflammatory diseases.

**Pharmacologic agents** that can lead to first-degree atrioventricular block include digoxin; calcium channel blockers such as nifedipine, amlodipine, verapamil, and diltiazem; and beta-blockers.

The condition is characterized by prolonged PR interval (greater than 200 msec), which can also occur as a normal variant in some individuals.

### Symptoms

Individuals who present with first-degree atrioventricular block have few or no **symptoms** and typically are not at risk of developing other comorbid conditions. Diagnosis is typically made during routine physical examination or when being examined for another complaint. In patients with first-degree atrioventricular block, heart rate and rhythm are typically normal, and there may be nothing wrong with the heart. However, some patients may present with fainting and syncope, bradycardia, left ventricular systolic dysfunction, and comorbid congestive heart failure.

Many well-trained athletes may present with first-degree atrioventricular block but do not present with symptoms.

### Complications and Prognosis

**Complications associated with first-degree atrioventricular block** include progression of condition to a higher degree of atrioventricular block, reduction in left ventricular stroke volume and cardiac output leading to left ventricular systolic dysfunction, and pacemaker syndrome. Patients who progress usually progress to Mobitz type I, second-degree atrioventricular block, but sometimes progress to complete atrioventricular block.

The **prognosis** associated with first-degree atrioventricular block is excellent, especially in patients with asymptomatic disease. First-degree atrioventricular block does not present with increased mortality or morbidity. However, patients who present with comorbid intranodal blocks have an increased risk of developing complete atrioventricular block, which comes with a high risk of serious complications, including death.

## Second-Degree Atrioventricular Block Types I and II

**Second-degree atrioventricular block type I,** also known as Wenckebach or Mobitz I, is also an asymptomatic dysrhythmia. The condition typically occurs in adults as post myocardial infarction or with inferior wall ischemia.

**Second-degree atrioventricular block type II** also known as Mobitz II is an intermittent failure of conduction of impulses below the AV node. The condition is often associated with HIS-Purkinje system cardiac disease, which can lead to complications such as complete heart block or ventricular asystole. It occurs most often in adults and is associated with a high mortality rate.

### *Type I*

#### Causes and Risk Factors

Second-degree atrioventricular block type I can occur due to the presence of structural heart disease. However, structural heart disease does not have to be present for the disease to occur. The condition may also occur due to a normal variant or autosomal dominant trait, making the individual genetically predisposed.

**Pharmacologic agents** that slow conduction through the atrioventricular node have been shown to cause second-degree atrioventricular block type I. These agents include cardioactive drugs such as digoxin, beta-blockers, calcium channel blockers, and certain antiarrhythmic drugs such as sodium channel blockers (procainamide).

Other disorders that can lead to second-degree atrioventricular block type I include inflammatory diseases such as endocarditis, myocarditis, Lyme disease, and acute rheumatic fever; infiltrative diseases such as amyloidosis, hemochromatosis, and sarcoidosis; metabolic disorders such as hyperkalemia, hypermagnesemia, and Addison's disease; and vascular diseases such as ankylosing spondylitis, dermatomyositis, rheumatoid arthritis, scleroderma, lupus, and Reiter syndrome. Also, acute myocardial infarction has been associated with second-degree atrioventricular block type I.

#### Diagnosis and Screening

Physical examination, patient history, and diagnostic screening tools are used to **diagnose** second-degree atrioventricular block type I. The condition is often hard to diagnose, as patients typically present with few or no symptoms. Many individuals go undiagnosed due to lack of symptoms.

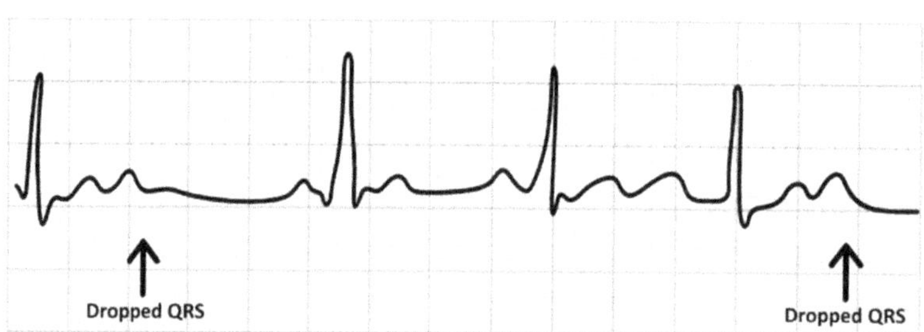


The condition is diagnosed on electrocardiogram by progressive lengthening of PR interval followed by a P wave without an associated QRS complex. A Holter monitor or event recorder can be used to diagnose outpatients. Laboratory tests including serum electrolyte and magnesium levels, serum digoxin levels, and thyroid function tests may be used to find the cause. Other imagining tests may be performed, depending on the patient's symptoms and presence of comorbid cardiovascular conditions. Diagnostic electrophysiologic testing may be necessary to determine the site of block and need for a pacemaker.

### Symptoms

Individuals who present with second-degree atrioventricular block type I have few or no **symptoms** and typically are not at risk of developing other comorbid conditions. Diagnosis is typically made during routine physical examination or when being examined for another complaint. In patients with second-degree atrioventricular block type I, heart rate and atrial rhythm are typically abnormal due to atrioventricular node dysfunction. However, some patients may present with lightheadedness, dizziness, decreased cardiac output, activity intolerance, shortness of breath, chest pain, hypotension, bradycardia, heart failure, stroke, and syncope.

However, symptoms in patients diagnosed with second-degree atrioventricular block type I can vary greatly, depending on the overall health and physical conditioning of the patient as well as presence of other comorbid conditions.

### Complications and Prognosis

**Second-degree atrioventricular block type I** is typically a benign condition that does not require immediate treatment. The **complications** associated with more mild forms of the condition are minimal except in patients with poor health or other cardiovascular comorbid conditions.

Patients undergoing treatment with agents that have the potential to induce second-degree atrioventricular block type I should be monitored closely, and doses should be adjusted if the condition is induced by the medication.

The **prognosis** of second-degree atrioventricular block type I depends on the extent and degree of the block. Atrioventricular nodal blocks, which make up most of the type I blocks, carry a better prognosis than intra- or infra- bundle blocks. Intra- and/or infra- bundle blocks can progress to higher degrees of atrioventricular block, including complete atrioventricular block.

## *Type II*

**Second-degree atrioventricular block type II,** also known as Mobitz II, is an intermittent failure of conduction of impulses below the AV node. The condition is often associated with HIS-Purkinje system cardiac disease, which can lead to complications such as complete heart block or ventricular asystole. It occurs most often in adults and is associated with a high mortality rate, as the condition can progress rapidly to a complete heart block.

The condition is highly associated with infra- and intranodal blocks, which indicate the location of the blocks. A small percentage of second-degree atrioventricular block type II occurs due to underlying structural disease. The condition occurs in adults and equally in men and women. There is no correlation between ethnicity and/or race and second-degree atrioventricular block type II. The condition is less common than second-degree atrioventricular block type I. Second-degree atrioventricular block type II is associated with a high mortality rate when it occurs with comorbid anterior wall myocardial infarction.

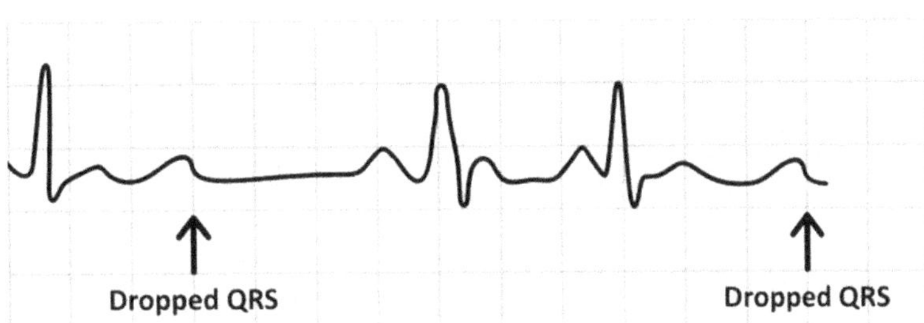

### Diagnosis and Screening

Physical examination, patient history, and diagnostic screening tools are used to **diagnose** second-degree atrioventricular block type II. The condition is typically associated with significant underlying conduction system conditions. Patients often present with hypotension, diaphoresis, and pauses in pulse caused by decreased cardiac output.

The condition is diagnosed by electrocardiogram, Holter monitor, or event recorder. Not every P wave has an associated QRS complex (1:3, etc.), and there is NO progressive prolongation of PR interval. Lab tests and echocardiography may be necessary to further elucidate the underlying cause. Also, diagnostic electrophysiologic testing may be necessary to determine the site of the block and need for a pacemaker.

### Causes and Risk Factors

Second-degree atrioventricular block type II can occur due to the presence of structural heart disease. However, structural heart disease does not have to be present for the disease to occur. The condition may also occur due to a normal variant or autosomal dominant trait, making the individual genetically predisposed.

**Pharmacologic agents** that slow conduction through the AV node have been shown to cause second-degree atrioventricular block type II. These agents include cardioactive drugs such as digoxin, beta-blockers, calcium channel blockers, and certain antiarrhythmic drugs such as sodium channel blockers (procainamide).

Other disorders that can lead to second-degree atrioventricular block type II include inflammatory diseases such as endocarditis, myocarditis, Lyme disease, and acute rheumatic fever; infiltrative diseases such as amyloidosis, hemochromatosis, and sarcoidosis; metabolic disorders such as hyperkalemia, hypermagnesemia, and Addison's disease; and vascular diseases such as ankylosing spondylitis, dermatomyositis, rheumatoid arthritis, scleroderma, lupus, and Reiter syndrome. Also, acute myocardial infarction, congestive heart failure, coronary artery disease, and primary diseases have been associated with second-degree atrioventricular block type II.

### Symptoms

Some patients may present with lightheadedness, dizziness, decreased cardiac output, activity intolerance, shortness of breath, chest pain, hypotension, bradycardia, diaphoresis, pauses in pulse, heart failure, stroke, and/or syncope or fainting.

However, **symptoms** in patients diagnosed with second-degree atrioventricular block type I can vary greatly, depending on the overall health and physical conditioning of the patient as well as presence of other comorbid conditions.

### Complications and Prognosis

The **prognosis for patients with second-degree atrioventricular block type II** is not as good as the prognosis for patients with second-degree atrioventricular block type I. Typically, second-degree atrioventricular block type II progresses to complete heart block and carries risk of syncope, stroke, myocardial infarction, and congestive heart failure. In particular, intra- and/or infra- bundle blocks can progress to higher degrees of atrioventricular block, including complete atrioventricular block.

Patients undergoing treatment with agents that have the potential to induce second-degree atrioventricular block type II should be monitored closely, and doses should be adjusted if the condition is induced by the medication.

## Third-Degree Atrioventricular Block

**Third-degree atrioventricular block,** also known as complete heart block, involves complete dissociation of impulses between the atria and ventricles. The condition is not well tolerated and is most common in adults but can also occur in adolescents with congenital heart disease. The condition can occur intermittently or consistently, depending on the underlying cause of the condition.

In the United States, the prevalence of third-degree atrioventricular block is approximately 0.02%. The **incidence** of third-degree atrioventricular block increases with age but may also occur in infants or adolescents due to congenital complete heart block.

### *Causes and Risk Factors*

The most common **causes** of third-degree atrioventricular block include drugs that target the atrioventricular node such as beta-blockers, calcium channel blockers, quinidine, and procainamide; degenerative diseases such as Lenègre disease and Lev disease; infectious causes such as Lyme disease, rheumatic fever, myocarditis, and Chagas disease; rheumatic diseases such as ankylosing spondylitis, Reiter syndrome, relapsing polychondritis, rheumatoid arthritis, and scleroderma; infiltrative processes such as amyloidosis, sarcoidosis, tumors, Hodgkin's disease, and multiple myeloma; neuromuscular disorders such as Becker muscular dystrophy and myotonic muscular dystrophy; ischemia or infarction; and metabolic causes such as hypoxia and hyperkalemia.

### *Symptoms*

Most patients diagnosed with third-degree atrioventricular block present with **symptoms**. However, some patients present with few or no symptoms. Additionally, third-degree atrioventricular block may be an underlying condition in patients who present with sudden cardiac death.

The symptoms associated with third-degree atrioventricular block include fainting or syncope, near-syncope, lightheadedness, fatigue, dyspnea, and chest pain. Patients diagnosed with third-degree atrioventricular block typically present with a series of P waves and QRS complexes that do not relate to one another. Additionally, atrial heart rate is normal, but ventricular heart rate is abnormal.

### *Diagnosis and Screening*

Physical examination, medical history, and diagnostic screening tools are used to **diagnose** third-degree atrioventricular block. Electrocardiogram (ECG), Holter monitor, and event recorders are used to diagnose. On the ECG, there is no association between P waves and QRS complexes. Further tests including echocardiography, and lab tests may be necessary to fully elucidate the source of the block.

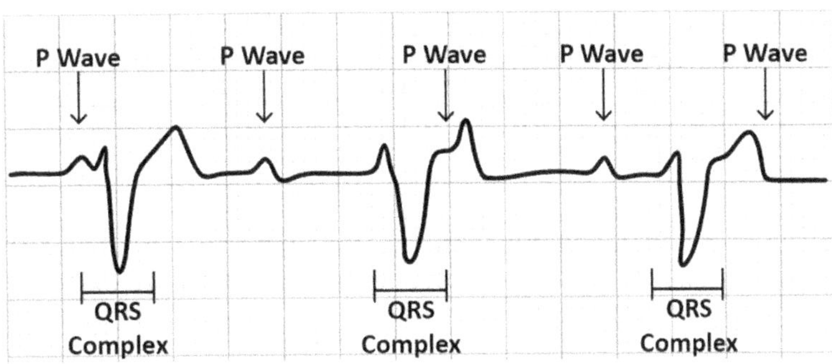

### Complications and Prognosis

The **prognosis of third-degree atrioventricular block** is excellent for patients who receive treatment with permanent pacing. However, patients who are untreated or seek treatment too late are at higher risk for serious complications. Patients who have other comorbid cardiovascular health conditions and/or are in poor health have a poorer prognosis. Patients diagnosed with third-degree atrioventricular block are at high risk for stroke, congestive heart failure, and myocardial infarction.

Patients undergoing treatment with agents that have the potential to induce third-degree atrioventricular block should be monitored closely, and doses should be adjusted if the condition is induced by the medication.

> **Review Video: AV Heart Blocks**
> Visit mometrix.com/academy and enter code: 487004

## Cardiogenic Shock

**Cardiogenic shock** is a condition characterized by inadequate perfusion from cardiac dysfunction. It is an emergency situation and requires immediate treatment. Cardiogenic shock is the most common cause of mortality in patients who experience a myocardial infarction.

In the United States, cardiogenic shock occurs in approximately 8.6% of patients experiencing ST-segment elevation myocardial infarction, with about 29% of those presenting to the hospital already in shock. Cardiogenic shock occurs in a smaller percentage of patients with non-ST segment elevation myocardial infarction, occurring in approximately 2% of patients.

**Mortality rates** vary from one race to another, with Hispanics at highest risk, followed by African Americans and then Caucasians and Asians. Women comprise 42% of all patients with cardiogenic shock.

### Diagnosis and Screening

Physical examination, medical history, and diagnostic screening tools are used to **diagnose** cardiogenic shock. The condition is treated on an emergency basis, requires prompt attention, and is typically diagnosed in the emergency room setting. It is typically diagnosed when a patient has been admitted to the emergency room for a myocardial infarction.

Diagnostic screening tools used to diagnose cardiogenic shock include blood pressure monitoring, electrocardiogram, echocardiogram, chest x-ray, and coronary angiography. Laboratory blood tests that may be performed include arterial blood gas measurement, electrolyte levels, cardiac enzyme levels, renal function, liver function, lactate levels, and thyroid function tests.

### Causes and Risk Factors

The most common **cause** of cardiogenic shock is myocardial infarction. However, not every patient who experiences a myocardial infarction goes into cardiogenic shock. The individuals at highest risk for cardiogenic shock include patients who have experienced a myocardial infarction, those of older age, and those with a history of congestive heart failure, diabetes, dysrhythmia, and/or coronary artery disease.

Common causes of cardiogenic shock include ventricular septal rupture, papillary muscle infarction or rupture, myocarditis, endocarditis, arrhythmias, pericardial tamponade, and pulmonary embolism.

Other causes of cardiogenic shock include beta-blocker overdose, calcium channel blocker overdose, myocardial contusion, respiratory acidosis, hypocalcemia, hypophosphatemia, ventricular hypertrophy, restrictive cardiomyopathies, aortic stenosis, hypertrophic cardiomyopathy, dynamic outflow obstruction, aortic coarctation, malignant hypertension, mitral stenosis, endocarditis, mitral or aortic regurgitation, atrial myxoma, tamponade, and cardiotoxic drugs such as doxorubicin.

### *Symptoms*

The **symptoms** associated with cardiogenic shock vary depending on the patient and presence of underlying comorbid conditions. Younger patients in good health tend to present with fewer symptoms than older patients with other comorbid cardiovascular conditions.

The common symptoms associated with cardiogenic shock include confusion, lack of alertness, loss of consciousness, palpitations, sweating, fainting or syncope, pale skin, weak pulse, rapid breathing, shortness of breath, decreased or no urine output, cold hands and/or feet, anxiety, nervousness, weakness, lethargy, fatigue, loss of ability to concentrate, decreased mental status, restlessness, agitation, coma, dizziness, and lightheadedness.

### *Complications and Prognosis*

**Complications associated with cardiogenic shock** include cardiopulmonary arrest, dysrhythmia, renal failure, multisystem organ failure, ventricular aneurysm, thromboembolic disease, stroke, congestive heart failure, and death.

The **prognosis** for patients diagnosed with cardiogenic shock is very poor. Approximately 50% of patients who experience cardiogenic shock do not survive. The reason that patients diagnosed with cardiogenic shock are able to survive is prompt treatment with pharmacologic agents and/or surgical intervention. The ability to restore blood flow to vital organ systems improves outcomes and prognosis. Patients who undergo treatment promptly with pharmacologic intervention or surgical intervention have an improved prognosis. Evidence of right ventricular dilation on echocardiogram may indicate worse prognosis than other underlying causes of the condition.

# Patient Interview

## Elements of the Patient Interview

The **patient interview** should include:

- **History**: Includes biographic data, reason for seeking medical care, present health condition, history of present illness or chief complaint, past health (including major childhood illnesses, accidents, surgeries, obstetric history, vaccinations), and current medications (including supplements, herbal medications). Important medications to be aware of in the cardiac patient include blood pressure medications and blood thinners (in addition to the patient's compliance with these medications and the last time they were taken).
- **Chief complaint**: Include location, character, severity, timing, aggravating and alleviating factors, timing (onset, duration), associated symptoms, and effects on activities/daily living. Adults often present with a myriad of health problems, so a problem-based assessment focusing on finding a solution to chief complaints and current health problems can be effective. Once a problem is identified, then differential diagnoses are determined. With adults, there may be a combination of physical and psychosocial elements to a problem.
- **Allergies**: Both the allergen and the reaction should be noted as well as adverse effects to medications, foods, or other substances that may suggest sensitization.

## Social Determinants of Health

Social determinants of health refer to the non-medical elements of a person's social environment that have a direct impact on his or her physical health and tendencies. The heavy influence of this component of health is reflected in its being listed as one of the five main sections of *Healthy People 2030,* an initiative of the US Department of Health and Human Services (HHS) that aims to allow people to have longer and healthier lives, to reduce health disparities, to create environments that promote health, and to improve the quality of life and health across all age groups. According to HHS, social determinants of health are "the conditions in the environments where people are born, live, learn, work, play, worship, and age that affect a wide range of health, functioning, and quality-of-life outcomes and risks." Heart health can directly be influenced by these social determinants, so screening of lifestyle, home environment, work environment, and other factors should be built into the patient interview.

## Pain Assessment

The following are qualities of pain that should be assessed in a thorough patient history:

1. **Quality**: Have the patient describe the quality of the pain using words such as dull, stabbing, sharp, aching, throbbing, and burning.
2. **Severity**: Pain can be rated on a scale of 1–10, or another assessment tool can be used.
3. **Location**: Where on the body is the pain located? Does it radiate or shift?
4. **Timing**: When did the pain begin? Is it constant, or does it come and go with a predictable or random frequency?
5. **Causative factors**: Ask whether or not the patient is able to pinpoint a precipitating event prior to the onset of pain.
6. **Aggravating factors**: Does the quality or severity of pain change with activity, position, stress level, or other varying conditions?
7. **Alleviating factors**: What effect do medication, position, or other noninvasive treatment interventions have on the amount of pain?
8. **Related symptoms**: Is the pain accompanied by nausea, dizziness, shortness of breath, or other closely related symptoms?

## Age-Related Cardiovascular Changes in Older Patients

**Age-related cardiovascular changes** include the following:

- The risk for blockage by constriction of the vessels or blood clots increases with age, as does a tendency toward pooling blood in the legs and feet.
- Cardiac output is reduced. Cardiac tissue and vessels can become hardened or brittle or become narrowed from plaque and inflammation buildup, all of which reduce cardiac efficiency and restrict blood flow.
- Exercise endurance and oxygen perfusion is reduced. Many of these factors can be mitigated by maintaining an active lifestyle with a focus on endurance training as the patient ages.

## Obtaining Accurate, In-Depth Personal History

The following are methods of questioning that encourage the patient to give an accurate, in-depth personal history:

- **Open discussion**: This promotes patient comfort by encouraging questions and feedback during the interview.
- **Ask leading questions**: Ask questions that require more than a "yes" or "no" answer and give clear permission for the patient to speak freely about their health.
- **Restate and summarize provided information in another way**: This technique allows you to verify that your understanding of given information is correct.
- **Focus**: Assist the patient to concentrate on identifying their highest healthcare needs or making connections between healthcare behavior and higher priorities.
- **Order and sequence**: Verify cause and effect and timing of the events given in a patient history.
- **Encourage self-evaluation**: Allow the patient to draw their own conclusions regarding information. Do not judge or try to educate at this point.
- **Make observations**: Provide commentary on the patient's physical, mental, and emotional demeanor to help them focus, and give permission to discuss further aspects of their health or immediate needs.

# Cardiovascular Assessment

## Comprehensive Cardiovascular Patient Assessment

The four basic components of a **comprehensive cardiovascular assessment** include the following:

1. **Patient history**: The best source of information about the history of their condition is the patient. Other resources might include past medical records and involved family members.
2. **Physical exam**: Execute a full, head-to-toe symmetrical exam including inspection, palpation, percussion, and auscultation methods as appropriate.
3. **Laboratory results**: Typical laboratory tests include cardiac enzymes, clotting function, cholesterol levels, and therapeutic medication levels.
4. **Diagnostic tests**: Diagnostic tests can include x-ray, computed tomography (CT) scan, magnetic resonance imaging (MRI), electrocardiogram (ECG), echocardiography (ECHO), myocardial perfusion imaging, and cardiac catheterization.

## Physical Examination Procedure

The general order of procedure for a physical examination is described below:

1. **Inspection**: visual inspection with the naked eye and specialized equipment such as an ophthalmoscope to view physical features such as height, body mass, skin condition and color, breath frequency and quality, hair distribution, balance, gait, and presence of tremors or physical injuries
2. **Palpation**: examination by touch for pulses, organ size and location, pain response, temperature, and distinguishable masses
3. **Percussion**: further touch intervention, utilizing the fingers to create sound
4. **Auscultation**: auditory assessment with and without the assistance of a stethoscope, generally focusing on the cardiac, respiratory, and digestive systems. Other useful tools might include the use of Doppler to locate pulses that were difficult to palpate.

This general procedure varies slightly during assessment of the abdomen, placing auscultation before palpation and percussion. Other systems may not require the use of all four examination elements.

**Review Video: Cardiovascular Assessment**
Visit mometrix.com/academy and enter code: 323076

**Review Video: Functions of the Circulatory System**
Visit mometrix.com/academy and enter code: 376581

**Review Video: Heart Blood Flow**
Visit mometrix.com/academy and enter code: 783139

**Review Video: Mnemonics for Heart Anatomy and Physiology**
Visit mometrix.com/academy and enter code: 849489

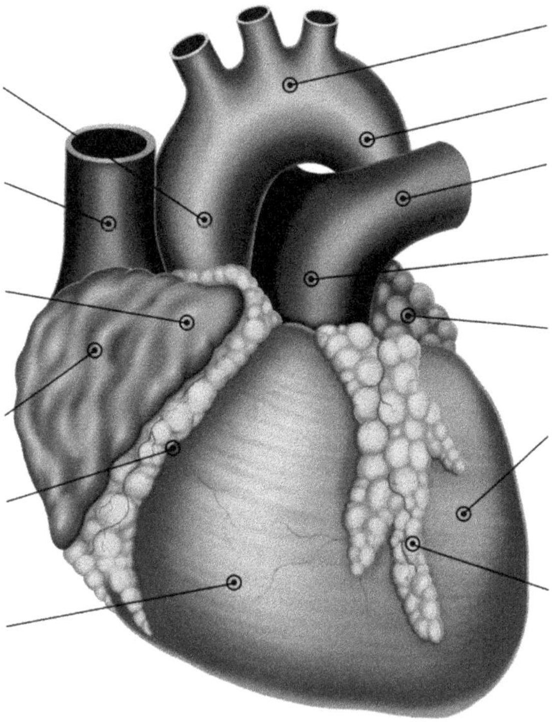


## ASSESSMENT OF PULSES AND USE OF CHEST X-RAY

With each contraction of the heart, a volume of blood (stroke volume) is pumped into the arteries, resulting in a pressure wave that is felt in the peripheral arteries as a **pulse**. Both apical and peripheral pulses should be assessed. The difference between the apical and peripheral pulse is the pulse deficit, which may indicate weak pulse or dysrhythmia:

- **Rate**: Normally, the rate ranges from 60 to 100 bpm in the adult.
- **Rhythm**: The rate should be regular, although children and young adults often exhibit a sinus arrhythmia (increased rate with inspiration and decreased with expiration).
- **Force**: The force may vary with the stroke volume and resultant pulse pressure:
  - 0: Absent pulse
  - 1+: Weak, thready pulse
  - 2+: Normal pulse
  - 3+: Strong, bounding pulse

**Chest x-rays** may be used to evaluate the structure (including size and shape) of the chest and the organs inside, including the heart, major vessels, and lungs, and may aid in the diagnosis of heart failure and cardiomyopathy. This method of assessment can also identify fluid in the lungs that may indicate congestive heart failure (CHF). The chest x-ray may also be used to help determine the most appropriate placement of implantable devices, such as a pacemaker, and to monitor the devices after implantation.

## NIHSS

The **National Institutes of Health Stroke Scale** (NIHSS) is a standardized tool used to grade the deficits resulting from a stroke. It is administered with careful attention to directions. Generally, the NIHSS should be administered as close to the onset of symptoms as possible and then in frequent intervals thereafter (based on physician orders and facility policy) in order to closely monitor the progression of stroke symptoms. The NIHSS is also an important assessment scale when administering tPA to treat an ischemic stroke as a method of measuring the effectiveness of the tPA and the potential complication of a hemorrhagic stroke from the tPA. The examiner should record the answers and avoid coaching or repeating requests, although demonstration may be used with aphasic patients. The scale comprises 11 sections, with scores for each section ranging from 0 (normal) to 2–4:

- Level of consciousness: responds to stimulation (0–3), responds with month and age (0–2), open/close eyes, grip/release with unaffected hand (0–2)
- Best gaze: tracking eye movement (0–2)
- Visual: visual fields (0–3)
- Facial palsy: symmetry when patient shows teeth, raises eyebrows, and closes eyes (0–3)
- Motor, arm: drift while arm is extended with palms down (0–4)
- Motor, leg: leg drift at 30° while patient is supine (0–4)
- Limb ataxia: finger-nose and heel-shin (0–2)
- Sensory: grimace or withdrawal from pinprick (0–2)
- Best language: describes action of pictures (0–3)
- Dysarthria: reads or describes words on list (0–2)
- Extinction and inattention: visual spatial neglect (0–2)

## Borg Scale in Patient Evaluation

Frequently used in outpatient and community exercise programs, the **Borg scale** is a method to evaluate patient exertion based on breath quality and perceived exhaustion. The subjective data—perceived increases in heart rate, respirations, sweating, and muscle endurance—are rated on an ascending scale of 6–20. A mild physical effort would produce a lower number; extreme exertion would correlate with a higher number. This scale number also provides a fairly accurate estimate of the patient's actual pulse rate when multiplied by 10 (i.e., a rating of 9 [mild exertion] would correlate to a generalized pulse rate of 90). This method can be taught to the patient in order to assess their exertion level outside of a monitored, therapeutic environment.

## Physical Examination with Known or Suspected PAD

**Physical assessment** for a patient with suspected **peripheral arterial disease (PAD)** includes the following:

- Obtain blood pressure results from both arms as well as notations regarding hypertension and medications used to treat it.
- Assess carotid, femoral, and extremity pulses for presence, intensity, and bruit.
- Perform abdominal auscultation and palpation for bruits or pulsation.
- Conduct a thorough skin examination, including bare feet, assessing color, temperature, perfusion, integrity, nail changes, and hair distribution.
- Gather a subjective history, including smoking, diabetes, extremity pain, numbness, exertion fatigue, reports of past slow-healing wounds, abdominal pain after eating, and family history of PAD or abdominal aortic aneurysm.
- Gather laboratory values for cholesterol levels and clotting times. Anticipate ultrasound evaluation of any abnormalities.

### Types of Congenital Heart Disease in Adult Patients

The following are the most common types of congenital heart disease that might be encountered in adult patients:

- **Atrial septal defects**: The most common congenital deformity is created from the incomplete closure of the patent foramen ovale after birth, leaving a small opening that increases the risk of the patient forming emboli that may lead to cerebrovascular incidents or peripheral artery blockage. This deformity may be repaired with a transseptal patch or left untreated if it is small enough. Patients with septal defects are generally only treated for embolisms if they become symptomatic.
- **Marfan syndrome**: This is a genetic connective tissue disorder that affects cardiac tissue, causing deformity of the valves and/or weakness of vessels that can cause aortic aneurysm. Physical signs might include unusually elongated limbs and a deformity of the chest area (either appearing sunken in or protruding outward).

# Data Collection and Interpretation

## Qualitative vs. Quantitative Methods of Data Collection

**Qualitative**: Seeks to identify generalities and answer initial questions regarding a situation or incident. Its focus is on exploring and observing to gain information. Answers and information are expressed in words and theory. Data gathered and conclusions made can be more subjective than quantitative data. It is generally used as a first step or in conjunction with more strictly defined quantitative studies.

**Quantitative**: Answers specific questions, tests theories, establishes cause and effect relationships, gauges impact and outcome of various conditions, and can be translated into mathematical answers. Quantitative studies are generally easier to duplicate for credibility.

## Placing Patients on Continuous Cardiac Monitoring

The criteria according to the AHA for placing a patient on continuous cardiac (telemetry) monitoring is described below:

- **Class I**: These patients are under the highest risk for immediate, life-threatening cardiac events. They require continuous monitoring under the supervision of a practitioner highly skilled in both ECG interpretation and defibrillation. This level of care suggests intensive care treatment.
- **Class II**: This is a lower risk classification suggested for patients on cardiac medications, minor surgical interventions such as angioplasty, or pacemaker lead placement. These patients are normally found on a cardiac step-down or intermediate cardiac care unit.
- **Class III**: These patients carry the lowest risk for cardiac events but require a short interval of increased monitoring, such as surgical and labor patients.

## Diagnostic Tools

Uses of chest x-ray, computed tomography (CT) scan, and magnetic resonance imaging (MRI) are described below:

- **Chest x-ray** is used for initial evaluation, x-ray provides a cursory view of the chest organs including size and position of the heart and health of the lungs.
- **CT scan**, without the use of contrast dye, is still considered a noninvasive procedure utilizing concentrated x-rays. CT scans are useful for expanding the available view of an organ to a more 3-dimensional picture.
- **MRI** uses a magnetic field to create a computerized 3-dimensional image without the use of harmful radiation; however, it is consequently the most expensive of the three procedures. MRI provides the most accurate and detailed information regarding the status of the soft tissue organs.

## Expected Pattern of CK Results Following an MI

**Creatine kinase (CK) and CK-MB levels** are evaluated every 6–8 hours in a suspected myocardial injury. Total CK and CK-MB (specific to cardiac cells) initially rise within the first 4–6 hours of an MI. A normal range would be 30–180 IU/L for CK and CK-MB totaling 0–5% of the CK level.

Assuming no further damage is sustained, peak levels (in excess of 6 times the normal range) are reached 12–24 hours after the injury. CK levels will return to normal within 3–4 days of the event. Small spikes in CK level might also occur following invasive cardiac procedures.

## Troponin I and T

**Troponin**, which is found in cardiac and skeletal muscle, is a type of protein. Both troponin I and T (isolates of troponin) are found in the myocardium, but troponin T is also found in skeletal muscle, so it is less specific than troponin I. Troponin I, therefore, may be used to detect a myocardial infarction after non-cardiac surgery and to detect acute coronary syndrome. Troponin is released into the bloodstream when injury to the tissue (such as the myocardium) occurs, causing damage to the cell membranes as occurs with myocardial injury.

| | |
|---|---|
| **Troponin I (<0.05 ng/mL)** | Appears in 2–6 hours, peaks at 15–20 hours, and returns to normal in 5–7 days. Exhibits a second but lower peak at 60–80 hours (biphasic). |
| **Troponin T (<0.2 ng/mL)** | Increases 2–6 hours after MI and stays elevated. Returns to normal in 7 days. (Less specific than troponin I) |

## Doppler Ultrasound

**Doppler ultrasound** is used when assessing a patient's cardiac and vascular system:

- **Aortic blood flow/Cardiac output**: These are assessed with esophageal Doppler monitoring (EDM) for evaluation of hypoperfusion (hypovolemia or septic shock), major organ dysfunction (renal or liver failure), hypotension, heart failure, cardiogenic shock, ruptures within the heart, mitral regurgitation, or tamponade. EDM may be used before, during, or after cardiac surgery. Doppler ultrasound technology is used to monitor both the function of the left ventricle and the patient's fluid status.
- **Intraarterial blood pressure monitoring**: Before catheter insertion, collateral circulation must be assessed by Doppler or the Allen test (used for the hand).
- **Ankle-brachial index (ABI)**: Doppler is used to evaluate peripheral arterial disease of the lower extremities.
- **Radial artery graft**: The adequacy of collateral vessels and circulation to the hand by the ulnar artery must be assessed preoperatively per the Allen test and Doppler flow measurements.
- **Pseudoaneurysm (AKA false aneurysm)**: Diagnosis is per Doppler ultrasound or color flow imaging.
- **IABP**: Distal ischemia is the most common complication, so distal pulses/Doppler signals must be assessed routinely.

## Echocardiograms and Ejection Fraction

**Echocardiograms** (**ECG**) are used to assess various cardiac structures (chambers of the heart, valves, prosthetic valves, septum, pericardium), cardiac conditions (cardiomyopathy, coronary artery disease, tumors/masses, foreign bodies emboli source, bacterial endocarditis), cardiac output, and ejection fraction. Various types of echocardiograms with Doppler imaging are utilized in cardiovascular assessment:

- **Stress testing**: Increases accuracy of exercise/dobutamine testing and helps to identify areas of hypoperfusion and infarction.
- **Transthoracic**: Records the size, shape, and functions of the heart and takes different views of the heart.
- **Transesophageal**: Images are obtained from within the stomach or esophagus, so they are generally of higher quality than transthoracic images.

The **ejection fraction** is equal to the stroke volume divided by the end-diastolic volume and represents the percentage of the total ventricular volume that is ejected during each contraction of the heart, providing an indication of the functioning of the ventricles:

- Normal: 55–70% (usually about 65%). Some heart failure (HF) may be present in this range.
- Below normal: 40–54%. HF may remain asymptomatic.
- Moderately below normal: 35–39%. Mild HF is evident.
- Severe below normal: <35%. Moderate to severe HF is indicated.

## Typical Changes on ECG Indicating Heart Disease

In a normal **ECG**, P waves are no taller than 0.25 mV and no wider than 0.11 seconds. A normal PR interval is 0.12–0.20 seconds. A normal QRS is 0.04–0.10 seconds. T waves gently curve upright and are no taller than 5 mm (10 mm in chest leads). U waves, when visible, are also upright in the presence of myocardial injury. T waves turn upside down or become markedly tall. Higher T waves may be thinner than normal or longer and followed by an inverted U wave.

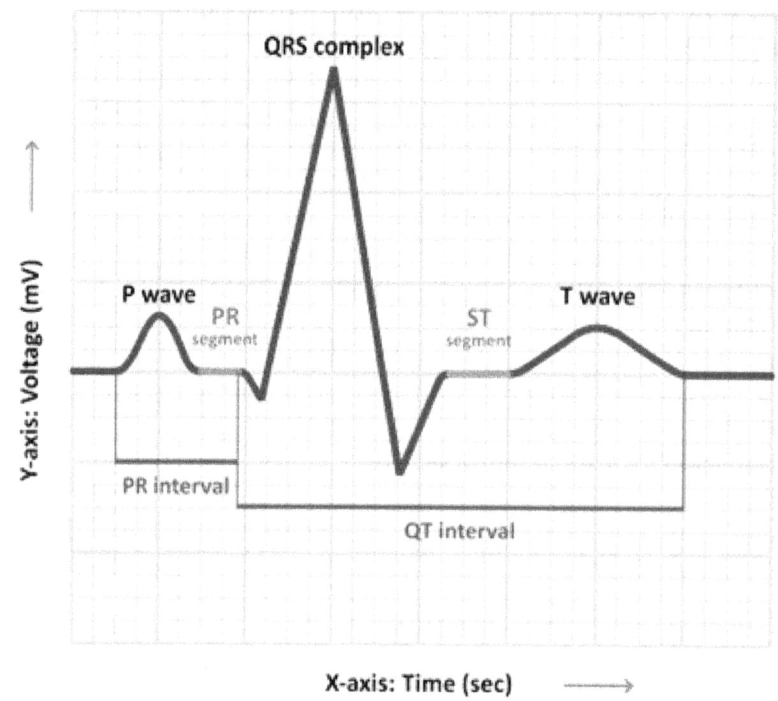


ST segment drops below the baseline or measures wider than 0.12 seconds. The ST segment might not have a return to the baseline between S and T.

Q waves may measure greater than 0.03 seconds.

## Sinus Node Arrhythmias as Seen on ECG

The sinus node is the primary pacemaker for the heart, setting a normal rhythm of 60–100 bpm.

- **Sinus arrhythmia**: ECG rate falls within normal limits, but there is a slight change in rhythm correlating to breathing (increased pulse with inspiration, slowing with expiration).

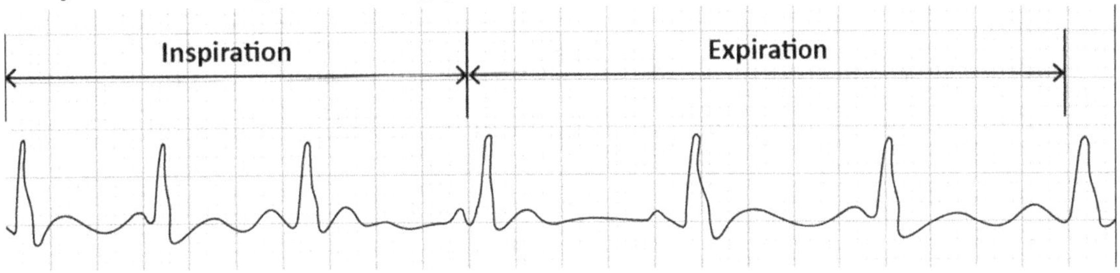


- **Sinus bradycardia**: Rhythm is normal, all parts of the ECG appear normal, but rate is below 60 bpm.

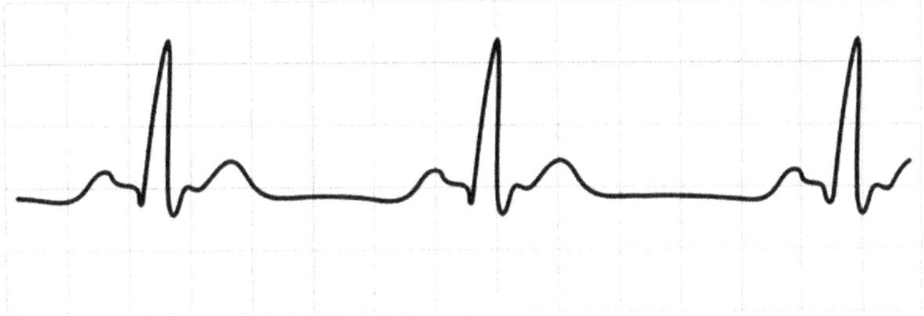

- **Sinus tachycardia**: Rhythm is normal, ECG is normal, but rate is greater than 100 bpm.

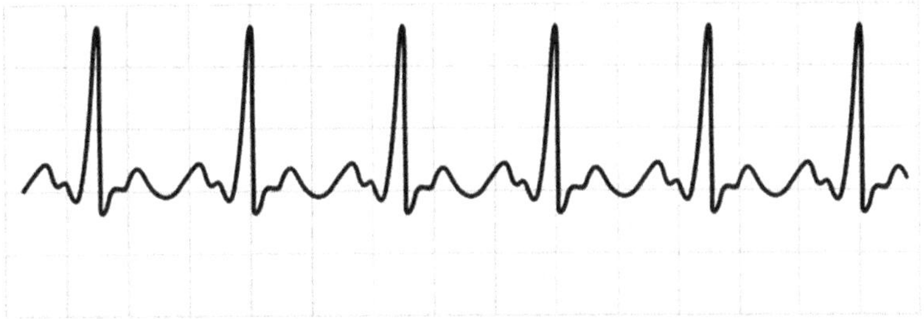

- **Sinus arrest**: Rate is normal, but rhythm is interrupted by occasional missing PQRST complexes. This is referred to as a sinus pause if only one or two beats are dropped; sinus arrest refers to three or more missing complexes.

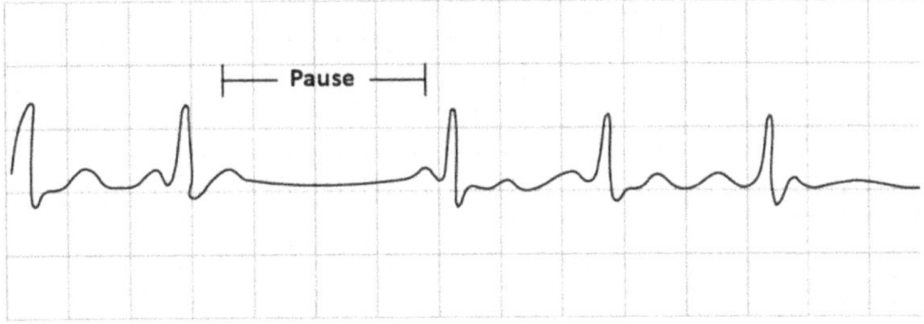


- **Sick sinus syndrome**: Rhythm is irregular, with the waves and complexes varying instead of forming a predictable pattern.

## Junctional Arrhythmias as Seen on ECG

Junctional arrhythmias as seen on ECG are discussed below:

- **Premature junctional contraction (PJC)**: Rate and rhythm are fundamentally regular with occasional early, inverted P wave and following QRS complex.

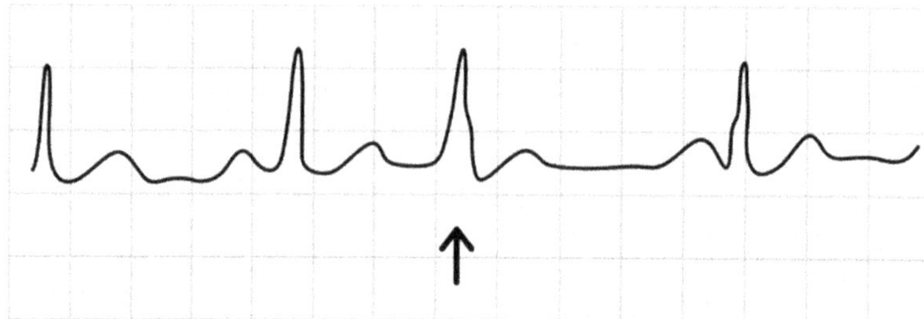

- **Junctional escape rhythm**: Regular rate and rhythm appear to be normal sinus rhythm except for inverted P waves.

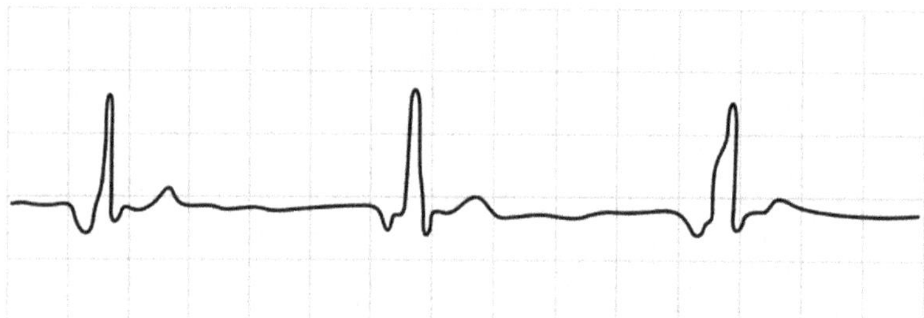

- **Accelerated junctional rhythm**: Regular rhythm of 60–100 bpm. P wave may be absent or appear inverted before or after the QRS complex. Everything else appears normal.
- **Junctional tachycardia**: Regular rhythm with a rate of 100–200 bpm. P wave is inverted and occurs after the QRS complex.

## Ventricular Arrhythmias as Seen on ECG

Ventricular arrhythmias as seen on ECG are discussed below:

- **Premature ventricular contraction (PVC)**: Underlying regular rate and rhythm, with occasional early, wide, and bizarre-looking QRS complex.

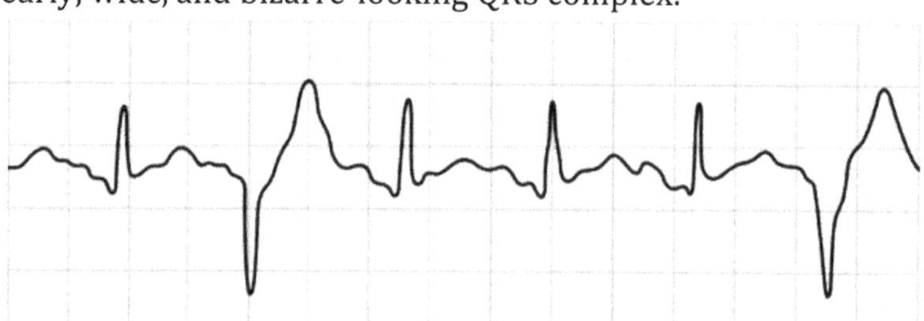

- **Ventricular tachycardia**: No P wave, wide and bizarre QRS complex with rapid rate of 100–200 bpm.

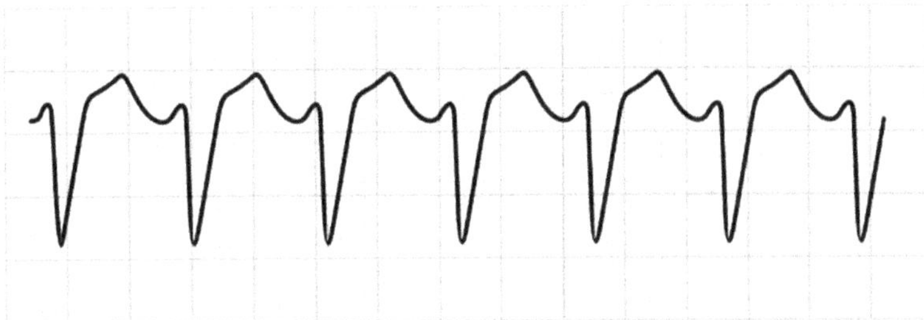

- **Ventricular fibrillation**: No identifiable rhythm, no identifiable wave forms. ECG shows only a fine or coarse, chaotic wavy line. Patient is unresponsive and pulseless.

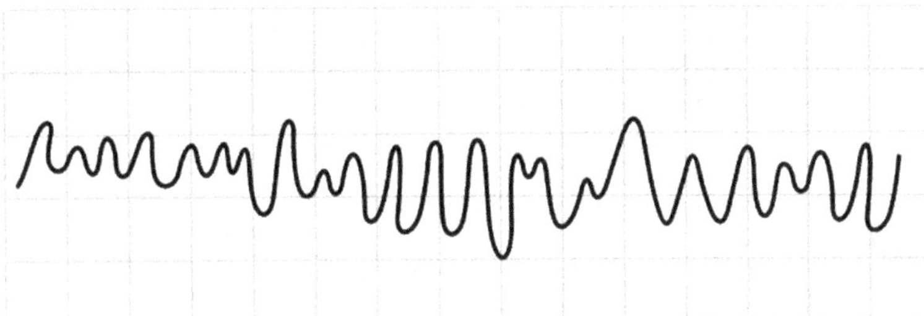

- **Idioventricular rhythms**: Ventricular rate of 20–40 bpm, independent or no P wave (PR interval unmeasurable) with bizarre-looking QRS complex longer than 0.12 seconds.

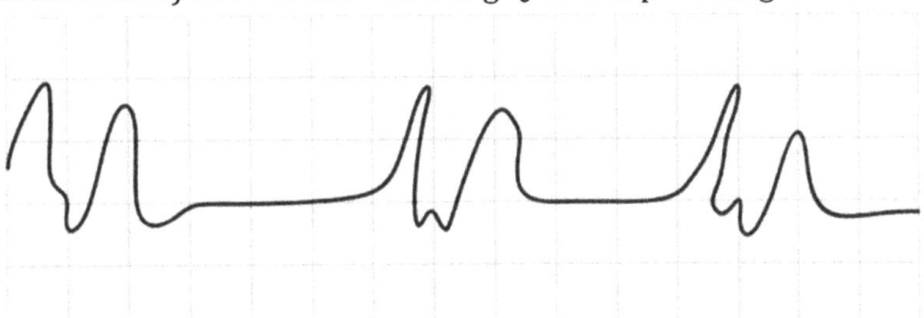

- **Asystole**: No electrical conduction, displayed as an almost flat line only disturbed by medical interventions such as CPR. Patient is unconscious and pulseless.

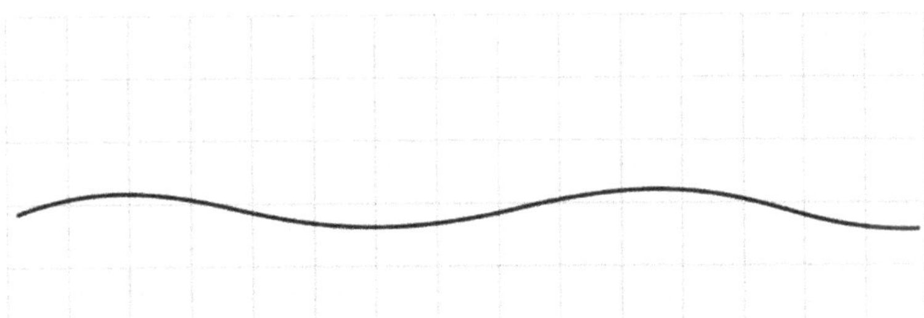

## Heart Block as Seen on ECG

The types of heart block as seen on ECG are discussed below:

- **First-degree AV block**: Rhythm is regular and appears very similar to a normal sinus rhythm. The only difference is a PR interval longer than 0.20 seconds.

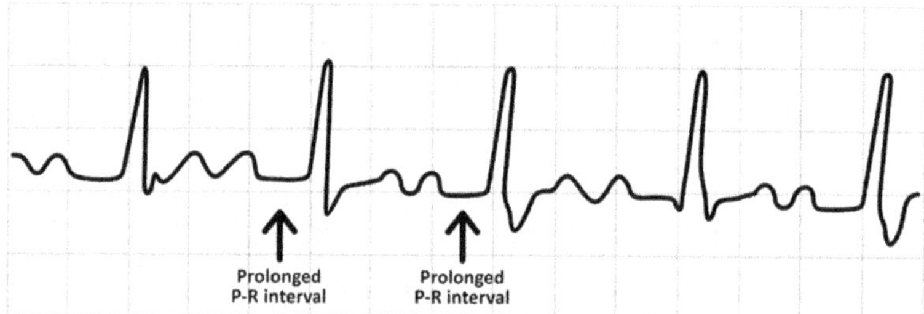


- **Type I second-degree AV block**: Atrial rhythm is regular with a repeating pattern of progressively longer PR intervals until a QRS complex no longer appears behind the P wave.

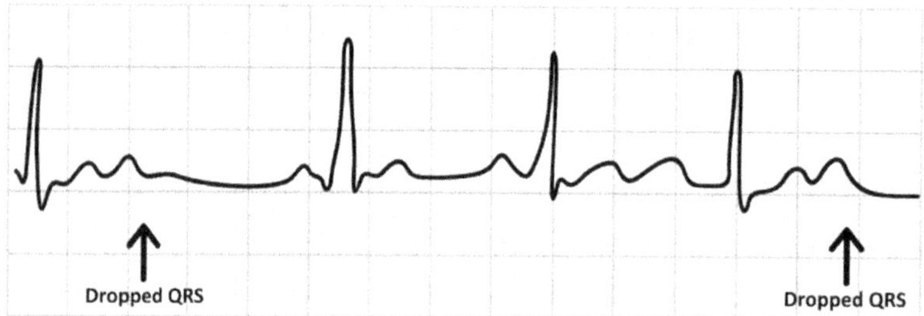


- **Type II second-degree AV block**: Atrial rhythm is regular; ventricular rhythm may be either regular or irregular. Look for missing QRS complexes.

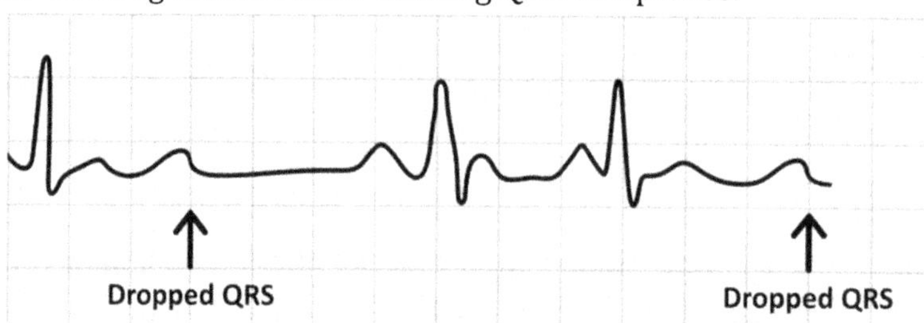


- **Third-degree AV block**: Atrial and ventricular rates are regular but independent of each other. PR interval will vary.

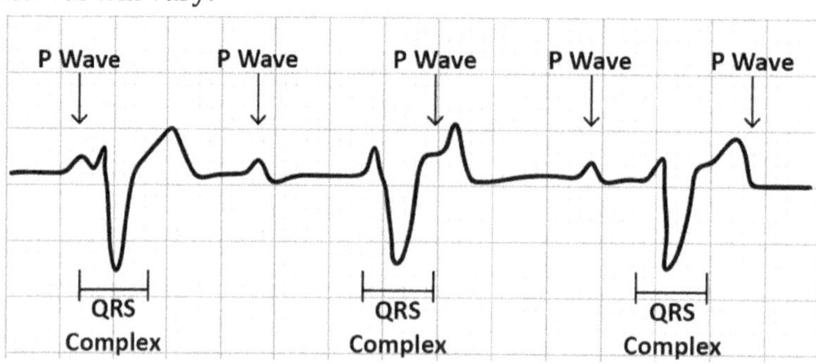

- **Left bundle-branch block**: Normal or inverted P waves are noted, but the QRS complex may be widened with a deep S wave and an interval of >0.12 seconds (in lead V1) that resembles a "W."

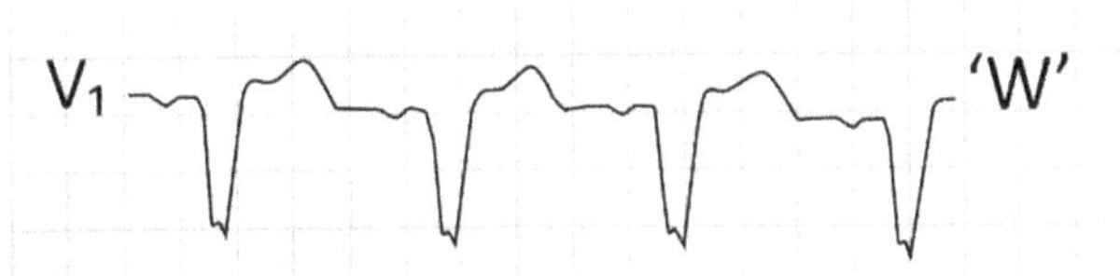


- **Right bundle-branch block**: QRS complex is wider than 0.12 seconds and has an unusual appearance (may look like rabbit ears or the letter M). T wave is inverted.

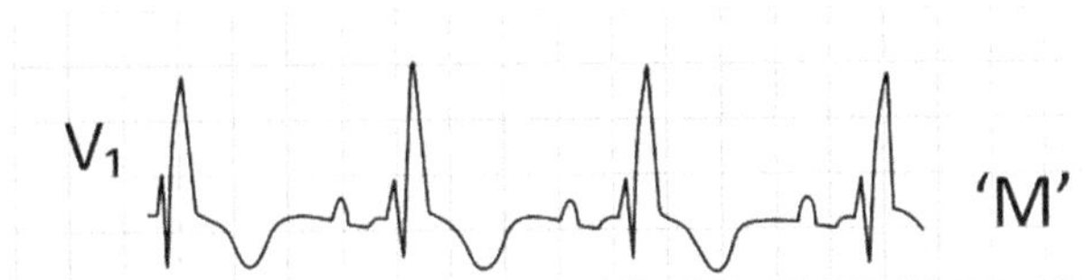


## Pulmonary Artery Pressure (PAP) Monitoring

The patient with a **pulmonary artery (PA) catheter** requires intensive monitoring due to the presence of a critical condition such as significant cardiac disease, multiple organ dysfunction, shock, or trauma. When the catheter is appropriately positioned, the monitor should show a waveform grouped with two small hills that correspond to the ECG waveforms. The two hills are represented by *a* and *v*. Left ventricular end-diastolic pressure is marked at *a* (normally measuring 1–6 mmHg). Left atrial filling is represented by the *v* wave (with a normal reading of less than 5 mmHg). Monitor and document the PA line for appropriate waveforms, infection at the insertion site, position of the stopcocks, secure connections, and proper line labeling. Balloon inflation required for a pulmonary artery wedge pressure (PAWP) reading requires no more than 1.5 cc of air, and the line is flushed after each reading. Normal results for a PAWP measurement should be 6–12 mmHg.

## Intraarterial Blood Pressure Monitoring

**Intraarterial blood pressure monitoring** is done for systolic, diastolic, and mean arterial pressure (MAP) for conditions that decrease cardiac output, tissue perfusion, or fluid volume. A catheter is inserted into an artery, such as the radial, dorsalis pedis, femoral, or axillary, percutaneously or through a cut-down. The radial approach is most preferred and frequently used due to the risk of infections in the alternate locations. Before catheter insertion, collateral circulation must be assessed by Doppler or the Allen test (used for the hand). In the Allen test, both the radial and ulnar artery are compressed, and the patient is asked to clench the hand repeatedly until it blanches. Then, one artery is released, and the tissue on that side should flush. Then the test is repeated, releasing the other artery. The MAP is most commonly used to evaluate perfusion, as it shows pressure throughout the cardiac cycle. Systole is one-third of the normal cardiac cycle, and diastole is two-thirds. The MAP for a blood pressure of 120/60 is calculated below (normal range 70–100 mmHg):

$$MAP = \frac{\text{Diastole} \times 2 + \text{Systole}}{3} = \frac{60 \times 2 + 120}{3} = \frac{240}{3} = 80$$

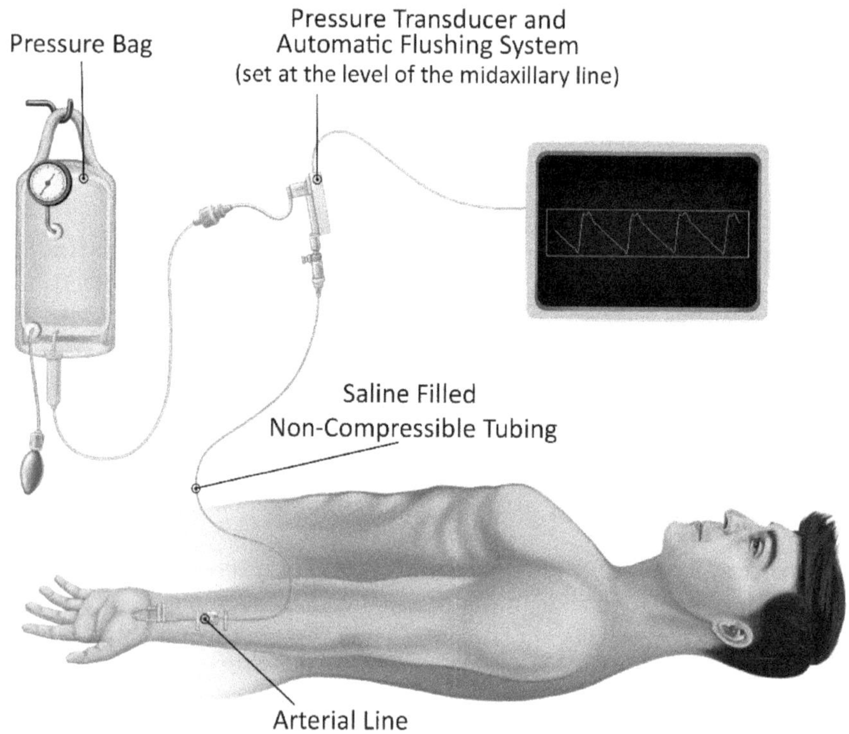


## CVP Monitoring

**Central venous pressure (CVP)**, the pressure in the right atrium or vena cava, is used to assess function of the right ventricles, preload, and flow of venous blood to the heart. Normal pressure ranges from 2–5 mmHg but may be elevated after surgery to 6–8 mmHg. The catheter is inserted into a vein, and the tip is advanced to (or near to) the right atrium. Incorrect catheter placement or malfunctioning can affect readings. CVP is most often used to monitor hemodynamic therapy:

- **Increased CVP** is related to overload of intravascular volume caused by decreased function, hypertrophy, or failure of the right ventricle; increased right ventricular afterload, tricuspid valve stenosis, regurgitation, or thrombus obstruction; or shunt from left ventricle to right atrium. It can also be caused by arrhythmias or cardiac tamponade.
- **Decreased CVP** is related to low intravascular volume, decreased preload, or vasodilation.

# Planning and Implementation

## Evidence-Based Guidelines and Quality Improvement

### ACC/AHA Guidelines for Quality Measures

Evidence-based research is the use of current research and patient values in practice to establish a plan of care. **Evidence-based practice guidelines** are general guidelines that can apply to specific groups of patients (such as those with atrial fibrillation) based on evidence-based research. The process of establishing evidence-based practice guidelines must be done systematically to ensure quality. The American College of Cardiology/American Heart Association (ACC/AHA) has utilized scientific evidence in the development of clinical practice guidelines to improve the care of patients with cardiovascular disease and overall cardiovascular health. The goal of the ACC/AHA is to provide clinical guidelines that focus on patient care recommendations and flow diagrams to guide care. The guidelines are standardized and presented in the modular knowledge chunk format, which bundles related recommendations. ACC/AHA provides supplementary information about the guidelines online. Each recommendation includes the class (strength) of the recommendation (ranging from Class I, strong, to Class III, harm) and the quality of evidence (Level A, high quality, to Level C-EO, based on expert opinion). Examples of clinical practice guidelines include *Primary Prevention* (2019), *Blood Cholesterol* (2018), and *Heart Failure (Focused Update)* (2017).

### CHEST/AHA Guidelines for Anticoagulation Administration

**CHEST guidelines** promote the use of a systematic protocol for anticoagulation therapy, including daily monitoring of the international normalized ratio prothrombin time (INR-PT/INR) to evaluate dosing levels. Optimal therapeutic INR range while on anticoagulants should be tightly controlled between 2.0 and 3.0. This method requires a high level of accountability in coordinating care and communication with treatment team members, as well as with the patient, regarding test results and rationale behind current dosing levels. The patient should be continuously instructed regarding self-management skills in anticipation for self-care. Anticoagulant therapy is contraindicated in the critically ill patient with active—or at a high risk for—bleeding. These recommendations are also sanctioned by the **American Heart Association.**

### AHA Guidelines Regarding Chronic Heart Failure

AHA identifies heart disease by four stages: A, B, C and D:

- **Stage A** (patients at high risk but without established heart disease) and **stage B** (patients with measurable damage to the heart who are still currently without symptoms) are the stages where progression to further disease is still preventable. Care is focused on education and prevention measures. ACE inhibitors may be added to the care of patients in stage B.
- **Stage C** (patients with heart disease and symptom complaints) would increase pharmaceutical treatments to also include diuretics. Dietary intervention might include low-salt diets and/or restricted fluid intake.
- **Stage D** (patients who have escalated to end-stage heart disease and require extreme medical measures or end-of-life care) may require surgical interventions on a case-by-case basis, including valve surgery, ventricular assist device (VAD), or transplant. Most patients at this stage do not qualify for such interventions and will enter into care focused on end-of-life comfort.

## Continuous Quality Improvement

Continuous quality improvement is a multidisciplinary management philosophy that can be applied to all aspects of an organization, whether related to such varied areas as the cardiac unit, purchasing, or human resources. The skills used for epidemiologic research (data collection, analysis, outcomes, action plans) are all applicable to the analysis of multiple types of events, because they are based on solid scientific methods. Multi-disciplinary planning can bring valuable insights from various perspectives, and strategies used in one context can often be applied to another. All staff, from housekeeping to supervising, must be alert to not only problems but also opportunities for improvement. Increasingly, departments must be concerned with cost-effectiveness as the costs of medical care continue to rise, so the quality professional in the cardiovascular unit is not in an isolated position in an institution but is just one part of the whole, facing similar concerns as those in other disciplines. Disciplines are often interrelated in their functions.

# Scope and Standards of Practice

## Licensure vs. Certification

**Licensure** is the meeting of legal parameters established by the government to identify that an individual has met a minimum standard of competence and safety in their profession. No one is allowed to practice in that profession without qualifying to do so under the laws of the state in which they intend to practice.

**Certification** is a step above and beyond licensure that is pursued by the individual nurse or required by an institution for employment in specialty areas. Guidelines and testing for certification are established by the profession with the backing of independent agencies to ensure standards of quality. Certification implies a higher level of competency within a specialized area of care.

## Leadership and Leadership Styles

**Leadership** is the personal characteristics or qualities that an individual uses to influence others to achieve set goals. Key characteristics and qualities associated with a leader include working well with others, facilitating communication, and motivating others. Leadership styles include autocratic, participative, laissez-faire, transactional, and transformational:

- **Autocratic leadership** uses power to influence members of a team.
- **Participative leadership** uses a democratic process for decisions among team members.
- **Laissez-faire leadership** involves minimal guidance from a leader and provides little feedback to team members.
- **Transactional leadership** focuses on daily activities and is comfortable with the status quo.
- **Transformational leadership** involves a vision and commitment to meet a team's goals.

## Qualities Promoting Positive Leadership

Qualities promoting positive leadership include the following:

- The leader works well in a group/team setting and is able to coordinate patient care with multiple groups and areas of healthcare.
- The leader promotes communication between all members of the group, streamlining and coordinating care (participative leader).
- The leader appropriately motivates the team toward common goals, emphasizing and rewarding productive work environments (transactional leader).
- The leader appropriately motivates the team toward positive change as needed (transformational leader).
- The leader provides respect, support, and encouragement to all contributors and listens to all voices before making final decisions.

Of the generally recognized leadership styles, those possessing a participative or transformational style appear to have the best outcomes in healthcare and interdisciplinary settings. Unfavorable leadership methods tend to be autocratic (firm control with little group input) and laissez-faire (hands-off, unmotivated leadership).

## Assertiveness in Communication

**Assertiveness** should not be confused with aggression, a negative communication method used to manipulate and control interactions rather than collaborate and share respect. Assertiveness empowers the communicator to feel comfortable speaking freely and defending their own thoughts and feelings in a given situation, using "I" statements. The assertive communicator also processes others' opinions and uses "you" statements in a positive manner. They are not passive or silent when there is a need to speak out, but they use positive language that is appropriate to the situation and those who will be listening and trying to understand.

## DELEGATION

There are five basic **responsibilities associated with delegating**:

1. **Right task**: The task must be clearly defined and achievable.
2. **Right circumstances**: Can the task be completed in a timely manner? Are the needed tools easily accessible?
3. **Right person**: Is the person giving direction within their scope of practice to delegate the task, and is the person being asked to complete the task able to complete it within their own scope of practice?
4. **Right communication**: Are the task and the expected outcome clearly outlined so that both parties understand what needs to be done?
5. **Right supervision**: Appropriate monitoring, intervention, and accountability need to be maintained regardless of who is ultimately assigned the task.

## POSITIVE ATTRIBUTES OF A MENTOR

A **mentor** is a role model and a guide to successful care and skill-building experiences. They exhibit higher knowledge and experience than the individual they are guiding. The mentor is not in a leadership role over the student but is seen as a more experienced equal. They do not take over and make decisions for the student; rather, they provide options and information to help the student make positive decisions on their own. The mentor is honest and trustworthy, supportive, has effective communication and teaching skills, and is respected by those they are leading to higher skill levels.

# Legal and Ethical Considerations

## Provisions of the ANA's Code of Ethics for Nurses

The **ANA's Code of Ethics for Nurses** includes nine key points:

1. The nurse practices with compassion and respect for the inherent dignity, worth, and unique attributes of every person.
2. The nurse's primary commitment is to the patient, whether an individual, family, group, community, or population.
3. The nurse promotes, advocates for, and protects the rights, health, and safety of the patient.
4. The nurse has authority, accountability, and responsibility for nursing practice; makes decisions; and takes action consistent with the obligation to provide optimal patient care.
5. The nurse owes the same duties to self as to others, including the responsibility to promote health and safety, preserve wholeness of character and integrity, maintain competence, and continue personal and professional growth.
6. The nurse, through individual and collective effort, establishes, maintains, and improves the ethical environment of the work setting and conditions of employment that are conducive to safe, quality healthcare.
7. The nurse, in all roles and settings, advances the profession through research and scholarly inquiry, professional standards development, and the generation of both nursing and health policy.
8. The nurse collaborates with other health professionals and the public to protect human rights, promote health diplomacy, and reduce health disparities.
9. The profession of nursing, collectively through its professional organizations, must articulate nursing values, maintain the integrity of the profession, and integrate principles of social justice into nursing and health policy.



## Patient Care Partnership

In 2003, the AHA replaced its *Patient's Bill of Rights* with the ***Patient Care Partnership***, a brochure that outlines what each patient should expect from the hospital stay in terms of rights and involvement of care. The key components outlined in this brochure include the following:

1. High quality hospital care
2. A clean and safe environment
3. Involvement in your care: discussing your medical condition and information about medically appropriate treatment choices; discussing your treatment plan; getting information from you; understanding your healthcare goals and values; understanding who should make decisions when you cannot
4. Protection of your privacy
5. Preparing you and your family for when you leave the hospital
6. Help with your bill and filing insurance claims

## Informed Consent

Patients or guardians must provide **informed consent** for all treatment the patient receives. This includes a thorough explanation of all procedures, treatments, and associated risks. The American Medical Association has established guidelines for informed consent:

- Explanation of diagnosis
- Nature of and reason for treatment or procedure
- Risks and benefits
- Alternative options (regardless of cost or insurance coverage)
- Risks and benefits of alternative options
- Risks and benefits of not having a treatment or procedure

Providing informed consent is a requirement of all states.

## Advance Directives

In accordance with federal and state laws, individuals have the right to self-determination in healthcare, including decisions about end-of-life care through **advance directives** such as living wills and the right to assign a surrogate person to make decisions through a **durable power of attorney**. Patients should routinely be questioned about an advanced directive, as they may present at a healthcare organization without the document. Patients who have indicated they desire a **do-not-resuscitate** (DNR) order should not receive resuscitative treatments for terminal illness or conditions in which meaningful recovery cannot occur.

## Patient Advocacy

The American Nurses Association (ANA) regards **patient advocacy** as a basic cornerstone that helps define the profession of nursing. Advocacy denotes the nurse's commitment to promoting optimal health and safety for their patient (whether that is an individual, group, or community). Nurses assume the responsibility of preserving a patient's basic rights for informed care that promotes the highest quality of life. This standard is maintained in communication and cooperation with all healthcare team members providing treatment, education, pain relief, comfort, and safety while avoiding harm to the patient.

## Approaches Toward Promoting Change

Consumerism, paternalism, and patient advocacy approaches toward promoting change are explained below:

- **Consumerism**: This impersonal view presents the patient with the cost-effectiveness and anticipated outcomes of various treatments but does not take into account personal belief systems.
- **Paternalism**: The care provider or another influential person in the patient's life assumes the role of parent and tries to dictate the patient's healthcare decisions for them.
- **Patient advocacy**: The healthcare provider works directly with the patient, involving them in making decisions about what is best at any given time and respecting these wishes. Being an advocate involves creating a therapeutic relationship, presenting options, and promoting understanding that allows the patient to make an informed decision and, as needed, defending the patient's decisions to other care providers or individuals in their life who might question or try to negate the power to be in control of their own health.

## Ethical Decision-Making

The most important aspect of **ethical decision-making** is the fact that these decisions are not made by just one person. When an ethical dilemma exists, the problem is brought to the attention of a committee of which the nurse and the patient, or their representative if the patient is incapacitated, are members. Questions addressed would include an in-depth analysis of all the facts; then options are presented and prioritized. Consideration for the patient's wishes should be paramount to any decision made. Once a decision is reached, the nurse must act as a patient advocate and facilitate actions related to that decision regardless of their personal feelings about the dilemma.

## Building Trust in Obtaining Information

The following are steps that can be taken to build a relationship of trust with your patient in order to obtain the highest quality of information during a health interview:

- Before beginning, review prior records and notes to avoid causing patient frustration and duplicating information.
- Ensure that the interview environment is quiet, comfortable, and private. Interviews should be conducted with the patient alone whenever possible. If needed, further information can be obtained from family members or others at a separate time.
- Assess for communication restrictions such as hearing difficulties or slurred speech from cerebral vascular injury.
- Minimize interruptions and show priority attentiveness to the patient while watching and listening to both verbal and nonverbal communication efforts.
- Avoid judgmental statements or an appearance of superiority. Place yourself on the same level physically. Show respect for cultural and personal belief systems that might affect healthcare decisions.



## Helpful and Therapeutic Nurse-Patient Relationship

The nurse and patient should be actively working together on a common goal regarding the patient's healthcare and recovery. The plan of action, means, and evaluation of the intervention are completed jointly.

The patient should feel respected by the nurse and understand that their privacy will be protected in order to encourage an involvement in their own care.

Emotional bonds may form but should be kept in proper context and boundaries. There will always be a beginning, middle, and end to a nurse-patient relationship.

The nurse must be prepared on all levels—mental, physical, and emotional—to be a positive, patient, and helpful influence in the relationship.

## Role of Listening

**Listening** is often overlooked as an important communication skill because it seems natural to many. It is actually a learned skill that allows the communicator to overcome barriers such as stress, anger, and distraction to truly process all aspects of the message being conveyed by the other party. It enables problem identification and sensitivity to emotions, relieves stress, and facilitates problem solving. Active listening is a two-way process that allows both parties to express their thoughts and feelings with the knowledge that they will be heard and that the other person truly wants to understand the message and work for resolution.

## Providing Competent and Culturally Sensitive Care

The following are the four basic keys to providing competent and culturally sensitive nursing care:

- Care should always be specifically geared to the individual patient. Do not make assumptions about their needs or wishes based on personal views or previous interactions and circumstances.
- Take time to identify the patient's unique cultural values and belief systems before establishing care goals.
- Nursing interventions enable and include the patient as the primary decision maker about their own care, according to their cultural values and belief system.
- Nurses and the care they provide should never reflect a personal judgment regarding the patient's culture or unique beliefs.

## Kleinman Model in Teaching Environments

The **Kleinman model** relies on a series of questions to help a nurse prepare to teach a patient from an unfamiliar cultural background. These questions allow the patient to define their own healthcare beliefs and problems. The questions include:

- The patient's name for a problem or condition
- The patient's perception of the problem's cause and initiating events as well as their timing
- How the problem is affecting the patient—what problems result from the illness or variance in health
- The patient's beliefs regarding the severity of the problem and its anticipated progression
- The patient's confidence in various treatments
- What the patient hopes intervention will accomplish for them
- The patient's fears regarding the illness and the proposed treatments

## End-of-Life Care

If treatments fail to control the patient's heart failure, it is possible for the disease to progress to a point where even a heart transplant is no longer an option. At this point, it is time to educate the patient and family regarding their **end-of-life care options**. Many patients choose the support of hospice. This option allows for care at home, surrounded by family and friends. Those involved in the care might include nurses, nursing aides, social workers, and even trained volunteers to help ease the passage from life to death by giving support to all facets of a person's life: health, social, mental, emotional, and spiritual. Other options might be continued care within the hospital or transfer to a chronic care facility. Discussions must be held regarding end-of-life care parameters and wishes, and these decisions must be documented and expressed to family and friends.

## Legal Regulation of Nursing Practice

**Legal regulation of nursing practice** protects the health, safety, and welfare of patients. All states require nurse licensing, and most states require additional accreditation for advanced nursing practice. Nursing practice acts are state laws that grant the right to practice nursing to individuals who meet predetermined standards. Regulatory boards are responsible for determining eligibility for licensing and relicensing, approving and supervising educational programs, enforcing statutes, and writing rules and regulations. Licensing requirements, state statutes and monitoring, advisory boards, and guidelines effectively protect patients and aim to ensure optimum care by nurses.

### Negligence and Malpractice

**Negligence and malpractice** are classified as unintentional torts (wrongful acts). Negligence refers to harm caused by carelessness or failure to act. Malpractice is a specific form of negligence that results from harm caused by not meeting reasonable standards of care set within the profession of nursing. Malpractice cases can be pursued if the wronged party is able to prove that the nurse in question was responsible for performing, or not performing, an intervention within their scope of practice. It must be reasonably proven that this action by the nurse was directly related to the harm and suffering of the patient.

Some of the most common areas of nursing malpractice include medication errors, inadequate assessment or monitoring of the patient (including allowing a patient to fall), performing activities for which the nurse has not been trained, and failure to communicate and document events or follow proper procedure.

## HIPAA

**HIPAA** expands on a patient's basic right to know that their personal health information is held in confidence and only shared on a "need to know" basis that is clearly defined for the patient. If knowledge of the patient's information is required for those outside of the patient's direct care, it cannot be provided without their specific consent. HIPAA requires all persons and institutions with access to this information to practice high levels of protection for that information. Every healthcare institution is required by law to establish and enforce policies and procedures that ensure patient confidentiality.

### CARE and Conflict/Confrontation

The **CARE approach** stands for Clarify, Articulate, Request and Encourage:

- **Clarify**: Be specific in identifying the problem that needs to be addressed.
- **Articulate**: Clearly define the reason(s) why a particular behavior or attitude is a problem.
- **Request**: Define an acceptable means of change that will help resolve the problem.
- **Encourage**: Offer support and respect toward others as you work together on creating change and resolving conflict.

Regardless of the other party's behavior, it is the nurse's personal responsibility to act with calm respect and dignity in the face of confrontation in order to facilitate positive change rather than contributing further to the problem.

### Win-Win Conflict Resolution

The following are the steps toward win-win conflict resolution:

1. Identify the need that is not being met rather than placing blame for dissatisfaction and frustration. Be specific in defining problem parameters.
2. Acknowledge differences of opinion and attempt to see the problem from all perspectives.
3. Involve all parties that are affected by the problem while searching for a solution.
4. Remember that win-win solutions may not always be what one person considers the easiest or most obvious. Base the solution on what reaches the greatest compromise and satisfaction for all concerned.
5. Agree on the action to be taken with all other involved parties.
6. Plan for the success of the solution with goals and definitions of roles and expectations.
7. Review the effectiveness of the plan and solution after it has been carried out to identify areas of further improvement or recognize the need to re-address the problem.

# Cardiovascular Procedures and Surgeries

## Coronary Atherectomy

An **atherectomy procedure**, also known as a Rotablator procedure, is a technique that involves a catheter with a grinding/cutting tool at the end of the device that is used to clear plaque build-up within diseased coronary arteries. An atherectomy procedure can be done in combination with percutaneous transluminal catheter angioplasty and/or stent procedure.

The procedure involves the use of a catheter introduced through the femoral, brachial, or radial artery into the diseased coronary artery. The catheter has a grinding/cutting tool at the end of the device, used to reduce plaque buildup in the diseased vessel.

There are **three atherectomy procedures** currently available: directional coronary atherectomy, rotational atherectomy, and transluminal extraction atherectomy.

- **Directional coronary atherectomy** is a procedure that involves the use of a catheter with a balloon and cutting tool at the end of the catheter. During the procedure, the catheter is inserted into the diseased tissue, the balloon is inflated to remove or disrupt the plaque, and the cutting tool is used to remove the rest of the plaque.
- **Rotational atherectomy** is a procedure (also catheter-based) that uses a metal cutting tool coated with diamonds, which breaks up the plaque into tiny particles to be removed.
- **Transluminal extraction atherectomy** is a procedure involving the use of a hollow tube with a cutting tool at the end of the device. The hollow tube also has suction bottles that collect removable plaque buildup.

### *Role of Practicing Clinician*

**Prior** to a coronary atherectomy procedure, practicing clinicians should take the patient's medical history, perform a physical examination, and evaluate the patient's overall health. Patients should be screened for drug-drug interactions; allergies; vital signs such as heart rate and blood pressure; and cardiovascular blood indicators such as potassium levels, prothrombin time, and hematocrit and creatinine levels. Patients should also undergo an electrocardiogram and echocardiogram prior to the procedure.

**During** the procedure, patients should only receive medications via an intravenous route, except for aspirin, which is given orally prior to the procedure. Pharmacologic agents used during the procedure include heparin, nitroglycerin, and/or a glycoprotein IIb/IIIa receptor inhibitor.

**After** the coronary atherectomy procedure, practicing clinicians should perform an electrocardiogram, echocardiogram, and physical assessment; monitor peripheral blood flow; look for swelling; and evaluate cardiac pain. Hospital protocols for aftercare should be followed. Prior to patient release, practicing clinicians should perform additional physical assessments and laboratory tests such as hematocrit, potassium levels, creatinine levels, and cardiac enzymes. Cardiac stress testing should be completed 2–6 months post procedure.

### *Indications, Contraindications, and Complications*

**Directional coronary atherectomy is indicated** for bifurcation lesions, ostial lesions, and eccentric lesions.

**Rotational atherectomy is indicated** for calcified lesions, ostial lesions, lesions 15–25 mm in length, and in-stent restenosis.

**Transluminal extraction atherectomy is indicated** for lesions that require removal of thrombus or debris, which can occur in patients with unstable angina, acute myocardial infarction, and failed thrombolytic therapy.

**Contraindications** for coronary atherectomy include high-risk coronary anatomy, severe coronary artery disease, bleeding disorder, and/or multiple episodes of percutaneous transluminal coronary angioplasty restenosis.

**Complications** associated with coronary atherectomy include abrupt closure of the diseased coronary artery, periprocedural myocardial infarction, coronary restenosis, bleeding, or hematoma at catheter introduction site, arterial embolism, pseudoaneurysm, retroperitoneal bleeding, vascular spasm, distal embolization, vessel perforation, and sudden death.

## PTCA Procedure and Procedure Indications

The goal of **percutaneous transluminal coronary angioplasty (PTCA)** is to increase blood flow to the coronary arteries by reducing plaque buildup. The procedure involves the use of a catheter introduced through the femoral, brachial, or radial artery into the diseased coronary artery. The catheter has a balloon at the end of the device to be used to tamponade plaque in the diseased vessel. Once the catheter is inserted, balloon pressure is applied to the area of plaque formation to decrease plaque size and/or stretch the vessel wall. The balloon is threaded over a wire after the wire is placed properly in the diseased vessel through angiography. A stent is often placed after ballooning opens the vessel.

Percutaneous transluminal coronary angioplasty is indicated for patients with refractory angina, unstable angina, evidence of cardiac ischemia, acute myocardial infarction, angina post coronary bypass surgery, unsuitable coronary anatomy for coronary bypass surgery, and restenosis after successful percutaneous transluminal coronary angioplasty or stent placement.

### *Role of Practicing Clinician*

**Prior** to percutaneous transluminal coronary angioplasty, practicing clinicians should take the patient's medical history, perform a physical examination, and evaluate the patient's overall health. Patients should be screened for drug-drug interactions, allergies, vital signs such as heart rate and blood pressure, and cardiovascular blood indicators such as potassium levels, prothrombin time, and hematocrit and creatinine levels. Patients should also undergo electrocardiogram and echocardiogram prior to procedure.

**During** the procedure, patients should only receive medications via intravenous access, except for aspirin, which is given orally prior to procedure. Pharmacologic agents used during the procedure include heparin, nitroglycerin, and/or glycoprotein IIb/IIIa receptor inhibitors.

**After** the percutaneous transluminal coronary angioplasty, practicing clinicians should perform electrocardiogram, echocardiogram, and physical assessment; monitor peripheral blood flow; look for swelling; and evaluate cardiac pain. Hospital protocols for aftercare should be followed. Prior to patient release, practicing clinicians should perform additional physical assessment and laboratory tests such as hematocrit, potassium levels, creatinine levels, and cardiac enzymes. Cardiac stress testing should be completed 2–6 months post procedure.

### *Contraindications and Complications*

**Contraindications** for a percutaneous transluminal coronary angioplasty procedure include high-risk coronary anatomy, severe coronary artery disease, bleeding disorder, and/or multiple episodes of percutaneous transluminal coronary angioplasty restenosis.

**Complications** associated with percutaneous transluminal coronary angioplasty include abrupt closure of diseased coronary artery, periprocedural myocardial infarction, coronary restenosis, bleeding or hematoma at catheter introduction site, arterial embolism, pseudoaneurysm, retroperitoneal bleeding, and sudden death. Bleeding from the site of catheter insertion (usually the femoral artery) and anaphylaxis to the dye used are also major risk factors.

Other complications may occur due to the patient's overall health, allergies, and other comorbid conditions. Therefore, practicing clinicians need to take a careful medical history and perform a physical examination prior to the procedure.

## Stents

A **stent** is defined as a small mesh tube that is inserted into a diseased cardiac vessel that is narrowed or weakened to increase blood flow and restore cardiac function. Stents are typically implanted during an angioplasty procedure. Stents can be made of metal such as stainless steel, tantalum, cobalt alloy, platinum or nitinol, fabric, and may also be drug-coated to prevent restenosis.

A **stent procedure** is very similar to a percutaneous transluminal coronary angioplasty. There are several types of stent procedures, including balloon-expandable and self-expanding stent procedures. With balloon-expanding stents, the stent is placed over the balloon and is placed once the balloon is expanded at the plaque site within the diseased coronary vessel. Self-expanding stents are covered by a sheath that allows the stent to expand when removed.

### *Indications, Contraindications, and Complications*

Stent procedures are **indicated** for patients with refractory angina, unstable angina, evidence of cardiac ischemia, acute myocardial infarction, angina post coronary bypass surgery, unsuitable coronary anatomy for coronary bypass surgery, focal de novo lesions, stenosis of previously placed saphenous vein grafts, and restenosis after successful percutaneous transluminal coronary angioplasty or stent placement.

**Contraindications** for a stent procedure include high-risk coronary anatomy, severe coronary artery disease, bleeding disorder, and/or multiple episodes of percutaneous transluminal coronary angioplasty restenosis. If glycoprotein IIb/IIIa inhibitors are used, other contraindications include gastrointestinal bleeding, inability to take antiplatelet agents, intracranial hemorrhage, recent surgery, or trauma.

**Complications** associated with stent procedures include abrupt closure of diseased coronary artery, periprocedural myocardial infarction, coronary restenosis, bleeding, or hematoma at catheter introduction site, arterial embolism, pseudoaneurysm, retroperitoneal bleeding, and sudden death.

### *Role of Practicing Clinician*

**Prior** to a stent procedure, practicing clinicians should take a patient's medical history, perform a physical examination, and evaluate the patient's overall health. Patients should be screened for drug-drug interactions, allergies, vital signs such as heart rate and blood pressure, and cardiovascular blood indicators such as potassium levels, prothrombin time, hematocrit, and creatinine levels. Patients should also undergo electrocardiogram and echocardiogram prior to procedure.

**During** the procedure, patients should only receive medications via an intravenous route, except for aspirin, which is given orally prior to the procedure. Pharmacologic agents used during the procedure include heparin, nitroglycerin, and/or a glycoprotein IIb/IIIa receptor inhibitor.

**After** the stent procedure, practicing clinicians should perform electrocardiogram, echocardiogram, and physical assessment; monitor peripheral blood flow; look for swelling; and evaluate cardiac pain. Hospital protocols for aftercare should be followed. Prior to patient release, practicing clinicians should perform additional physical assessment and laboratory tests such as hematocrit, potassium levels, creatinine levels, and cardiac enzymes. Cardiac stress testing should be completed 2–6 months post procedure.

## Percutaneous Transluminal Angioplasty of the Lower Extremity

**Percutaneous transluminal angioplasty of the lower extremity** is a procedure used for the treatment of peripheral arterial disease. The procedure involves balloon angioplasty of the diseased peripheral vessel to improve blood flow to extremities. The procedure is similar to percutaneous transluminal coronary angioplasty. The catheter has a balloon at the end of the device, used to reduce the plaque in the diseased vessel. Once the catheter is inserted, balloon pressure is applied to the area of plaque formation to decrease plaque size and/or stretch the vessel wall. The procedure can be done with stents, thrombolytic agents, and with arthrectomy approaches.

### *Types*

The **types of percutaneous transluminal angioplasty of the lower extremity** include aortoiliac percutaneous transluminal angioplasty and stenting and femoropopliteal percutaneous transluminal angioplasty.

- **Aortoiliac percutaneous transluminal angioplasty** is a procedure that involves access through a retrograde approach or an iliac crossover approach. The catheter has a balloon at the end of the device, used to reduce plaque buildup in the diseased vessel. Once the catheter is inserted, balloon pressure is applied to the area of plaque formation to cause plaque rupture, endothelial disruption, and/or stretching of the vessel wall.
- **Femoropopliteal percutaneous transluminal angioplasty** is a procedure that involves access through an antegrade femoral approach or a femoral crossover approach. The role of stents in this approach is dependent on the length of the lesion.

### *Role of Practicing Clinician*

**Prior** to a percutaneous transluminal angioplasty of lower extremity, practicing clinicians should take the patient's medical history, perform a physical examination, and evaluate the patient's overall health. Patients should be screened for drug-drug interactions; allergies; vital signs such as heart rate and blood pressure; and cardiovascular blood indicators such as potassium levels, prothrombin time, and hematocrit and creatinine levels. Patients should also undergo an electrocardiogram and echocardiogram prior to the procedure.

**During** the procedure, patients should only receive medications via an intravenous route, except for aspirin, which is given orally prior to the procedure. Pharmacologic agents used during the procedure include heparin, nitroglycerin, and/or a glycoprotein IIb/IIIa receptor inhibitor.

**After** the percutaneous transluminal angioplasty of the lower extremity, practicing clinicians should perform an electrocardiogram, echocardiogram, and physical assessments; monitor peripheral blood flow; look for swelling; and evaluate ischemic pain. Hospital protocols for aftercare should be followed.

**Prior** to patient release, practicing clinicians should perform additional physical assessments and laboratory tests such as hematocrit, potassium levels, creatinine levels, and cardiac enzymes.

#### *Indications, Contraindications, and Complications*

Percutaneous transluminal angioplasty of the lower extremity is **indicated** for symptoms of severe claudication and critical limb ischemia. Percutaneous transluminal angioplasty of the lower extremity can be done in combination with surgical bypass surgery.

Percutaneous transluminal angioplasty of the lower extremity is **contraindicated** in patients who are medically unstable or who have long arterial occlusions, poor distal runoff, or diabetes.

**Complications** associated with percutaneous transluminal angioplasty of the lower extremity include vasospasm, thrombus formation, arterial dissection, vessel perforation, compartment syndrome, arterial dissection, restenosis, and sudden death. Other complications may occur due to the patient's overall health, allergies, and other comorbid conditions. Therefore, practicing clinicians need to take a careful medical history and perform a physical examination prior to the procedure.

### Percutaneous Transluminal Angioplasty of the Carotid Artery

**Percutaneous transluminal angioplasty of the carotid artery** is a procedure that involves increasing blood flow by reducing plaque buildup within the brain. The procedure can be done alone or in combination with stenting. Vascular approaches include accessing the internal carotid artery through the femoral artery, but access through the axillary and brachial arteries can also be done. During the procedure, a wire is guided from the vascular access to the site within the carotid artery, and a stent is put into place. Balloon angioplasty may be done prior to wire access to dilate the blood vessel and reduce plaque buildup.

#### *Indications, Contraindications, and Complications*

Percutaneous transluminal angioplasty of the carotid artery is **indicated** for stenosis of the internal carotid artery, stenosis associated with transient ischemic attacks, bilateral stenosis, contralateral carotid artery occlusion, previous neck irradiation, radial neck dissection, increased operative risk such as severe coronary artery disease, and systemic restenosis.

Percutaneous transluminal angioplasty of the carotid artery is **contraindicated** in patients with major thrombus formation and thick circular or semicircular stenosis. **Complications** associated with percutaneous transluminal angioplasty of the carotid artery include transient ischemic attacks, stroke, cerebral hemorrhage, amaurosis fugax, stent restenosis, cranial nerve injury, and sudden death.

#### *Role of Practicing Clinician*

**Prior** to percutaneous transluminal angioplasty of the carotid artery, practicing clinicians should take the patient's medical history, perform a physical examination, and evaluate the patient's overall health. Patients should be screened for drug-drug interactions; urine output; allergies; vital signs such as heart rate and blood pressure; and cardiovascular blood indicators such as potassium levels, prothrombin time, and hematocrit and creatinine levels. Patients should also undergo an electrocardiogram and echocardiogram prior to the procedure. Also, patients are premedicated with heparin, atropine, and nifedipine.

**During** the procedure, patients should only receive medications via an intravenous route, except for aspirin, which is given orally prior to procedure. Pharmacologic agents used during the procedure include heparin, nitroglycerin, and/or a glycoprotein IIb/IIIa receptor inhibitor.

**After** the percutaneous transluminal angioplasty of the carotid artery, practicing clinicians should perform an electrocardiogram, echocardiogram, and physical assessments; monitor peripheral blood flow; look for swelling; and evaluate cardiac pain. Hospital protocols for aftercare should be followed. Prior to patient release, practicing clinicians should perform additional physical assessments and laboratory tests such as hematocrit, potassium levels, creatinine levels, and cardiac enzymes. Follow-up examination one week post procedure is completed to check neurological status. Additionally, Doppler ultrasound is performed every 3–6 months and then every year. Magnetic resonance imaging will be performed three months post procedure as well.

## PERCUTANEOUS TRANSLUMINAL ANGIOPLASTY OF RENAL ARTERY

**Percutaneous transluminal angioplasty of the renal artery** is a procedure that involves increasing blood flow to the kidney, decreasing associated secondary hypertension, and improving renal function. Percutaneous transluminal angioplasty of the renal artery is typically done for fibromuscular dysplasia, but stenting can be used as an adjunctive approach for atherosclerotic plaque formation.

The procedure involves the use of a catheter introduced through the femoral or brachial arteries into the renal artery. The catheter has a balloon at the end of the device, used to reduce plaque buildup in the diseased vessel. Once the catheter is inserted, balloon pressure is applied to the area of plaque to decrease size and/or stretch the vessel wall.

### *INDICATIONS, CONTRAINDICATIONS, AND COMPLICATIONS*

Percutaneous transluminal angioplasty of the renal artery is **indicated** for renovascular hypertension-caused atherosclerotic disease, renal transplant artery stenosis, renal artery or vein bypass graft stenosis, and renal insufficiency with more than 50% renal artery stenosis.

Percutaneous transluminal angioplasty of the renal artery is **contraindicated** for borderline lesions, long section of occlusion, aortic plaque extending to renal artery, and other unstable comorbid medical conditions.

**Complications** of percutaneous transluminal angioplasty include vascular access complications, worsening of renal failure, thrombus, nonocclusive dissection, embolism to peripheral artery, rupture of artery, and sudden death.

### *ROLE OF PRACTICING CLINICIAN*

**Prior** to percutaneous transluminal angioplasty of the renal artery, practicing clinicians should take the patient's medical history, perform a physical examination, and evaluate the patient's overall health. Patients should be screened for drug-drug interactions; urine output; allergies; vital signs such as heart rate and blood pressure; and cardiovascular blood indicators such as potassium levels, prothrombin time, hematocrit, and creatinine levels. Patients should also undergo electrocardiogram and echocardiogram prior to procedure.

**During** the procedure, patients should only receive medications via an intravenous route, except for aspirin, which is given orally prior to the procedure. Patients undergoing the procedure with stent placement may receive clopidogrel post procedure.

**After** the percutaneous transluminal angioplasty of the renal artery, practicing clinicians should perform an electrocardiogram, echocardiogram, and physical assessment; monitor peripheral blood flow; look for swelling; and evaluate cardiac pain. Hospital protocols for aftercare should be followed. Prior to patient release, practicing clinicians should perform additional physical assessment and laboratory tests such as hematocrit, potassium levels, creatinine levels, and cardiac enzymes. Cardiac stress testing should be completed 2–6 months post procedure.

## Percutaneous Balloon Valvuloplasty

**Percutaneous balloon valvuloplasty** is a procedure that involves restoring blood flow and cardiac function by opening a constricted heart valve. There are two types of percutaneous balloon valvuloplasty: percutaneous balloon mitral valvuloplasty and percutaneous balloon aortic valvuloplasty.

- The **percutaneous balloon mitral valvuloplasty** procedure involves the use of a catheter introduced through the femoral, brachial, or radial artery into the diseased valve. Transeptal catheterization is performed, and a large balloon catheter is placed over the mitral valve. Once the catheter is inserted, balloon pressure is applied to the area of the mitral valve. Please note that two balloon catheters can be used for this procedure as well.
- The **percutaneous balloon aortic valvuloplasty** involves the use of a catheter introduced through the femoral, brachial, or radial artery into the diseased valve. Transeptal catheterization is performed, and a large balloon catheter is placed over the aortic valve. Once the catheter is inserted, balloon pressure is applied to the area of aortic valve.

### *Role of Practicing Clinician*

**Prior** to percutaneous balloon valvuloplasty, practicing clinicians should take the patient's medical history, perform a physical examination, and evaluate the patient's overall health. Patients should be screened for drug-drug interactions; allergies; vital signs such as heart rate and blood pressure; and cardiovascular blood indicators such as potassium levels, prothrombin time, and hematocrit and creatinine levels. Patients should also undergo electrocardiogram and echocardiogram prior to procedure.

**During** the procedure, patients should only receive medications via an intravenous route, except for aspirin, which is given orally prior to the procedure. Pharmacologic agents used during the procedure include heparin, nitroglycerin, and/or a glycoprotein IIb/IIIa receptor inhibitor.

**After** the percutaneous balloon valvuloplasty, practicing clinicians should perform an electrocardiogram, echocardiogram, and physical assessment; monitor peripheral blood flow; look for swelling; and evaluate cardiac pain. Hospital protocols for aftercare should be followed. Prior to patient release, practicing clinicians should perform additional physical assessments such as the patient's heart sounds and laboratory tests such as hematocrit, potassium levels, creatinine levels, and cardiac enzymes. Patients should follow up with their practicing clinician one week post procedure and should undergo an echocardiogram 3–6 months post procedure.

### *Indications, Contraindications, and Complications*

Percutaneous balloon **mitral valvuloplasty** is **indicated** for symptomatic mitral valve stenosis with or without valvular disease, with a small degree of mitral valve regurgitation, and nonsurgical candidates with severely calcified or fused mitral valves.

Percutaneous balloon **aortic valvuloplasty** is **indicated** for short-term relief of valve surgery candidates, left ventricular dysfunction, and symptomatic patients subject to undergo noncardiac surgery.

**Contraindications** associated with percutaneous balloon valvuloplasty include atrial thrombus, severely fused or calcified leaflets, severe coronary artery disease, and severe aortic regurgitation.

**Complications** associated with percutaneous balloon valvuloplasty include periprocedural myocardial infarction, emergency coronary artery bypass surgery, coronary restenosis, bleeding or hematoma at catheter introduction site, arterial embolism, pseudoaneurysm, retroperitoneal bleeding, hemopericardium or tamponade, mitral regurgitation, atrial septal defects, and sudden death.

## Artificial Pacemakers

**Artificial pacemakers** provide electrical stimulation to the cardiac muscle when the heart is not able to keep up with the demands of the body. This occurs when the intrinsic heart rate is not able to provide enough cardiac output. The artificial pacemaker is made up of a pulse generator and either a unipolar or bipolar lead and is implanted in the right atrium or ventricle in contact with the cardiac walls.

The **types of pacemakers** include permanent pacemakers and temporary pacemakers. Temporary pacemakers include transvenous pacing, transcutaneous pacing, epicardial pacing, and transthoracic pacing. Other types of pacing include single chamber pacing, dual chamber pacing, rate modulating pacing, atrial overdrive pacing, and antitachycardia pacing.

### *Temporary Artificial Pacing*

In **transvenous pacing**, vascular access is gained by percutaneous puncture of the internal jugular, subclavian, antecubital, or femoral vein. Access can also be gained by venous cutdown in an antecubital vein. A bipolar, transvenous pacing lead is usually placed and maintained.

**Transcutaneous pacing** requires a nonsurgical approach where electrodes are attached to the anterior and posterior chest walls and connected to an external generator. This approach is typically used during emergency situations.

In **epicardial pacing**, surgery is done to attach leads to the atria and/or ventricle. The other end of the lead is connected externally to a generator.

In **transthoracic pacing**, a long needle is used to thread a lead to the right ventricle, which is then connected to an external generator. This approach is reserved for emergency situations.

### *Generic Pacemaker Code*

Pacemakers are classified using a **5-position code**, which encodes the type of pacemaker and its functions:

- Position one (I) indicates the chamber or chambers being paced.
- Position two (II) indicates the chamber or chambers being sensed.
- Position three (III) indicates the device's response to sensing.
- Position four (IV) indicates the programmability and rate of modulation function.
- Position five (V) is only used for tachycardia functions.

Each position has additional subsets to describe the function taking place. For example, for position III, response to sensing, O=none, T=triggered, I=inhibited, and D=dual (triggered and inhibited). In positions I and II, there will be an A (atrial), V (ventricle), or D (dual) for the chamber(s) paced and sensed.

### *Types of Pacing*

**Single chamber pacing** involves either the atrium or ventricle being paced but not both chambers in combination. However, **dual chamber pacing** involves both the atria and ventricles being paced together.

**Rate-modulated pacing** involves the pacing of the atria and ventricles based on physiological stress with increased heart rate. This type of pacing uses sensors to modulate pacing. Upon muscle or body movement, the sensor responds and modulates pacing.

**Atrial overdrive pacing** is a technique used to treat atrial flutter and tachycardia by providing atrial pacing rates of 200–500 impulses per minute.

**Antitachycardia pacing** is a technique that sends impulses to the heart to disrupt tachycardia. This approach can be used with implantable cardioverter defibrillators.

### *Permanent and Temporary Pacemakers*

**Permanent pacing** is indicated for third-degree atrioventricular block, second-degree atrioventricular block with symptomatic bradycardia, intermittent third-degree atrioventricular block, type II second-degree atrioventricular block, sinus node dysfunction with symptomatic bradycardia or third-degree heart block, symptomatic chronotropic incompetence, persistent second-degree atrioventricular block with bilateral bundle branch, or third-degree atrioventricular block, transient advanced second- or third-degree infranodal atrioventricular block and associated bundle block, ventricular tachycardia, recurrent syncope caused by carotid sinus stimulation, and symptomatic recurrent supraventricular tachycardia.

**Temporary pacing** is indicated for symptomatic bradycardia after acute myocardial infarction or associated hyperkalemia and/or drug toxicity, prior to permanent pacing, bradycardia nonresponsive to atropine or isoproterenol, bifascicular bundle block, alternating bundle branch block associated with acute myocardial infarction, transient right bundle block, and post cardiovascular surgery to address bradycardia.

### *Operating Settings*

**Operational settings for pacemakers** are described based on rate, output, and sensitivity.

- **Rate** is defined as the number of times per minute that the pacemaker will fire when the patient's rate goes below that of the set rate.
- **Output** is described as the intensity of the electrical stimulus used to depolarize the cardiac tissue.
- **Sensitivity** is defined as the ability of a pacemaker to sense the patient's intrinsic heart rate. The sensitivity of the pacemaker increases as the number decreases.

The operational settings vary based on the type of pacemaker and whether it is for permanent pacing or temporary pacing.

### *Contraindications and Complications*

**Contraindications** for implantation of pacemakers include first-degree atrioventricular block, asymptomatic second-degree atrioventricular block, transient atrioventricular block, atrioventricular block due to interior wall myocardial infarction, asymptomatic sinus node dysfunction, and suppression of ventricular tachycardia.

**Complications** associated with pacemaker implantation can vary depending on whether permanent or temporary pacing is being used. Complications associated with permanent pacing include pneumothorax, hemothorax, inadvertent entry into an artery, perforation of cardiac tissue or vein, damage to cardiac valve, inadequate or improper connection to leads, pain or infection in pacemaker pocket, migration of pacemaker, intravascular thrombus, bradycardia, tachycardia, endocarditis, and manual disruption of pacing.

Complications associated with temporary pacing include malfunction of the pacing system; ventricular tachycardia; thromboembolism; endocarditis; infection; phlebitis; failure to capture or sense properly; pneumothorax; hemothorax; perforation of atria, ventricle, or cardiac tissue/vessels; and cardiac tamponade.



### Permanent Pacemaker Implantation

#### Role of Practicing Clinician

Practicing clinicians need to understand how the pacemaker works in terms of operational settings as well as programming so they will be able to intervene if a problem arises.

**Prior** to permanent pacemaker implantation, practicing clinicians should take a patient's medical history, perform a physical examination, and evaluate overall health. Patients should be screened for drug-drug interactions; allergies; vital signs such as heart rate and blood pressure; and cardiovascular blood indicators such as potassium levels, prothrombin time, and hematocrit and creatinine levels. Patients should also undergo electrocardiogram and echocardiogram prior to the procedure. Additionally, they should take prophylactic antibiotic therapy.

**After** permanent pacemaker implantation, practicing clinicians should perform an electrocardiogram, echocardiogram, and physical assessment; monitor peripheral blood flow; look for swelling; and evaluate cardiac pain. Hospital protocols for aftercare should be followed. Prior to patient release, practicing clinicians should perform additional physical assessments, such as assessing the patient's heart sounds, and performing laboratory tests such as hematocrit, potassium levels, creatinine levels, and cardiac enzymes. Chest x-ray should also be performed pre and post pacemaker placement.

### Temporary Pacemaker Implantation

#### Role of Practicing Clinician

Practicing clinicians need to understand how the pacemaker works in terms of operational settings as well as programming so they will be able to intervene if a problem arises.

**Prior** to temporary pacemaker placement, a sterile environment needs to be established. A clean insertion site needs to be established to prevent infection. Guidelines for care of central venous catheters and dressing should be followed for this procedure.

**After** temporary pacemaker placement, daily iodine cleaning of areas where leads exit the body should be performed. Electrical safety is necessary in the care of these patients. Practicing clinicians should always wear gloves when handling pacing and/or wiring, insulate exposed metal ends of pacing leads, keep dressing dry, and make sure all other electrical equipment in the room is grounded.

### Required Follow-Up

Patients should be instructed to **follow up** with their practicing clinician one week post permanent pacemaker placement and then follow up every 3–6 months to check programming and settings of the device. Elderly patients should be checked on a regular basis for risk of infection, heart sounds, and cardiac risk factors. Patients at risk for other cardiovascular complications should be monitored on a regular basis.

Some patients may be followed via telephone for pacemaker battery status with transtelephonic monitoring. This method of monitoring sends a telephone transmission of a rhythm strip that allows the pacemaker battery status to be measured.

## Implantable Cardioverter Defibrillator

**Implantable cardiac defibrillators** are used to treat life-threatening irregular heartbeat. They are small devices implanted in the chest or abdomen to control heart rate and cardiovascular function. The device consists of a pulse generator and lead system, which is available for pacing, sensing, and shocking.

The implantation of a cardiac defibrillator is very similar to that of permanent pacemakers. The transvenous lead system is inserted into the right ventricle and then connected to the pulse generator. Also, a patch is connected from the ventricle to the pulse generator. However, some systems may have more than one lead and more than one patch.

Implantable cardiac defibrillators are capable of defibrillation, cardioversion, antitachycardia pacing, and antibradycardia pacing.

### *Indications, Contraindications, and Complications*

Implantable cardiac defibrillators are **indicated** for cardiac arrest due to ventricular fibrillation or ventricular tachycardia, sustained ventricular tachycardia, undetermined syncope or fainting, nonsustained and inducible ventricular tachycardia due to coronary heart disease, left ventricular dysfunction or previous myocardial infarction, hypertrophic cardiomyopathy with high risk for sudden death, and prolonged QT syndrome.

**Contraindications** associated with implantable cardiac defibrillators include myocardial ischemia, electrolyte abnormalities, terminal illness with short life expectancy, and ventricular tachycardia or ventricular fibrillation due to dysrhythmia.

### *Role of Practicing Clinician*

Practicing clinicians need to understand how the implantable defibrillator works in terms of operational settings as well as programming so they will be able to intervene if a problem arises.

**Prior** to implantable defibrillator placement, practicing clinicians should take the patient's medical history, perform a physical examination, and evaluate the patient's overall health. Patients should be screened for drug-drug interactions; allergies; vital signs such as heart rate and blood pressure; and cardiovascular blood indicators such as potassium levels, prothrombin time, and hematocrit and creatinine levels. Patients should also undergo electrocardiogram and echocardiogram prior to procedure. Additionally, they should take prophylactic antibiotic therapy.

**After** implantable defibrillator placement, practicing clinicians should perform an electrocardiogram, echocardiogram, and physical assessment; monitor peripheral blood flow; look for swelling; and evaluate cardiac pain. Hospital protocols for aftercare should be followed. Prior to patient release, practicing clinicians should perform additional physical assessments, such as assessing the patient's heart sounds, and laboratory tests such as hematocrit, potassium levels, creatinine levels, and cardiac enzymes. Chest x-ray should also be performed pre and post implantable defibrillator placement to assess for pneumothorax.

### *Required Follow-Up*

Patients should be instructed to **follow up** with their practicing clinician one week post implantable defibrillator placement and then follow up every 3–6 months to check programming and settings of the device. Practicing clinicians should assess stored data and provide any treated episodes of dysrhythmia. Elderly patients should be checked on a regular basis for risk of infection, heart sounds, and cardiac risk factors. Other patients at risk for cardiovascular complications should be monitored on a regular basis.

Chest x-rays should be done annually to evaluate the implantable cardioverter. If the implantable defibrillator discharges, the patient should notify the provider. Emergency services should be contacted if the device discharges multiple times and/or the patient feels ill.

## Coronary Artery Bypass Graft Surgery

**Coronary artery bypass graft surgery** is a procedure that uses a vessel graft to treat ischemic areas of cardiac tissue. Surgical revascularization uses vessel grafts including internal mammary artery, saphenous vein graft, gastroepiploic artery, and radial artery.

The procedure is performed under general anesthesia and requires opening of the sternum and putting the patient on cardiopulmonary bypass while the procedure is being completed. During the procedure, the cardiac muscle is arrested using a pharmacologic agent and hypothermia.

The procedure can also be performed minimally invasively as well as without the assistance of cardiopulmonary bypass.

### *Indications, Contraindications, and Complications*

Coronary artery bypass graft is **indicated** for angina refractory to drugs and other surgical interventions, significant left cardiac main disease, triple vessel coronary artery disease, acute myocardial infarction, and left ventricular failure due to cardiogenic shock or congestive heart failure.

**Contraindications** associated with coronary artery bypass graft include lack of adequate graft; small coronary arteries; severe aortic stenosis and severe left ventricular failure; and coexisting peripheral vascular, renal, and pulmonary disease.

**Complications** associated with coronary artery bypass graft procedures include postoperative bleeding such as heparin-induced thrombocytopenia, disseminated intravascular coagulopathy and diluted anemia, myocardial depression, cardiac tamponade, perioperative myocardial infarction, dysrhythmia including atrial tachycardia or atrial fibrillation, pulmonary edema, pulmonary atelectasis, pneumothorax, renal impairment, abdominal distension, cerebral ischemia, postcardiotomy delirium, peripheral neurological deficits, postpericardiotomy syndrome, wound infection, and sudden death.

### *Role of Practicing Clinician*

**Prior** to coronary artery bypass graft procedure, practicing clinicians should take the patient's medical history, perform a physical examination, and evaluate the patient's overall health. Patients should be screened for drug-drug interactions; allergies; vital signs such as heart rate and blood pressure; and cardiovascular blood indicators such as potassium levels, prothrombin time, and hematocrit and creatinine levels. Patients should also undergo electrocardiogram and echocardiogram prior to procedure. Additionally, they should take prophylactic antibiotic therapy and undergo chest x-ray. Overall, a full cardiovascular workup should be conducted prior to the procedure.

**During** the procedure, patients should only receive medications via an intravenous route, except for aspirin, which is given orally prior to the procedure.

**After** coronary artery bypass graft, practicing clinicians should perform an electrocardiogram, echocardiogram, and physical assessment; monitor peripheral blood flow; look for swelling; and evaluate cardiac pain. Hospital protocols for aftercare should be followed. Prior to patient release, practicing clinicians should perform additional physical assessments, such as assessing patient's heart sounds and laboratory tests such as hematocrit, potassium levels, creatinine levels, and cardiac enzymes. Overall, a full cardiovascular workup should be conducted prior to releasing the patient.

### *Risk Factors and Complications*

**Risk factors and complications** associated with the CABG procedure include:

- Death
- Pain: incisional or related to new-onset myocardial infarction
- Bleeding: surgical trauma, thrombocytopenia, anemia, or disseminated intravascular coagulopathy (DIC)
- Myocardial depression: cardiac dysfunction
- Cardiac tamponade: increased pericardial fluid
- Myocardial infarction: additional injury occurring after surgery
- Dysrhythmia: most commonly atrial fibrillation
- Pulmonary complications: pulmonary edema, atelectasis, pneumothorax
- Renal impairment: mild to acute renal failure
- Neuropsychological problems: cerebral ischemia, infarction, emboli, postcardiotomy delirium (ranging from elation and denial to hallucinations and neurological symptoms), brachial plexus, or ulnar nerve injury
- Postpericardiotomy syndrome: autoimmune response to surgical injury
- Infection: wound, sepsis
- Gastrointestinal problems: distention, ileus, hepatic dysfunction, mesenteric ischemia

## CABG vs. MIDCAB

**Traditional coronary artery bypass graft (CABG)** surgery involves restoring cardiac blood flow by grafting in a new vein or artery to direct blood around a blockage in the coronary artery. This procedure requires a large incision, stopping the heart, and use of a heart-lung machine.

**Minimally invasive direct coronary artery bypass (MIDCAB)** uses a smaller incision and can be performed on a heart that is slowed but still beating. Prime candidates for this operation are patients with proximal left anterior descending lesion. This requires less time and therefore shorter exposure to anesthesia with earlier extubation. Initial pain during recovery may be greater than with CABG, but it is relieved more quickly. There are fewer risks associated with the procedure, and expenses are reduced. Patients receiving MIDCAB report better physical activity and sleeping conditions than those undergoing CABG.

## Valvular Replacement and Valvular Repair

**Valvular replacement** is a procedure that is used when repair will not be effective for fixing a dysfunctional valve. Two types of valvular replacements are currently available: mechanical valve replacements such as bileaflet, tilting-disk, and caged ball valves, and biologic valve replacements such as xenografts, homografts, or allografts.

The procedure can be performed through standard cardiovascular procedure with sternum access, minimally invasive approaches, or port access. However, cardiac arrest is required to perform the procedure; therefore, patients need to undergo general anesthesia and cardiopulmonary bypass. Valvular replacement may be performed for aortic stenosis and aortic insufficiency.

**Valvular repair** is a procedure that involves repair of calcified or nonfunctioning cardiac valves. Several types of valve repair procedures may be performed, including commissurotomy, annuloplasty, and chordoplasty. Commissurotomy is a procedure that separates fused leaflets of a cardiac valve. Annuloplasty is a procedure that repairs the junction between the cardiac valve leaflet and cardiac muscle. Two different approaches can be used to perform annuloplasty, including the use of a ring prosthesis and/or sutures. Chordoplasty is a procedure that involves the repair of an elongated or ruptured chordae tendinea.

The procedure can be performed open, through minimally invasive approaches, or through port access. However, cardiac arrest is required to perform the procedure; therefore, patients need to undergo general anesthesia and cardiopulmonary bypass. Valvular repair may be performed for mitral valve stenosis and mitral insufficiency.



### *Indications, Contraindications, and Complications*

Valvular repair or valvular replacements are **indicated** for aortic or mitral valve disease. **Contraindications** for valve repair and/or replacement include presence of other cardiovascular comorbidities or poor health status as well as those patients at high surgical risk.

**Complications** of valvular repair and/or valvular replacements include postoperative bleeding such as heparin-induced thrombocytopenia, disseminated intravascular coagulopathy and diluted anemia, myocardial depression, cardiac tamponade, perioperative myocardial infarction, dysrhythmia including atrial tachycardia or atrial fibrillation, pulmonary edema, pulmonary atelectasis, pneumothorax, renal impairment, abdominal distension, cerebral ischemia, postcardiotomy delirium, peripheral neurological deficits, postpericardiotomy syndrome, wound infection, and sudden death.

### *Mechanical vs. Biological Valve Replacements*

Two **types of valvular replacements** are currently available: mechanical valve replacements such as bileaflet, tilting-disk, and caged ball valves, and biologic valve replacements such as xenografts, homografts, or allografts. Mechanical valve replacements require life-long anticoagulation therapy due to risk of thrombosis.

- **Mechanical valves** last longer and are typically used for patients under 65 or patients over 65 who have a long life expectancy.
- **Biologic valves** deteriorate at a rate inversely proportional to the patient's age (they wear out faster in younger patients). Thus, biological valves are typically great for elderly patients in whom the expected lifespan is less than the life of the valve (15–20 years). Women who would like to become pregnant should also have biologic valves placed to avoid long-term teratogenic anticoagulants.

### *Role of Practicing Clinician*

**Prior** to valvular repair or replacement, practicing clinicians should take a patient's medical history, perform a physical examination, and evaluate a patient's overall health. Patients should be screened for drug-drug interactions; allergies; vital signs such as heart rate and blood pressure; and cardiovascular blood indicators such as potassium levels, prothrombin time, and hematocrit and creatinine levels. Patients should also undergo an electrocardiogram and echocardiogram prior to the procedure. Additionally, they should take prophylactic antibiotic therapy and undergo a chest x-ray. Overall, a full cardiovascular workup should be conducted prior to the procedure.

**During** the procedure, patients should only receive medications via an intravenous route, except for aspirin, which is given orally prior to the procedure.

**After** valvular repair or replacement, practicing clinicians should perform an electrocardiogram, echocardiogram, and physical assessment; monitor peripheral blood flow; look for swelling; and evaluate cardiac pain. Hospital protocols for aftercare should be followed. Prior to patient release, practicing clinicians should perform additional physical assessments, such as assessing the patient's heart sounds, and laboratory tests such as hematocrit, potassium levels, creatinine levels, and cardiac enzymes. Overall, a full cardiovascular workup should be conducted prior to releasing the patient.

## Arterial Bypass Surgery

In cases of severe ischemia or occlusion of cardiac blood vessels, bypass grafts may be used to reroute blood flow and improve cardiac function. Bypass vessels that can be used to reroute cardiac blood flow include femoral artery bypass grafting or axillofemoral reconstruction. Bypass grafts can be made from the patient's own tissue or may be made of synthetic nature. Synthetic graft materials include expanded polytetrafluoroethylene and woven or knitted Dacron.

Various approaches may be used to perform **arterial bypass surgery**, including aortobifemoral bypass, aortoiliac endarterectomy, or femoral to popliteal graft. Other approaches may be used, depending on the extent and degree of the patient's disease and/or presence of other comorbid conditions.

### *Indications, Contraindications, and Complications*

Arterial bypass surgery is **indicated** for severe unilateral or bilateral aortoiliac disease, distal aortic occlusion, and critical limb ischemia with diffuse disease and severe occlusion.

**Contraindications** for arterial bypass surgery include patients who are medically unstable and have poor distal runoff. **Complications** of arterial bypass surgery include thrombosis, embolization, bleeding, arterial dissection, infection, restenosis, compartment syndrome, mesenteric ischemic, mesenteric infarction, and/or sudden death. Other complications may arise due to the presence of other comorbid conditions such as diabetes and various cardiovascular conditions as well as due to the patient's overall health.

### *Role of Practicing Clinician*

**Prior** to arterial bypass surgery, practicing clinicians should take the patient's medical history, perform a physical examination, and evaluate the patient's overall health. Patients should be screened for drug-drug interactions; allergies; vital signs such as heart rate and blood pressure; and cardiovascular blood indicators such as potassium levels, prothrombin time, and hematocrit and creatinine levels. Patients should also undergo an electrocardiogram and echocardiogram prior to the procedure. Additionally, they should take prophylactic antibiotic therapy and undergo a chest x-ray. Overall, a full cardiovascular workup should be conducted prior to the procedure.

**During** the procedure, patients should only receive medications via an intravenous route, except for aspirin, which is given orally prior to the procedure.

**After** arterial bypass surgery, practicing clinicians should perform an electrocardiogram, echocardiogram, and physical assessment; monitor peripheral blood flow; look for swelling; and evaluate cardiac pain. Extremity swelling of legs and feet is typical after arterial bypass surgery and should be monitored and treated if it becomes severe. Additionally, patients should be evaluated for compartment syndrome and/or infection.

Pharmacologic management post surgery may include anticoagulants, antiplatelet agents, aspirin, and/or broad spectrum antibiotics.

Hospital protocols for aftercare should be followed. Hemodynamic blood flow should be monitored, and patients should be assessed for hemorrhagic shock. Doppler evaluation of vessels may also be completed. Prior to patient release, practicing clinicians should perform additional physical assessments, such as assessing the patient's heart sounds, and laboratory tests such as hematocrit, potassium levels, creatinine levels, and cardiac enzymes. Overall, a full cardiovascular workup should be conducted prior to releasing the patient.

## Aneurysm Repair

**Aneurysm repair** involves aneurysm resection and bypass grafting. Aneurysms can be categorized as abdominal, thoracic, aortic, subclavian, femoral, or popliteal. Aneurysm repair procedures may be done on an emergency basis or as a routine procedure to prevent other cardiovascular complications such as stroke, myocardial infarction, or congestive heart failure.

The procedure requires removal of the aneurysm by accessing the location of the aneurysm, clamping above and below the site, opening the aneurysm, and inserting a graft. Types of aneurysm repair procedures include endovascular grafting, abdominal aortic aneurysm grafting, and ascending thoracic aneurysm grafting.

### *Indications, Contraindications, and Complications*

Aneurysm repair is **indicated** for abdominal aortic aneurysms and thoracic aneurysms. **Contraindications** for aneurysm repair include patients who are medically unstable. However, in the case of dissection, emergency surgery may be performed.

**Complications** associated with aneurysm repair procedures include postoperative bleeding, cardiac tamponade, myocardial infarction, pulmonary complications such as pulmonary edema or embolism, renal impairment, gastrointestinal upset such as abdominal distension, ileus, hepatic dysfunction or mesenteric ischemia, hematoma, infection, endocarditis, ischemia, embolism, spinal cord ischemia, and/or sudden death. Other complications may arise due to the presence of other comorbid conditions such as diabetes and various cardiovascular conditions as well as due to the patient's overall health.

### *Role of Practicing Clinician*

**Prior** to aneurysm repair, practicing clinicians should take the patient's medical history, perform a physical examination, and evaluate the patient's overall health. Patients should be screened for drug-drug interactions; allergies; vital signs such as heart rate and blood pressure; and cardiovascular blood indicators such as potassium levels, prothrombin time, and hematocrit and creatinine levels. Patients should also undergo an electrocardiogram and echocardiogram prior to the procedure. Additionally, they should take prophylactic antibiotic therapy and undergo a chest x-ray. Overall, a full cardiovascular workup should be conducted prior to the procedure.

Practicing clinicians should also assess the patient for signs of impending aneurysm rupture. Symptoms associated with abdominal aneurysm that can lead to rupture include back or abdominal pain. Symptoms associated with thoracic aneurysm include severe chest, back, shoulder, or abdominal pain. Other associated symptoms include hypotension, congestive heart failure, and/or falling hematocrit.

**During** the procedure, patients should only receive medications via an intravenous route, except for aspirin, which is given orally prior to the procedure.

**After** aneurysm repair, practicing clinicians should perform an electrocardiogram, echocardiogram, and physical assessment; monitor peripheral blood flow; look for swelling; and evaluate cardiac pain.

Hospital protocols for aftercare should be followed. Hemodynamic blood flow should be monitored, and patients should be assessed for hemorrhagic shock. Doppler evaluation of vessels may also be completed. Prior to patient release, practicing clinicians should perform additional physical assessments, such as assessing a patient's heart sounds, and laboratory tests such as hematocrit, potassium levels, creatinine levels, and cardiac enzymes. Overall, a full cardiovascular workup should be conducted post surgery and prior to releasing the patient, including cardiac status, respiratory status, neurological status, peripheral vascular status, gastrointestinal status, pain status, psychosocial status, and potential high-risk complications associated with aneurysm repair.

## Carotid Endarterectomy

**Carotid endarterectomy** is a common procedure that removes plaque buildup within the carotid artery that serves cerebral blood flow. The procedure involves clamping of the carotid artery and then removal of the plaque buildup to restore blood flow. In an effort to monitor blood flow to the brain, Doppler and electroencephalogram may be used during the procedure.

Carotid endarterectomy is **indicated** for patients with severe asymptomatic or symptomatic carotid stenosis, ulcerated or intermediate degrees of stenosis that are not effectively treated with anticoagulation therapy, and severe stenosis with contralateral internal carotid occlusion.

### *Contraindications and Complications*

Carotid endarterectomy is **contraindicated** in patients with thick circular calcification, completely blocked arteries, and other cardiovascular comorbid conditions that may be better treated with percutaneous transluminal angioplasty or stent procedure.

**Complications** associated with carotid endarterectomy include thrombus formation, embolism, transient ischemic attack, stroke, cranial nerve injury, infection, hematoma, intracranial hemorrhage, restenosis, and/or sudden death. Other complications may arise due to the presence of other cardiovascular comorbid conditions such as diabetes, congestive heart failure, hypertension, or hyperlipidemia as well as due to the patient's overall health status. Elderly or severely ill patients with cardiovascular comorbid conditions should be monitored closely both before and after carotid endarterectomy.

### *Role of Practicing Clinician*

**Prior** to carotid endarterectomy, practicing clinicians should take a patient's medical history, perform a physical examination, and evaluate a patient's overall health. Patients should be screened for drug-drug interactions; allergies; vital signs such as heart rate and blood pressure; and cardiovascular blood indicators such as potassium levels, prothrombin time, and hematocrit and creatinine levels. Patients should also undergo an electrocardiogram and echocardiogram prior to the procedure. Additionally, they should take prophylactic antibiotic therapy and undergo a chest x-ray. Overall, a full cardiovascular workup should be conducted prior to the procedure. Additionally, the patient's neurological status should be assessed.

**During** carotid endarterectomy, patients should only receive medications via an intravenous route, except for aspirin, which is given orally prior to the procedure.

**After** carotid endarterectomy, practicing clinicians should perform an electrocardiogram, echocardiogram, and physical assessment; monitor peripheral blood flow; look for swelling; and evaluate cardiac pain. Neurological assessment including level of consciousness, vocal cord functioning, reflexes, motor strength, level of sensation, pupil size, and reaction to light should be made every 1–2 hours post surgery.

Hospital protocols for aftercare should be followed. Hemodynamic blood flow should be monitored, and patients should be assessed for hemorrhagic shock. Doppler evaluation of vessels may also be completed. Prior to patient release, practicing clinicians should perform additional physical assessments, such as assessing the patient's heart sounds, and laboratory tests such as hematocrit, potassium levels, creatinine levels, and cardiac enzymes. Overall, a full cardiovascular workup should be conducted post surgery and prior to releasing the patient.



### *Required Follow-Up*

Patients should be instructed to **follow up** with their practicing clinician one week post procedure, and another follow up should be done after three months. At three months, Doppler evaluation should be performed to assess artery patency. At six months and then yearly, Doppler evaluation should be performed to assess for restenosis. Elderly patients should be checked on a regular basis for risk of infection, heart sounds, and cardiac risk factors. Patients at risk for other cardiovascular complications should be monitored on a regular basis. Patients should also be assessed for other cardiovascular risk factors and managed for these risks.

## Peripheral Thromboembolectomy

**Peripheral thromboembolectomy** is a procedure that uses a balloon catheter to remove an arterial embolism and restore blood flow through the peripheral circulation. For aortic or iliac occlusions, bilateral ventricle groin incisions, followed by an embolectomy balloon catheter approach, are typically performed. The procedure can be performed on both legs once the initial clot is removed from the occlusion.

For femoral and popliteal occlusions, incisions in the distal common femoral artery, followed by an embolectomy balloon catheter approach, are typically performed. If thromboembolectomy fails, then adjuvant balloon dilatation and/or atherectomy may also be performed. However, anticoagulation therapy may be initiated prior to peripheral thromboembolectomy.

### *Indications, Contraindications, and Complications*

Peripheral thromboembolectomy is **indicated** for patients with acute symptomatic arterial occlusion as well as patients with gangrene to achieve lower-level amputation.

**Contraindications** of peripheral thromboembolectomy include advanced ischemia up to two days. Patients with advanced ischemia after 48 hours have a higher risk of amputation. Complications associated with peripheral thromboembolectomy include thrombus formation, vessel vasospasm, hemorrhage, bleeding, hematoma formation, artery dissection, compartment syndrome, venous thrombosis, edema, hyperkalemia, cardiac arrhythmia, renal failure, and rhabdomyolysis.

**Complications** may arise due to the presence of other cardiovascular comorbid conditions such as diabetes, congestive heart failure, hypertension, or hyperlipidemia as well as the patient's overall health status.

### Role of Practicing Clinician

**Prior** to peripheral thromboembolectomy, practicing clinicians should take a patient's medical history, perform physical examination, and evaluate overall health. Patients should be screened for drug-drug interactions; allergies; vital signs such as heart rate and blood pressure; and cardiovascular blood indicators such as potassium levels, prothrombin time, and hematocrit and creatinine levels. Patients should also undergo electrocardiogram and echocardiogram prior to the procedure. Additionally, they should take prophylactic antibiotic therapy and undergo a chest x-ray. Overall, a full cardiovascular workup should be conducted prior to the procedure. Additionally, patients should be administered heparin prior to the procedure.

**During** peripheral thromboembolectomy, patients should only receive medications via an intravenous route, except for aspirin, which is given orally prior to the procedure.

**After** peripheral thromboembolectomy, practicing clinicians should perform an electrocardiogram, echocardiogram, and physical assessment; perform pedal pulse assessment with Doppler and/or ankle brachial indices; monitor peripheral blood flow; look for swelling; and evaluate cardiac pain.

Hospital protocols for aftercare should be followed. Hemodynamic blood flow should be monitored, and patients should be assessed for hemorrhagic shock. Doppler evaluation of vessels may also be completed. Prior to patient release, practicing clinicians should perform additional physical assessments, such as assessing the patient's heart sounds, and laboratory tests such as hematocrit, potassium levels, creatinine levels, and cardiac enzymes. Overall, a full cardiovascular workup should be conducted post surgery, prior to releasing the patient.

### Required Follow-Up

Patients should be instructed to **follow up** with their practicing clinician one week post procedure, and then follow-up with Doppler and/or duplex ultrasound evaluation should be performed. Elderly patients should be examined on a regular basis for risk of infection, heart sounds, and cardiac risk factors. Other patients at risk for other cardiovascular complications should be monitored on a regular basis. Patient should also be assessed for other cardiovascular risk factors and managed for these risks. Patients should also be referred to a podiatrist or foot surgeon to address any additional limb and/or foot complications.

## Cardiac Transplantation

**Cardiac transplantation** involves the replacement of a patient's own heart with a donor heart. The procedure is performed in patients with progressive end stage cardiovascular disease. Cardiac transplantation is indicated for patients with class III or IV end stage cardiovascular disease and life expectancy of less than a year who are under 65 years of age, medically stable, and have no underlying comorbid conditions such as systemic infection, irreversible renal insufficiency, irreversible pulmonary insufficiency, irreversible hepatic insufficiency, active peptic ulcer, or recent pulmonary embolism.

Practicing clinicians and nurses need to work as a team to prepare a patient for cardiac transplantation. Preoperative care focuses on immunosuppression, acute renal failure, bradycardia, and right ventricular dysfunction.

**Long-term complications** associated with cardiac transplantation include rejection, infection, transplant coronary artery disease, nephrotoxicity, hypertension, hyperlipidemia, transplant lymphoproliferative disease, and malignancy. Long-term pharmacologic management to prevent these complications includes use of immunosuppressive agents, antibiotics, antihypertensive agents, diuretics, and lipid-lowering agents.

## VAD

A **ventricular assist device** (VAD) is a 1- to 2-pound pump, usually placed internally by the left ventricle. It is electrically controlled from outside the body. It re-routes the blood flow from the ineffective or damaged ventricle through a series of tubes that will pump the blood more efficiently than the body is able to do on its own. This treatment is not without significant risk, but the patient with chronic heart failure that can no longer be controlled with medication or pacemaker may be assessed for eligibility. The most likely candidate is a younger, healthy patient who is awaiting transplant.

### Risks Associated with Vascular Repair

**Vascular repair** procedures include aortic aneurysm repair, bypass grafting, vena cava filter insertion, and embolism removal.

**Postoperatively**, monitor for:

- **Bleeding**: external at incision site or internal, causing low blood pressure, increased heart rate, diminished respirations, restlessness, confusion, abdominal pain, increased girth, or rigidity
- **Occlusion**: diminished or absent peripheral pulses, abnormal sensation and/or pain, reduced oxygen saturation, and cyanosis
- **Infection**: fever; redness; warmth; drainage; pain; abnormal heart rate, respiration, or blood pressure; or cough and congestion
- **Renal impairment**: swelling, weight gain, low urinary output, and increased blood urea nitrogen (BUN) and creatinine levels



### Therapeutic Hypothermia

Targeted temperature management (previously referred to as therapeutic hypothermia) is used to reduce ischemic tissue damage associated with cardiac arrest, ischemic stroke, traumatic brain/spinal cord injury, neurogenic fever, and subsequent coma (3 on Glasgow scale). Reducing the body's temperature to below normal range has a neuroprotective effect by making cell membranes less permeable. Hypothermia should be initiated immediately after an ischemic event if possible, but some benefit remains up to 6 hours. Hypothermia to 33 °C may be induced by cooled saline through a femoral catheter, reducing temperature 1.5–2.0 °C/hr by an electronic control unit. Hypothermic water blankets covering ≥80% of the body's surface can also lower body temperature. In some cases, both a femoral cooling catheter and a water blanket are used for rapid reduction of temperature. Rectal probes are used to measure core temperature, but Foley temperature catheters are more common. Desflurane or meperidine is given to reduce the shivering response. Hypothermia increases risk of bleeding (decreased clotting time), infection (due to impairing leukocyte function and introducing catheters), arrhythmias, hyperglycemia, and DVT. Rewarming is done slowly at 0.5–1.0 °C/hr. through warmed intravenous fluids, warm humidified air, and/or warming blanket. The warming process is a critical time, as it causes potassium to be moved from extracellular to intracellular spaces and the patient's electrolyte levels must be monitored regularly.

## Pharmacologic Therapies

### Sympathomimetic Agents

**Sympathomimetic agents** stimulate both alpha- and beta-adrenergic receptors. Stimulation of alpha-adrenergic receptors induces vasoconstriction, and stimulation of beta-adrenergic receptors increases cardiac contraction and heart rate. Sympathomimetic agents also target dopamine receptors, which also increases cardiac contraction and dilates renal blood vessels. Therapeutic uses of sympathomimetic agents include treatment of hypotension and cardiogenic shock associated with myocardial infarction.

Adverse events associated with sympathomimetic agents include gastrointestinal side effects such as nausea and vomiting; cardiovascular events such as tachycardia, dysrhythmia, hypertension, palpitations, and angina; and central nervous system events such as throbbing headache and cerebral hemorrhage. Contraindications to sympathomimetic agents include tachydysrhythmia, ventricular fibrillation, and pheochromocytoma.

## Classes of Agents in the Adrenergic Group of Drugs

The **classes of agents** included in the **adrenergic group** of drugs include sympathomimetics such as dobutamine, isoproterenol, dopamine, metaraminol, epinephrine, and norepinephrine; alpha-1 selective adrenergic agonists such as methoxamine, phenylephrine, and midodrine; alpha-2 selective adrenergic agonists such as clonidine, guanfacine, guanabenz, and methyldopa; alpha-adrenergic antagonists such as doxazosin, prazosin, phenoxybenzamine, terazosin, phentolamine, and tolazoline; and beta-adrenergic antagonists such as acebutolol, atenolol, betaxolol, bisoprolol, carteolol, carvedilol, esmolol, labetalol, metoprolol, nadolol, penbutolol, pindolol, propranolol, sotalol, and timolol.

## Alpha-Adrenergic Antagonists

**Alpha-adrenergic antagonists** target both alpha-1 adrenergic and alpha-2 adrenergic receptors and block receptor action. Alpha-1 adrenergic receptors produce the effects of the sympathetic nervous system, while alpha-2 adrenergic receptors stimulate norepinephrine release. Drugs within this class of agents have different affinities for these receptors. Prazosin, terazosin, and doxazosin have more affinity for blocking alpha-1 receptors, while phenoxybenzamine and phentolamine have similar affinity for both alpha-1 and alpha-2 receptors.

Alpha-adrenergic antagonists decrease vascular tone, increase vasodilation, and decrease blood pressure. Therapeutic uses of alpha-adrenergic antagonists include hypertension, pheochromocytoma, and extravasation of tissue-toxic agents.

### *Adverse Events and Contraindications*

**Adverse events** associated with alpha-adrenergic antagonists include cardiovascular events such as postural hypotension, dysrhythmia, edema, congestive heart failure, and angina as well as central nervous system events such as dizziness, weakness, fatigue, drowsiness, and depression. Other adverse events include fainting and syncope up to 90 minutes post administration. Therefore, practicing clinicians should monitor patients, starting treatment with these agents to assess side effects and titrating the dose to get the desired effect with minimal adverse effects. Caution should be used when administrating these agents in patients with congestive heart failure, pregnancy, and renal failure.

## Alpha-1 Selective Adrenergic Agents

The **alpha-1 selective adrenergic agents** stimulate vascular smooth muscle by targeting alpha-adrenergic receptors. Stimulation of alpha-adrenergic receptors increases peripheral vascular resistance and also increases blood pressure through vasoconstriction. Therapeutic uses of alpha-1 selective adrenergic agents include the treatment of persistent hypotension, neurally-mediated hypotension, or orthostatic hypotension.

Adverse events associated with alpha-1 selective adrenergic agents include overstimulation that leads to high levels of blood pressure and profuse sweating. Contraindications of alpha-1 selective adrenergic agents include hypertension, tachycardia, vasospasm, and lactation.

These agents should not be stopped immediately, as sudden withdrawal could lead to reverse complications and sudden death. These agents should be tapered over a few days.

## Alpha-2 Selective Adrenergic Agents

The **alpha-2 selective adrenergic agents** stimulate the cardiovascular control centers of the central nervous system, activating alpha-2 receptors. Stimulation of alpha-2 receptors decreases blood pressure and heart rate. Therapeutically, alpha-2 selective adrenergic agents are used in the treatment of systemic hypertension.

Adverse events associated with alpha-2 selective adrenergic agents include central nervous system events such as depression, nightmares, sedation, drowsiness, fatigue, and headache as well as cardiovascular events such as hypotension, congestive heart failure, and bradycardia. Other adverse events include dry mouth, sexual dysfunction, and decreased urinary output. Contraindications of alpha-2 selective adrenergic agents include severe coronary artery disease, vascular disease, and chronic renal failure. Sudden discontinuation of these agents could lead to withdrawal reactions, so practicing clinicians should titrate down dosages upon discontinuation.



## Beta-Adrenergic Antagonists

**Beta-receptor antagonists** block beta-adrenergic receptor signaling. Beta-1 adrenergic receptors stimulate myocardial contraction and increase heart rate. Beta-2 receptors are found in vascular smooth muscle of lungs, blood vessels, and uterus and stimulate dilation and relaxation. Drugs within this class of agents have different affinities for these receptors, with most agents targeting both beta-1 and beta-2 receptors equally.

Beta-adrenergic antagonists decrease heart rate and blood pressure. Therapeutic uses include treatment of hypertension, ventricular dysrhythmia, chronic angina, prevention of reinfarction after myocardial infarction, congestive heart failure, supraventricular tachycardia, dysrhythmias, idiopathic hypertrophic subaortic stenosis, and pheochromocytoma.

### *Adverse Events and Contraindications*

**Adverse events** associated with **beta-adrenergic antagonists** include cardiovascular events such as bradycardia, heart block, congestive heart failure, hypotension, and peripheral vascular insufficiency; pulmonary events such as shortness of breath, coughing, and bronchospasm; and central nervous system events such as fatigue, dizziness, depression, paresthesia, sleep disturbances, memory loss, and disorientation. Other adverse events include nausea, vomiting, diarrhea, colitis, decreased libido, sexual dysfunction, vomiting, slowed recovery from hypoglycemia, and decreased exercise function.

**Contraindications** include cardiovascular conditions such as bradycardia or heart block and pulmonary conditions such as bronchospasm, chronic obstructive pulmonary disease, or acute asthma. These agents should be used with caution in patients with heart failure and/or diabetes. Sudden discontinuation of these agents could lead to withdrawal reactions, so practicing clinicians should titrate down dosages over a 2-week period.

## Ionotropic Group of Drugs

The classes of agents included in the **ionotropic group** of drugs include cardiac glycosides such as digitalis, digitoxin, and digoxin; phosphodiesterase inhibitors such as amrinone and milrinone; and sympathomimetics such as dopamine, dobutamine, isoproterenol, metaraminol, epinephrine, and norepinephrine.

## Cardiac Glycosides

**Cardiac glycosides** target the sodium/potassium pump, which maintains resting membrane potential of nerve and muscle cells of the heart. Cardiac glycosides allow for influx of calcium into myocardial cells during depolarization, which increases contraction of cardiac muscle, increases cardiac output, increases renal profusion, decreases heart rate, and decreases conduction velocity through the atrioventricular node. Therapeutically, cardiac glycosides are used to treat congestive heart failure, atrial flutter, atrial fibrillation, and paroxysmal atrial tachycardia.

Adverse events associated with cardiac glycosides include cardiovascular events such as premature ventricular contractions, dysrhythmia, and bradycardia; gastrointestinal events such as anorexia, nausea, and vomiting; and central nervous system events such as changes to visual field, headaches, fatigue, confusion, and depression.

### *Toxicity, Drug Interactions, and Contraindications*

Factors that can influence **toxicity** in patients undergoing treatment with cardiac glycosides include electrolyte imbalances such as decreased potassium levels as well as renal and hepatic insufficiency. Specifically, digitalis-related toxicities require treatment that includes decontamination, monitoring of plasma potassium levels, administration of anti-dysrhythmic agents, and digitalis antibodies.

Some **drugs** may decrease or increase the action of cardiac glycosides. Some specific examples include drugs that decrease the effect of digoxin, such as antacids, cholestyramine, neomycin, and sulfasalazine, and drugs that increase the effect of digoxin, such as albuterol, amiodarone, captopril, cyclosporine, diltiazem, erythromycin, nifedipine, omeprazole, tetracycline, and thyroxine.

**Contraindications** include ventricular tachycardia, ventricular fibrillation, atrioventricular block, idiopathic hypertrophic subaortic stenosis, myocardial infarction, and Wolff-Parkinson-White syndrome. Caution needs to be taken when administering cardiac glycosides, as their effective therapeutic dose is very close to their toxic dose.

## Phosphodiesterase Inhibitors

**Phosphodiesterase inhibitors** increase calcium levels within myocardial cells. These agents increase cardiac muscle contractions and cardiac output. However, these inhibitors have little impact on heart rate and blood pressure.

Phosphodiesterase inhibitors are typically prescribed over short periods due to a high degree of toxicity associated with these agents. They are used to treat decompensated congestive heart failure in patients who fail first-line treatment approaches. Adverse events associated with phosphodiesterase inhibitors include cardiovascular events such as dysrhythmia and gastrointestinal events such as nausea, vomiting, and liver enzyme changes. Other adverse events include thrombocytopenia and bone marrow toxicity. Contraindications include aortic or pulmonary valvular disease, myocardial infarction, and ventricular dysrhythmia.

## Anti-Dysrhythmic Group of Drugs

The **anti-dysrhythmic group** of drugs includes six classes of agents and two additional agents. The six classes of agents include classes IA, IB, IC, II, III, and IV.

- Examples of **class IA** agents include quinidine, procainamide, moricizine, and disopyramide.
- Examples of **class IB** agents include lidocaine, tocainide, mexiletine, and phenytoin.
- Examples of **class IC** agents include flecainide and propafenone.
- Examples of **class II** agents include propranolol, acebutolol, and esmolol.
- Examples of **class III** agents include bretylium, amiodarone, ibutilide, dofetilide, and sotalol.
- Examples of **class IV** agents include verapamil and diltiazem.

Other agents not categorized include digoxin and adenosine.

### *Mechanism of Action, Pharmacologic Effects, and Therapeutic Uses*

The mechanism of action, pharmacologic effects, and therapeutic uses for anti-dysrhythmic agents are discussed below:

- **Class I** anti-dysrhythmic **agents** inhibit sodium channels.
- **Class II drugs** include beta-adrenergic receptor antagonists, which slow heart rate and increase cardiac muscle contraction.
- **Class III drugs** inhibit potassium efflux during repolarization.
- **Class IV agents** include calcium channel blockers.
- **Unclassified agents** such as digoxin decrease conduction velocity, and adenosine activates adenosine receptors that play a role in potassium conductance.

**Therapeutic uses** of anti-dysrhythmic agents include atrial dysrhythmia, ventricular tachycardia, life-threatening ventricular dysrhythmias, ventricular dysrhythmias, sinus tachycardia, atrioventricular reentry, Wolff-Parkinson White syndrome, premature ventricular contractions, atrial fibrillation, atrial flutter, and atrial tachycardia.

### *Adverse Events and Contraindications*

**Adverse events associated with anti-dysrhythmic agents** include cardiovascular events such as new dysrhythmia, heart block, hypotension, vasodilation, and cardiac arrest. Noncardiac events include nausea, vomiting, hypersensitivity, hemolytic anemia, tinnitus, headache, blurred vision, arthralgia, arthritis, dizziness, euphoria, perioral numbness, agitation, disorientation, tremor, lightheadedness, slurred speech, seizures, bone marrow suppression, bronchospasm, photosensitivity, pulmonary fibrosis, liver enzyme dysfunction, thyroid dysfunction, constipation, lassitude, nervousness, peripheral edema, shortness of breath, flushing, and paresthesia. Specific agents within each class are more prone to certain adverse events than others, but all have potential for the above adverse events.

**Contraindications** include allergy, bradycardia, sick sinus syndrome, atrioventricular block, shock, hypotension, and respiratory depression. Caution should be used when administering these agents in patients with congestive heart failure.

## Nitrates/Nitrites

**Nitrates and/or nitrites** act directly on vascular smooth muscle and increase vasodilation. This class of agents increases blood flow and increases oxygen supply to myocardial cells. This class of agents has been shown to be ineffective in patients with coronary artery disease. Nitrates and/or nitrites are used to treat acute and chronic angina.

Adverse events associated with nitrates and/or nitrites include cardiovascular events such as hypotension, rebound tachycardia, bradycardia, flushing, and sweating and central nervous system events such as headache and dizziness. Other adverse events include nausea, vomiting, incontinence, and contact dermatitis. Contraindications include head trauma, cerebral hemorrhage, pregnancy, and lactation. Sublingual administration of nitrates/nitrites is the most preferred method of administration due to low bioavailability of these agents. Patients may develop resistance to these agents over time and may require higher doses to get the same effect.

### Vasodilator Group of Drugs

Classes of agents included in the **vasodilator group** include beta-blockers such as acebutolol, atenolol, betaxolol, bisoprolol, carteolol, carvedilol, esmolol, labetalol, metoprolol, nadolol, penbutolol, pindolol, propranolol, sotalol, and timolol; nitrates/nitrites, also known as anti-anginal vasodilators, such as amyl nitrate, isosorbide dinitrate, isosorbide mononitrate, and nitroglycerin; anti-hypertensive vasodilators such as diazoxide, minoxidil, fenoldopam, nitroprusside, hydralazine, and tolazoline; and calcium channel blockers such as amlodipine, bepridil, diltiazem, felodipine, isradipine, nicardipine, nifedipine, nimodipine, nisoldipine, and verapamil.

Beta-adrenergic inhibitors can also be classified as adrenergic agents. Beta-adrenergic inhibitors and calcium channel blockers indirectly act as vasodilators, whereas anti-anginal vasodilators and anti-hypertensive vasodilators directly act on vasodilator mechanisms.

### Calcium Channel Blockers

**Calcium channel blockers** act by antagonizing L-type calcium channels in vascular smooth muscle, which leads to reduced cardiac muscle contractility, decreased SA pacemaker rate, and decreased atrioventricular conduction velocity in cardiac tissue.

Therapeutic uses include angina, hypertension, congestive heart failure, bradycardia associated with angina, Raynaud's phenomenon, atrial tachycardia, atrial flutter, and subarachnoid hemorrhage. Adverse events associated with calcium channel blockers include headache, dysrhythmias, edema, bleeding gums, agranulocytosis, dizziness, nausea, fatigue, severe gastrointestinal upset, constipation, tachycardia, flushing, diarrhea, hypotension, and myocardial depression.

Patients on concomitant calcium channel blocker and beta-blocker and/or nitrate should have their blood pressure monitored by a practicing clinician due to increased risk of hypotensive episodes. Degree of vasodilation should be monitored due to increased risk of edema.

### Anti-Hypertensive Vasodilators

**Anti-hypertensive vasodilators** act directly on vascular smooth muscle and increase vasodilation. These agents decrease arteriolar resistance and decrease arterial blood pressure. Therapeutic uses include treatment of hypertension, hypertensive crisis, and pulmonary hypertension in newborns.

Adverse events associated with anti-hypertensive vasodilators include cardiovascular events such as sweating, flushing, edema, dizziness, hypotension, and reflex tachycardia and central nervous system events such as headache. Other adverse events include systemic lupus-like syndrome and hypertrichosis. Contraindications include pregnancy and lactation. Caution should be used when administering these agents in patients with peripheral vascular disease, coronary artery disease, congestive heart failure, and/or tachycardia. Practicing clinicians should take caution when administering nitroprusside in patients with renal failure.

## Anticoagulant, Anti-Thrombotic, and Thrombolytic Group of Drugs

The **classes of agents** within this group include anticoagulants, anti-thrombotic or anti-platelet agents, and thrombolytic or fibrinolytic agents. Anti-coagulants include anti-thrombin III; heparin; lepirudin; warfarin; danaparoid; and low molecular weight heparins such as ardeparin, dalteparin, enoxaparin and tinzaparin; argatroban; and bivalirudin. Anti-thrombotic or anti-platelet agents include aspirin, ibuprofen, sulfinpyrazone, clopidogrel, dipyridamole, eptifibatide, ticlopidine, and tirofiban. Thrombolytic or fibrinolytic agents include alteplase, streptokinase, anistreplase, urokinase, reteplase, and TNK t-PA.

This group of agents, which includes anticoagulants, anti-thrombotic or anti-platelet agents, and thrombolytic or fibrinolytic agents, prevents inhibition of platelet aggregation and clot formation.

### Anticoagulants

**Anticoagulants** prevent clot formation, but each of the agents included in this class have various mechanisms of action. These agents prevent clot formation by depleting clotting factors, inhibiting their activity, and/or prolonging clotting times.

Antithrombin III prevents clotting, while heparin is a protein that inhibits the conversion of prothrombin to thrombin, which prevents fibrinogen from being converted to fibrin. Lepirudin directly inhibits thrombin formation, while low molecular weight heparins block factors Xa and IIa, which inhibit thrombus and clot formation. Warfarin prevents clot formation by interfering with formation of vitamin K-dependent clotting factors in the liver.

#### *Administration Implications*

Practicing clinicians should not use warfarin during acute situations, as the onset of action is about 3 days and lasts for about 5 days. Heparin or low molecular weight heparins should be used during acute situations, but warfarin can be used over the long term due to the drug's long-lasting effects. Warfarin should be administered with caution, as the drug is contraindicated with a variety of drugs to treat a number of different conditions. Practicing clinicians should keep antidotes on hand in case of overdose, including protamine sulfate for heparin overdose and vitamin K for warfarin overdose.

#### *Therapeutic Uses, Adverse Events, and Contraindications*

**Therapeutic uses of anticoagulants** include prevention of deep venous thrombosis, pulmonary embolism, and clotting in blood samples; diagnosis and treatment of disseminated intravascular coagulation; treatment for hereditary antithrombin III deficiency with potential for thromboembolism, acute deep venous thrombosis, acute pulmonary embolism, atrial fibrillation with embolism, myocardial infarction, stroke, heparin-induced thrombocytopenia, artificial heart valves, and valvular damage; as well as use in dialysis and venous tubing.

**Adverse effects** associated with anticoagulants include bleeding complications, hemorrhage, nausea, gastrointestinal upset, thrombocytopenia, and hepatic dysfunction. **Contraindications** include hemorrhagic disorders, recent trauma, spinal puncture, gastrointestinal ulcers, recent surgery, intrauterine device placement, tuberculosis, indwelling catheters, and threatened abortion. More specifically, warfarin is contraindicated during pregnancy. Caution should be taken if anticoagulants are prescribed in patients with congestive heart failure, thyrotoxicosis, diarrhea, and fever.

### *HITTS*

**Heparin-induced thrombocytopenia and thrombosis syndrome** (HITTS) occurs in patients receiving heparin for anticoagulation. There are two types:

- **Type I** is a transient condition occurring within a few days and causing depletion of platelets (<100,000 $mm^3$), but heparin may be continued as the condition usually resolves without intervention.
- **Type II** is an autoimmune reaction to heparin that occurs in 3–5% of those receiving unfractionated heparin and also occurs with low-molecular-weight heparin. It is characterized by low platelets (<50,000 $mm^3$) that are ≥50% below baseline. Onset is 5–14 days but can occur within hours of heparinization. Death rates are <30%. Heparin-antibody complexes form and release platelet factor 4 (PF4), which attracts heparin molecules and adheres to platelets and endothelial lining, stimulating thrombin and platelet clumping. This puts the patient at risk for thrombosis and vessel occlusion rather than hemorrhage, causing stroke, myocardial infarction, and limb ischemia with symptoms associated with the site of thrombosis. Treatment includes:
    - Discontinuation of heparin
    - Direct thrombin inhibitors (lepirudin, argatroban)
    - Monitor for signs/symptoms of thrombus/embolus

## Antithrombotic or Anti-Platelet Agents

**Antithrombotic or antiplatelet agents** inhibit platelet aggregation. Specifically, tirofiban and eptifibatide are glycoprotein IIb/IIIa inhibitors that block platelet aggregation. Aspirin, ibuprofen, and sulfinpyrazone are cyclooxygenase inhibitors that inhibit the formation of thromboxanes, thereby blocking platelet aggregation. Clopidogrel and ticlopidine interfere with the ADP receptor blockade and prevent ADP from binding to platelets, thus inhibiting platelet aggregation. Dipyridamole is a phosphodiesterase inhibitor that increases cAMP, activating prostacyclin and inhibiting platelet aggregation.

Adverse events associated with antithrombotic or antiplatelet agents include bleeding, hemorrhage, gastrointestinal ulcerations, angina, dizziness, headache, syncope, rash, thrombocytopenia, neutropenia, nausea, and diarrhea.

### *Therapeutic Uses and Contraindications*

**Therapeutic uses of antithrombotic or antiplatelet agents** include percutaneous coronary intervention, risk reduction of recurrent TIAs in men, risk reduction of myocardial infarction or death in patients with history of cardiovascular disease, prevention of thromboembolism, reduction of embolization in rheumatic valve disease, and prevention of cardiac ischemic complications, as well as treatment for ischemia, atrial fibrillation, peripheral arterial disease, stroke, and acute coronary syndrome.

Caution should be taken when prescribing antithrombotic or antiplatelet agents in patients who have undergone recent surgery or who are at risk of excessive blood loss or closed head injuries. Patients undergoing treatment with antithrombotic or antiplatelet agents should avoid cutting themselves and contact sports.

## Thrombolytic or Fibrinolytic Agents

**Thrombolytic or fibrinolytic agents** open blood vessels and restore blood flow to dependent organ systems. These agents induce the production of plasmin through the digestion of fibrin, thereby degrading fibrin clots within blood vessels.

Specifically, streptokinase, urokinase, and anistreplase inhibit the formation of fibrin by disrupting the conversion of plasminogen to plasmin. Alteplase, tenecteplase, and reteplase activate the conversion of fibrin-bound plasminogen to plasmin.

Therapeutic uses of thrombolytic and fibrinolytic agents include lysis of thrombi in coronary arteries after myocardial infarction as well as treatment for stroke, pulmonary embolism, deep venous thrombosis, occluded cannulas in dialysis patients, and peripheral artery thrombosis.

#### *Adverse Events and Contraindications*

**Adverse effects associated with thrombolytic or fibrinolytic agents** include bleeding, bruising, anaphylaxis, and hematoma. **Contraindications** associated with use of thrombolytic or fibrinolytic agents include any condition that could be compromised by dissolution of clots such as recurrent surgery, hemorrhage, recent cerebrovascular accident, aneurysm, obstetric delivery, organ biopsy, serious gastrointestinal bleeding, major trauma, or hypertension.

#### *Aminocaproic Acid*

**Aminocaproic acid** inhibits fibrin formation and is typically administered to antagonize the action of thrombotic or fibrinolytic agents.

Patients should be monitored for blood loss. Also, practicing clinicians should initiate treatment with thrombolytic or fibrinolytic within three hours of experiencing an acute myocardial infarction to prevent further cardiovascular complications if percutaneous coronary intervention is not available.

### Agents That Influence the Renin-Angiotensin System

The **classes of drugs that influence the renin-angiotensin system** include angiotensin-converting enzyme inhibitors and angiotensin II antagonists. Angiotensin-converting enzyme inhibitors, also known as ACE inhibitors, include benazepril, moexipril, captopril, perindopril, enalapril, quinapril, fosinopril, ramipril, lisinopril, and trandolapril. Angiotensin II antagonists include candesartan, losartan, eprosartan, telmisartan, irbesartan, and valsartan.

Both angiotensin-converting enzyme inhibitors and angiotensin II antagonists induce vasodilation. However, angiotensin II antagonists are more specific in their mechanism of action than angiotensin-converting enzyme inhibitors. These drugs are mainly used for the treatment of hypertension but have other cardiovascular effects.

### Angiotensin II Antagonists

**Angiotensin II antagonists** are more specific in action than angiotensin-converting enzyme inhibitors. Angiotensin II antagonists block angiotensin II receptors by inhibiting a subtype of the angiotensin II receptor known as $AT_1$. Angiotensin II antagonists do not interfere with bradykinin metabolism. The pharmacologic effect of angiotensin II antagonists is decreased blood pressure caused by a decrease in both peripheral resistance and blood volume. Inhibition of the $AT_1$ receptors leads to inhibition of the pressor and aldosterone-releasing effects of angiotensin II, which causes the decrease in blood pressure.

Angiotensin II antagonists are mainly used to treat hypertension but also have effects on other cardiovascular conditions.

#### *Adverse Events and Contraindications*

**Adverse events associated with angiotensin II antagonists** include gastrointestinal upset, dry mouth, tooth pain, headache, dizziness, minor cough, dry skin, and alopecia. Since angiotensin II antagonists do not impact bradykinin metabolism, angiotensin II antagonists present with limited cough and fewer side effects when compared to angiotensin-converting enzyme inhibitors. Angiotensin II antagonists provide a more specific approach to the treatment of hypertension compared to angiotensin-converting enzyme inhibitors.

**Contraindications** associated with angiotensin II antagonists include pregnant women during their second and third trimesters due to risk of fetal malformations and death. Hypotension, potassium levels, and renal function should be monitored in patients undergoing treatment with angiotensin II antagonists.

## Angiotensin-Converting Enzyme Inhibitors

**Angiotensin-converting enzyme inhibitors** inhibit the converting enzyme that hydrolyzes angiotensin I to angiotensin II, which increases bradykinin, a potent vasodilator. By inhibiting the renin-angiotensin system, angiotensin-converting enzyme inhibitors prevent vasoconstriction by blocking angiotensin II formation, decreasing sodium and water reabsorption in the kidneys, and indirectly inducing bradykinin.

The pharmacologic effect of angiotensin-converting enzyme inhibitors is to decrease blood pressure through vasodilation and inhibiting salt reuptake through aldosterone. Therapeutic uses of angiotensin-converting enzyme inhibitors include treatment of hypertension, diabetic nephropathy, and congestive heart failure after myocardial infarction, as well as preservation of left ventricular function after myocardial infarction.

### *Adverse Events and Contraindications*

**Adverse events associated with angiotensin-converting enzyme inhibitors** include hypotension, glomerular damage, acute renal failure, hyperkalemia, dry cough, wheezing, angioedema, agranulocytosis, gastrointestinal upset, skin rash, and/or other hypersensitivities.

**Contraindications** of angiotensin-converting enzyme inhibitors include women during their second and third trimester of pregnancy due to risk of fetal hypotension, anuria, renal failure, fetal malformations, and/or death.

Patients with renal insufficiency should not be prescribed angiotensin-converting enzyme inhibitors due to elimination through the kidneys. However, fosinopril and moexipril are not eliminated through the kidneys and therefore can be administered in this patient population. Hypotension, potassium levels, and renal function should be monitored in patients undergoing treatment with angiotensin-converting enzyme inhibitors.

## Diuretic Group of Pharmacologic Drugs

The **classes of agents included in the diuretic group of pharmacologic agents** include thiazide diuretics such as bendroflumethiazide, benzthiazide, chlorothiazide, chlorthalidone, hydrochlorothiazide, hydroflumethiazide, indapamide, methyclothiazide, metolazone, polythiazide, quinethazone, and trichlormethiazide; loop diuretics such as bumetanide, ethacrynic acid, furosemide, and torsemide; potassium-sparing diuretics such as amiloride, spironolactone, and triamterene; and osmotic diuretics such as glycerin and mannitol.

Diuretics prevent reabsorption of sodium in the kidneys, with each class of diuretic working on a slightly different site within the nephron of the kidney. Each of these classes of diuretics has a slightly different mechanism of action.

### *Thiazide Diuretics*

**Thiazide diuretics** prevent the reabsorption of sodium within the nephron of the kidneys, which allows for sodium and other ions to be excreted in the urine and not reabsorbed in the blood stream. Specifically, thiazide diuretics inhibit sodium and chloride reabsorption in the nephron, resulting in excretion of potassium, chloride, and sodium in the urine. The excretion of sodium in the urine decreases the glomerular filtration rate and has been associated with moderate potassium loss, which needs to be monitored. Thiazide diuretic net effect is to decrease blood pressure, cardiac stroke volume, and cardiac output.

#### Therapeutic Uses, Adverse Events, and Contraindications

**Therapeutic uses** for thiazide diuretics include treatment of congestive heart failure, hypertension, and edema. The most common **adverse effects** associated with thiazide diuretics include electrolyte imbalance, fluid imbalance, hypotension, oliguria, anuria, dizziness, hypokalemia, hyponatremia, hypocalcemia, hyperglycemia, hyperuricemia, and gastrointestinal upset.

**Contraindications** of thiazide diuretics include patients with renal disease, hypokalemia, dysrhythmia, glucose intolerance, and gout. Thiazide diuretics should not be used prior to bedtime due to increased urine output. Caution should be used when using diuretics in combination with other antihypertensive agents. Practicing clinicians need to monitor electrolyte and renal function to prevent complications. Additionally, patients should monitor potassium intake due to potential for electrolyte imbalance and should supplement accordingly.

### *Loop Diuretics*

**Loop diuretics** prevent the reabsorption of sodium and chloride within the nephron of the kidneys, which allows for sodium, chloride, and potassium to be excreted in the urine and not reabsorbed in the blood stream. Loop diuretics are more powerful than thiazide diuretics and are associated with increased potassium loss. The loop diuretic net effect is to decrease blood pressure, cardiac stroke volume, and cardiac output.

Therapeutic uses of loop diuretics include treatment of congestive heart failure, pulmonary edema, hypertension, and edema associated with congestive heart failure, renal disease, or liver disease.

#### Adverse Events and Contraindications

The most common **adverse effects** associated with loop diuretics include electrolyte imbalance, fluid imbalance, hypotension, oliguria, anuria, dizziness, hypokalemia, hyponatremia, hypocalcemia, hyperglycemia, hyperuricemia, ototoxicity resulting in hearing loss, and gastrointestinal upset.

**Contraindications** of loop diuretics include patients with renal disease, hypokalemia, dysrhythmia, glucose intolerance, and gout. Loop diuretics should not be used prior to bedtime due to increased urine output. Caution should be used when using diuretics in combination with other antihypertensive agents. Practicing clinicians need to monitor electrolyte and renal function to prevent complications. Additionally, patients should monitor potassium intake due to potential for electrolyte imbalance and should supplement accordingly.

### *Potassium-Sparing Diuretics*

**Potassium-sparing diuretics** increase sodium excretion and decrease potassium secretion in the nephron of the kidneys, allowing for sodium and other ions to be excreted in the urine and not reabsorbed in the blood stream. However, potassium-sparing diuretics are associated with decreased potassium excretion compared to thiazide and loop diuretics, making potassium-sparing diuretics an attractive option. The potassium-sparing diuretics' net effect is to decrease blood pressure, cardiac stroke volume, and cardiac output.

Therapeutic uses of potassium-sparing diuretics include treating hypertension and edema from congestive heart failure, renal disease, or liver disease. In patients undergoing treatment with thiazide or loop diuretics who develop hypokalemia, potassium-sparing diuretics are another option.

#### ADVERSE EVENTS AND CONTRAINDICATIONS

The most common **adverse effects** associated with potassium-sparing diuretics include electrolyte imbalance, fluid imbalance, hypotension, oliguria, anuria, dizziness, hyperkalemia, some hyponatremia, glucose intolerance in diabetic patients, gynecomastia, and gastrointestinal upset.

Potassium-sparing diuretics should not be used prior to bedtime due to increased urine output. Caution should be exercised when using diuretics in combination with other antihypertensive agents. Practicing clinicians need to monitor electrolyte and renal function to prevent complications. Additionally, patients should monitor potassium intake due to potential for electrolyte imbalance and supplement accordingly, even though potassium levels are not impacted to the same degree as with thiazide or loop diuretics.

### *OSMOTIC DIURETICS*

**Osmotic diuretics** prevent the reabsorption of water within the permeable regions of the nephron because these nonabsorbable agents create an osmotic gradient favoring increased urine volume. The osmotic diuretic net effect is to decrease blood pressure, cardiac stroke volume, and cardiac output.

Therapeutic uses of osmotic diuretics include treatment of intracranial pressure and brain edema. The most common adverse effects associated with osmotic diuretics include electrolyte imbalance, fluid imbalance, hypotension, oliguria, anuria, and dizziness.

Osmotic diuretics should not be used prior to bedtime due to increased urine output. Caution should be exercised when using diuretics in combination with other antihypertensive agents. Practicing clinicians need to monitor electrolyte and renal function to prevent complications. Additionally, patients should monitor potassium intake due to potential for electrolyte imbalance and should supplement accordingly.

## ANTIHYPERLIPIDEMIC GROUP OF PHARMACOLOGIC DRUGS

The **classes of agents included in the antihyperlipidemic group of pharmacologic drugs** include resins, niacin, statins (also known as HMG-coenzyme A reductase inhibitors), and fibric acid derivatives. Drugs within the resin class of agents include cholestyramine, colestipol, and colesevelam. Drugs within the statins, or HMG-coenzyme A reductase inhibitors, include atorvastatin, pravastatin, fluvastatin, simvastatin, and lovastatin. Drugs within the fibric acid derivatives include clofibrate, fenofibrate, and gemfibrozil.

Antihyperlipidemic classes of agents directly or indirectly affect lipid and cholesterol levels by lowering low-density lipid levels, increasing high-density lipid levels, and decreasing triglyceride levels.

## RESINS

The pharmacologic effects of **resins** include decrease in low-density lipid levels, increase in high-density lipid levels, and decrease in triglyceride levels. The mechanism of action of these agents is to act as bile acid sequestrants, which increase liver low-density lipoprotein receptors, removing low-density lipids from circulation and oxidizing the cholesterol from low-density lipids to form bile acids.

Therapeutic uses for resins include treatment of hypercholesterolemia and hyperlipidemia. Resins are recommended only when a patient fails first-line therapy with diet modifications and exercise and their low-density lipid levels are above 160 mg/dL or above 130 mg/dL with more than two cardiovascular risk factors such as obesity, smoking, or high-density lipid levels below 40 mg/dL. The goal of treatment when prescribing resins in patients with coronary heart disease or at high risk for coronary heart disease is low-density lipid levels below 100 mg/dL. Resins may also be used in children between the ages of 11 and 20.

#### *Adverse Effects and Contraindications*

**Adverse effects** associated with resins include gastrointestinal upset, bloating, constipation, and malabsorption of vitamins A, D, and K. **Contraindications** associated with resins include hypertriglyceridemia, biliary obstruction, abnormal intestinal function, pregnancy, and lactation.

Practicing clinicians should inform patients that these agents should not be taken in dry powder form but should be mixed with fluids to be efficacious. Additionally, if resins in tablet form are prescribed, the tablets should not be cut, chewed, or crushed, as this will render them ineffective. Resins are designed to be broken down in the gastrointestinal tract and, if broken down sooner, the drugs will become ineffective.



### Niacin

The pharmacologic effects of **niacin** include a decrease in low-density lipid levels, increase in high-density lipid levels, and decrease in triglyceride levels. The mechanism of action of niacin is inhibition of lipolysis of triglycerides in fatty tissue, which decreases synthesis of triglycerides in the liver. In turn, decreased triglyceride synthesis decreases low-density lipid synthesis, decreasing low-density lipid levels. Niacin is the most effective agent for increasing high-density lipid levels, but it also has effects on lowering low-density lipid levels and triglyceride levels.

Therapeutic uses include hypertriglyceridemia, hypercholesterolemia, and hyperlipidemia. Niacin is recommended only when a patient fails first-line therapy with diet modifications and exercise and their low-density lipid levels are above 160 mg/dL or above 130 mg/dL with more than two cardiovascular risk factors such as obesity, smoking, or high-density lipid levels below 40 mg/dL. The goal of treatment when prescribing niacin in patients with coronary heart disease or at high risk for coronary heart disease is low-density lipid levels below 100 mg/dL.

#### *Adverse Events and Contraindications*

**Adverse events** associated with niacin include flushing, pruritus, abnormal glucose tolerance, and hyperuricemia. The most common adverse events associated with niacin include flushing and dyspepsia. These common adverse events decrease patient compliance and effectiveness of niacin treatment. However, flushing tends to decrease with treatment duration. Patients may also take aspirin 30 minutes prior to taking niacin to reduce flushing. They may also reduce hot beverage or alcohol intake to reduce extent and degree of flushing.

**Contraindications** associated with niacin treatment include pregnancy and gout. Patients should not take oral nicotinamide as treatment for hypertriglyceridemia, hypercholesterolemia, and hyperlipidemia because this source of niacin does not have any impact on lipid levels. The effective dose for antihypertensive treatment ranges between 1 and 2 grams per day or more.

### HMG Coenzyme A Reductase Inhibitors or Statins

**Statins** compete for inhibition of HMG coenzyme A reductase, which impacts cholesterol biosynthesis. Statins are well tolerated and effective agents for the treatment of hyperlipidemia and hypercholesterolemia. The pharmacologic effects of statins include decrease in low-density lipid levels, increase in high-density lipid levels, and decrease in triglyceride levels. Higher doses of more potent statins such as atorvastatin and simvastatin are more effective in reducing triglyceride levels.

Therapeutic uses of statins include hypertriglyceridemia, hypercholesterolemia, and hyperlipidemia. Statins are recommended only when a patient fails first-line therapy with diet modifications and exercise and their low-density lipid levels are above 160 mg/dL or above 130 mg/dL with more than two cardiovascular risk factors such as obesity, smoking, or high-density lipid levels below 40 mg/dL. The goal of treatment when prescribing statins in patients with coronary heart disease or at high risk for coronary heart disease is low-density lipid levels below 100 mg/dL.

#### *Adverse Effects and Contraindications*

**Adverse events** associated with **HMG coenzyme A reductase inhibitors or statins** include liver dysfunction, increase liver transaminases, myopathy, rhabdomyolysis associated with myalgia and fatigue, hypersensitivity, and renal failure. Due to risk of liver dysfunction and liver transaminases, practicing clinicians should monitor patients' alanine aminotransferase (ALT) levels. Measurements should be taken upon initiation of treatment and should be repeated every three months. Practicing clinicians should also monitor patients for cataract development, especially in elderly patients.

Additionally, due to increased risk for myopathy and rhabdomyolysis, practicing clinicians should instruct patients to tell them if they experience any muscle or joint pain, as that may be an early indication for rhabdomyolysis, which is a serious complication.

**Contraindications** associated with statins include liver disease and pregnancy. Statins should be administered prior to bedtime since the highest rates of cholesterol synthesis occur between the hours of midnight and 5:00 a.m.

### Fibric Acid Derivatives

The pharmacologic effects of **fibric acid derivatives** include decrease in low-density lipid levels, increase in high-density lipid, and decrease in triglyceride levels. However, the exact mechanism of action of fibric acid derivatives is unknown.

Therapeutic uses of fibric acid derivatives include treatment of hypertriglyceridemia primarily with minimal effect on hypercholesterolemia and hyperlipidemia. Fibric acid derivatives are recommended only when a patient fails first-line therapy with diet modifications and exercise and their triglyceride levels remain very elevated.

#### *Adverse Events and Contraindications*

**Adverse events** associated with fibric acid derivatives include gastrointestinal upset, rash, alopecia, fatigue, headache, impotence, anemia, and myositis flu-like syndrome.

**Contraindications** associated with fibric acid derivatives include renal failure and liver failure. Caution needs to be taken when prescribing fibric acid derivatives with other agents, as fibric acid derivatives also have anti-platelet effects. Gemfibrozil should not be administered with statins due to increased risk of rhabdomyolysis. However, if gemfibrozil is administered with a statin, practicing clinicians need to monitor patients very closely for the any indication of rhabdomyolysis. Therefore, due to increased risk for myopathy and rhabdomyolysis, practicing clinicians should instruct patients to tell them if they experience any muscle or joint pain, as that may be an early indication for rhabdomyolysis.

## ROLE OF HORMONE REPLACEMENT THERAPY

### *CORONARY HEART DISEASE*

The use of **hormone replacement therapy** to prevent acute myocardial infarction or recurrent myocardial infarction remains controversial. Initial observational studies have demonstrated the benefit of hormone replacement therapy in the prevention of acute myocardial infarction or recurrent myocardial infarction. However, the Women's Health Initiative (WHI) showed that although estrogen replacement has a beneficial effect on lipids, it may increase the risk of cardiovascular complications and, additionally, breast cancer.

Estrogen antagonists and selective estrogen receptor modulators may have similar impact, not reducing coronary heart disease as compared to estrogen or estrogen-progesterone combination. Currently, no evidence exists that demonstrates that estrogen antagonists and/or selective estrogen receptor modulators have any effect on coronary artery disease.

### *HYPERTENSION*

Recent data has demonstrated that the use of antihypertensive agents reduces cardiovascular complications such as risk for stroke, myocardial infarction, and congestive heart failure. In women undergoing treatment with hormone replacement therapy, these agents have been shown to have no effect on blood pressure or risk of stroke, but estrogen may improve compliance of large blood vessels. However, hormone replacement therapy with estrogen is contraindicated in postmenopausal women with a history of cardiovascular complications such as thromboembolic disorders.

Therefore, use of hormone replacement therapy for the treatment of hypertension and other cardiovascular complications remains controversial.



## ADVERSE REACTION OF HYPOTENSION

**Hypotension** (BP below 90/60, or 30 mmHg below baseline) may result in inadequate oxygenation of body tissues. The patient should be assessed for symptoms, such as signs of bleeding, palpitations, chest pain, dizziness, abdominal pain, and/or dyspnea. The patient's skin should be assessed for indications of shock or severe hypotension: color (pallor), temperature (cool, clammy), and moisture (sweating). If a paradoxical pulse is present, this may indicate pericardial tamponade. The patient may have abnormal heart sounds (gallops, murmurs, bradycardia, tachycardia, dysrhythmias) and abnormal lung sounds (crackles, wheezing). Patients who are on cardiac monitoring may exhibit a flattened waveform. While commonly associated with shock, hypotension may also be drug-induced or associated with severe infections, allergic reaction (anaphylaxis), and hypovolemia (dehydration, bleeding), so the cause must be determined in order to choose the most appropriate intervention, which may include transfusions for bleeding and LVAD for heart failure. However, immediate intervention to increase BP typically includes IV fluids and inotropic and/or vasopressor agents as well as oxygen.

> **Review Video: Different Types of Lung Sounds**
> Visit mometrix.com/academy and enter code: 765616

# Non-Pharmacologic and Complementary Therapies

## Alternative Therapies

**Alternative therapies** are sought by approximately 36% of all cardiovascular patients. Those seeking out complementary therapies are generally younger patients, those of female gender or Asian descent, and those with higher education and income than the general population.

These individuals most often utilize herbal remedies such as echinacea, garlic, ginseng, ginkgo biloba, and glucosamine to treat conditions unrelated to their cardiovascular disease.

Herbs are closely followed by physical interventions such as meditation, relaxation, and deep breathing to improve mind-body connections and promote cardiac wellness and recovery. Interventions such as meditation and tai chi may be safely and effectively recommended for stress reduction. At this time, not enough research supports positive cardiovascular health changes associated with acupuncture or chelation (removal of heavy metals).

Regardless of the type of therapy used, the majority of those seeking complementary or alternative treatments report that they found the treatments helpful.

## Stress Management Techniques

**Stress reduction and management** can help reduce an individual's cardiac risk. Stress reduction methods that might be employed by a patient can include:

- **Autogenics**: ritualistic deep relaxation that focuses on relieving tension within the muscles, regulating breathing, and training thoughts
- **Cognitive restructuring**: redirecting negative thoughts and emotions into more positive outlets
- **Imagery**: placing the mind into an imagined place of relaxation and safety
- **Relaxation**: progressive, conscious muscle relaxation, relieving tension and creating awareness of the body and its stress responses
- **Meditation**: deep relaxation technique that focuses on clearing the mind and settling the emotions
- **Exercise**: aerobic and repetitive exercises that can reduce stress and anxiety and relieve depressive or destructive moods

## EECP

**Enhanced external counterpulsation (EECP)** is a pain control method that may be effective for patients with recurring stable angina. Treatment involves sequential compression of the patient's entire leg length to promote blood flow and increase cardiac output. The patients who might receive the most benefit from this type of treatment are those who refuse invasive treatment measures, have not responded to medication and revascularization efforts, or are not candidates for such treatments. EECP should be used cautiously in the patient with preexisting decreased left ventricular ejection fraction or heart failure.

## Alternative and Supplemental Approaches to Hyperlipidemia

**Omega-3 supplements** from oily fish can help raise HDL and lower LDL cholesterol and are safe to use in conjunction with other medications.

**Stanols and sterols** in a recommended dosage of 2–3 grams a day interfere with the intestinal uptake of cholesterol and reduce LDL.

**Dietary intake** of foods such as almonds, walnuts, cranberry juice, pomegranate juice and black teas can also be helpful in reducing LDL while raising HDL.

## Care Coordination

### Case Manager

The American Nurses Credentialing Center defines a **nursing case manager** as someone who provides a dynamic, orderly, efficient, and cooperative approach to client care that improves healthcare continuity and provides the patient with quality care options. The case manager is responsible for coordinating efforts between multiple care professions to make sure the patient's needs are met in a timely, efficient, and cost-effective manner. They ensure that health education needs are met to allow for informed care decisions while acting as a patient advocate and facilitator of effective healthcare relationships between patient, family, and significant others as well as the healthcare team.



### Facilitating Collaboration and Coordination

Tools developed for this specific purpose in a healthcare setting include practice guidelines to help define each participant's role in care and clinical protocols or pathways to focus care and clarify procedures and strategies to be followed. The goal is to create a team where the members understand their own and each other's roles within the group, understand the goals of the team, share responsibility, reach collective decisions, and actively include the patient and their family in the care process. An effective collaboration effort includes all stages of care, from assessment of needs to action, communication, and evaluation of goals upon completion. A primary key is streamlined communication and respect for each individual's unique contributions. The nurse often plays a primary role as mediator and advocate for the patient, making sure they understand the purposes and joint goals of the group and its members.

### Subacute Care Facilities

The following are the four types of subacute care facilities that might be available for the patient who faces hospital discharge but is still too ill for home or nursing home care:

- **General**: Patients discharged to this level of care are stable and healing well but still require skilled care for such things as long-term intravenous treatments.
- **Chronic**: Chronic care facilities are for terminal and end-of-life patients who cannot be cared for in an at-home setting because of choice or complexity of care such as ventilator dependency.
- **Transitional**: At this level, patients still need complex medical and nursing care, such as deep wound management.
- **Long-term transitional**: At this level, patients require continued complex medical care that is expected to have an extended treatment time.

### Collaborative Team Members

Inflammation caused by myocarditis results in fatigue, fever, trouble breathing, palpitations and complaints of soreness in the chest. It requires close monitoring for signs of heart failure, effective communication, and a **collaborative effort** that might include the cardiologist, surgeon, infection control specialists (to determine origin and best treatment practices for causative agent), nephrologist, and physical and occupational therapists. It may also include referrals for alcohol treatment and extended cardiac rehabilitation. Care is focused on decreased activity levels to allow for cardiac muscle healing and antibiotics to treat bacterial infections.

## Need for Expanded Teaching and Discharge Planning

**Red flags requiring expanded teaching prior to discharge** include:

- Patients older than 70
- Anyone living alone, in another state or country, or whose housing arrangements are in question
- Anyone suspected of being abused or neglected
- Patients with multiple admissions
- Patients transferring from other care centers
- Patients with new or multiple diagnoses
- Anyone with a terminal illness or diseases requiring long-term intensive treatments and other significant life changes
- Patients with known or potential financial burdens related to care or basic needs
- Patients with few visitors or family/support system problems
- Those with little or no English-speaking ability or with learning disabilities
- Substance abusers

# Interventions

## Aneurysms

### *Treatment*

**Treatment recommendations for aneurysms** are based on the size and location of the aneurysm. Typically, aneurysms found early can be treated with aggressive risk factor modification including cessation of smoking, lowering cholesterol, treating hypertension, diet, exercise, and treatment with anti-platelet agents. However, surgery is often necessary if an aneurysm is large and at risk for rupture.

Once an aneurysm has ruptured, the goals of treatment are to surgically stop the bleeding, reestablish blood flow to prevent permanent end organ damage, and to reduce the risk of recurrence. Although repair of a ruptured aneurysm is possible, the likelihood of survival in patients with ruptured cerebral, abdominal, or thoracic aneurysms remains low.

### *Treatment by Aneurysm Location*

Treatment of a **cerebral aneurysm** is dependent on the size and location of the aneurysm in the brain. If the aneurysm is small and not causing symptoms, follow-up screening is recommended. However, surgery is recommended for large, symptomatic aneurysms due to their risk of rupture and stroke. Currently there are two surgical approaches for brain aneurysms: surgical clipping or endovascular coiling. If an aneurysm is infected, pharmacologic treatment is necessary.

#### Clipping

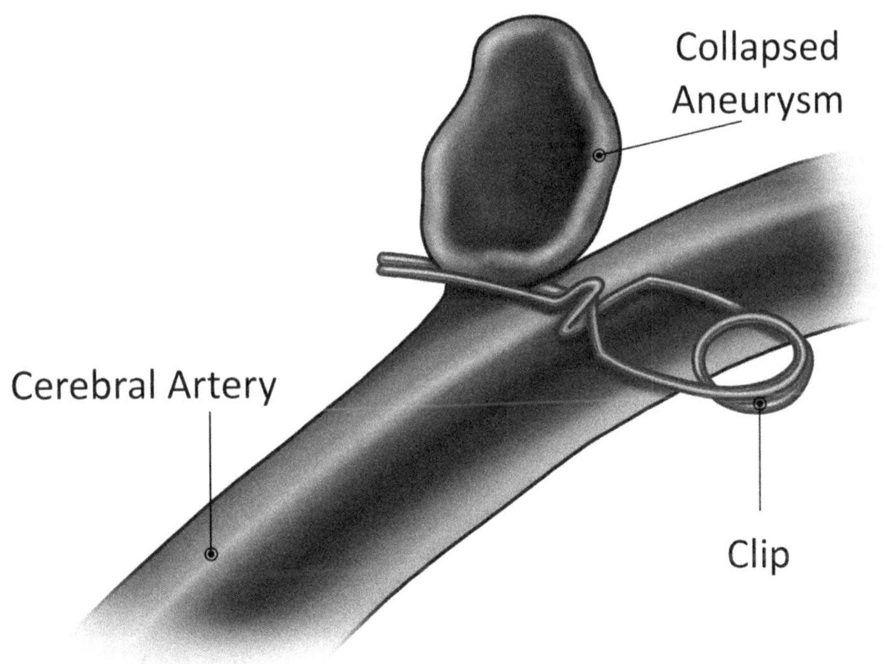

<u>Coiling</u>

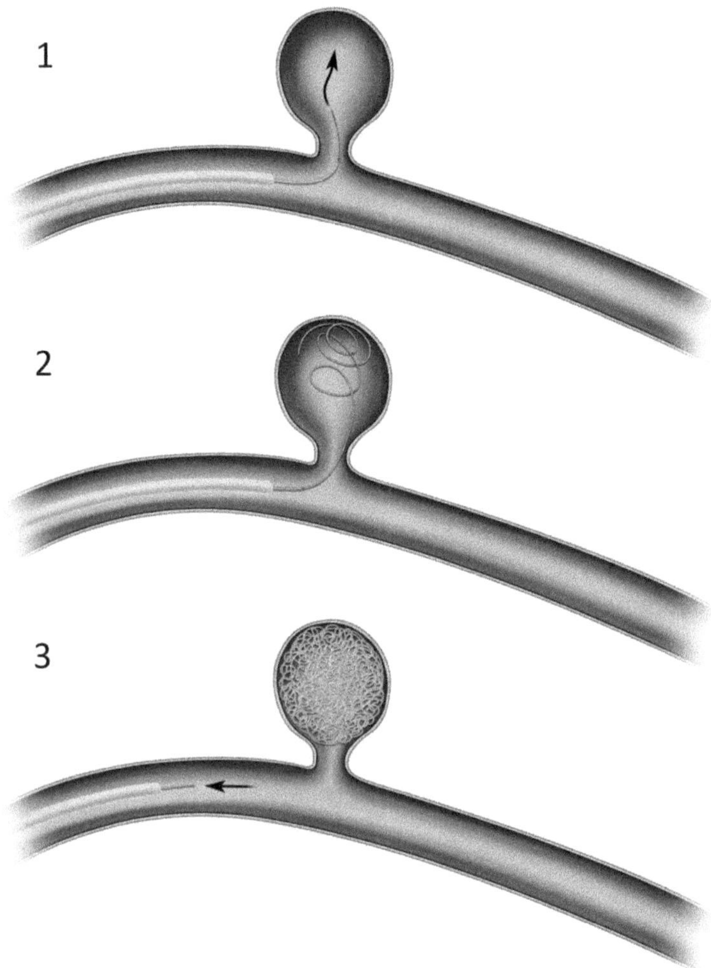


For **thoracic or abdominal aneurysms** less than 5 cm in diameter and not causing symptoms, pharmacologic approaches are typically used in combination with continuous monitoring. Surgical or interventional repair are options reserved for large unruptured aneurysms where the risk of rupture exceeds the risk of surgery.

**Peripheral aneurysms** in the extremities are typically asymptomatic and do not require treatment due to their low risk of rupture. Treatment of peripheral aneurysms depends on the presence of symptoms, the location of the aneurysm, and whether the blood flow through the artery is blocked.

### *Treatment by Aneurysm Size*

Treatment of aneurysms also involves management with pharmacologic agents such as anti-hypertensive, anti-coagulant, and anti-arrhythmia agents targeted at decreasing blood pressure, and/or heart rate. By decreasing blood pressure and heart rate, practicing clinicians can manage the patient's risk of stroke, heart attack, and death.

The guidelines used for the treatment of aneurysms depend on the **size** of the aneurysm and the types of symptoms the patient is experiencing.

For patients with an abdominal or thoracic aortic aneurysm with a diameter less than 3 cm and no symptoms, follow-up screening should be conducted within 5–10 years. For patients with an aorta of 3–4 cm in diameter, follow-up screening should be performed on a yearly basis.

For patients with a diameter of greater than 4 cm, careful follow-up needs to be performed on a biyearly basis. If a patient presents with an aorta with a diameter greater than 5 cm, surgery is recommended, which would include abdominal or open chest repair or endovascular repair.

#### *Prevention*

Few options are available for the **prevention of aneurysms**, but individuals should maintain proper blood pressure control, avoid smoking and stimulant drugs, avoid straining, use caution with aspirin use, exercise regularly, and maintain proper cholesterol levels.

Factors that put individuals at higher risk for aneurysms but cannot always be prevented or controlled include family history of aneurysms, hypertension or high cholesterol, natural aging, and diabetes. Secondary types of hypertension that could put an individual at high risk for aneurysms include renal disease, pheochromocytoma, Cushing syndrome, thyroid or pituitary dysfunction, and/or pregnancy.



### Atherosclerosis

#### *Pharmaceutical Approaches to Treatment*

Treatment recommendations for **atherosclerosis** are based on the size and location of the plaque. Typically, plaques found early can be treated successfully with pharmacologic approaches. Pharmacologic agents are typically used first line to decrease blood viscosity and reduce the risk of detachment or plaque size.

Pharmacologic agents used for the treatment of the disease include cholesterol-lowering medications such as statins. Anti-platelet medications such as aspirin, ticlopidine, and clopidogrel are also used. In situations where the atherosclerotic plaque is unstable, anticoagulants like heparin and warfarin are used. Concomitant risk factors are also treated: antihypertensives (beta-blockers, calcium channel blockers, angiotensin-converting enzyme [ACE] inhibitors) for hypertension, anti-diabetic medications for diabetes, and pharmacological agents for smoking cessation.

#### *Prevention*

**Preventing** the onset of atherosclerotic plaque formation and/or progression of atherosclerosis includes stress reduction, smoking cessation, maintaining a diet low in saturated fats and sodium, and physical exercise, as well as maintaining proper body mass index, blood pressure, blood sugar, and cholesterol levels. Patients should also reduce their homocysteine levels.

Patients with multiple risk factors should consult a practicing clinician to prophylactically reduce the risk of developing cardiovascular disease or experiencing heart attack and/or stroke.

Factors that put individuals at higher risk for plaque formation but cannot always be prevented or controlled include family history and natural aging.

#### *Lifestyle Modifications and Surgical Approaches*

**Lifestyle modifications** include physical exercise, healthy diet, dietary supplementation, smoking cessation, and treatment of comorbid conditions.

However, surgery may be performed if a plaque is large, inhibiting blood flow, and/or at risk for embolizing. Surgery or other procedures are used for individuals who present with more severe symptoms such as end organ dysfunction. Surgical approaches include angioplasty, endarterectomy, thrombolytic therapy, and bypass surgery. These approaches are used to physically expand narrowed arteries or create new, additional blood supply connections.

## Buerger's Disease

### *Treatment*

The main **treatment** for patients with **Buerger's disease** is smoking cessation, which will halt progression of the disease. Individuals who continue to smoke with Buerger's disease will likely have their digits amputated. Patients who need help to quit smoking should consult with their practicing clinician for alternatives like nicotine gum or patches.

Other options for the treatment of Buerger's disease include anti-coagulation agents or anti-platelet agents to improve blood flow, surgery to cut nerves in painful infected areas, and digit amputation due to extensive infection or gangrene. Experimental therapies with prostaglandins and thrombolytics have been used experimentally with some success.

Patients with Buerger's disease should dress any cuts or scrapes in the affected areas to prevent infection. Any cuts or scrapes that do not heal properly or in a timely manner should be addressed by a clinical practitioner.

### *Prevention and Prognosis*

The cause of Buerger's disease remains unclear but has been strongly linked to cigarette smoking and tobacco use. Therefore, smoking cessation is essential to **preventing** the onset and progression of the disease. Overall, the underlying mechanism of Buerger's disease is immunologic but remains unknown.

Buerger's disease is typically not life-threatening, but the death rate is higher in patients who continue to smoke or have other comorbid conditions such as emphysema or cancer. The disease is associated with amputation in up to 36% of patients. Major amputations are nearly twice as common in patients who continue to smoke.

## Raynaud's Phenomenon

### *Treatment*

**Treatment** of **Raynaud's phenomenon** involves self-care for patients with mild forms of the phenomenon, including keeping hands and feet warm and avoiding trauma to digits. However, in more moderate to severe cases, pharmacologic management can be used to reduce the degree and extent of the condition as well as to prevent tissue damage and treat any underlying causes of the condition.

Pharmacologic agents used in the treatment of Raynaud's phenomenon include calcium channel blockers to dilate blood vessels, alpha-blockers to counteract the constriction of blood vessels, and vasodilators to dilate and relax blood vessels.

Patients diagnosed with Raynaud's phenomenon should avoid over-the-counter agents such as cold remedies that contain pseudoephedrine, beta-blockers, and oral contraceptives due to their impact on blood circulation. They should also avoid stress and occupational hazards, such as tools that vibrate the hands.

Other options for patients with severe primary or secondary Raynaud's phenomenon include nerve surgery to reduce frequency and duration of symptoms, chemical injection to block sympathetic nerves affected, and/or amputation due to the development of infection or gangrene.

#### *Prevention*

Patients diagnosed with the condition should dress warmly in cold climates, take precautions outdoors, and consider moving to a warmer climate.

**Self-care approaches** that can reduce the degree and frequency of Raynaud's phenomenon include smoking cessation, physical activity, stress management, avoidance of vasoconstrictors such as caffeine, maintaining hands and feet carefully, and avoiding stress triggers and occupational hazards.

In order to avoid complications, individuals having a Raynaud's attack should move to a warmer area; wiggle fingers and toes to stimulate blood circulation; place hands/feet behind kneecaps, under armpits, or under warm water; and/or massage hands and feet. Also, relaxation techniques such as cognitive behavior therapy, biofeedback, breathing techniques, or meditation may also improve Raynaud's symptoms when stress triggers the attack.



### Cardiomyopathy

#### *Treatment*

Treatment of **cardiomyopathy** depends on the type, extent, and degree of disease. Patients with mild disease may only require lifestyle modifications and short-term pharmacologic treatment, whereas patients with more moderate to severe disease may require pharmacologic management and/or surgery. Lifestyle modifications include smoking cessation, diet low in saturated fats and sodium, physical activity, alcohol and drug cessation, weight loss in overweight individuals, resting, reducing stress, and treating underlying comorbidities such as diabetes and high blood pressure. The goals of cardiomyopathy management include treatment of comorbid conditions such as diabetes and congestive heart failure, controlling symptoms, preventing disease progression, and reducing associated risks and complications. Pharmacologic agents used for the treatment of cardiomyopathy include diuretics, ACE inhibitors, beta-blockers, calcium channel blockers, anticoagulants, antiarrhythmic agents, antibiotics, and corticosteroids. Surgical approaches include septal myectomy, surgically implanted devices such as left ventricular devices or implantable cardioverter defibrillators, and heart transplant. Another nonsurgical approach used by clinical practitioners is alcohol septal ablation, which uses ethanol to shrink thickened tissue in the myocardium.

#### *Treatment by Type of Disease*

**Dilated cardiomyopathies** can be treated with a combination of pharmacologic agents and/or surgical approaches. Pharmacologic agents used for treatment of this condition include angiotensin-converting enzyme (ACE) inhibitors, angiotensin-receptor blockers, and beta-blockers. For more serious cases of dilated cardiomyopathies, implantable cardioverter defibrillators (ICDs) or pacemakers may be implanted to coordinate the contractions between the left and right ventricles and reduce the chance of sudden cardiac death.

**Hypertrophic cardiomyopathy** can also be treated with a combination of pharmacologic agents and/or surgical approaches. Pharmacologic agents include beta-blockers and calcium channel blockers. Other surgical options include implantation of ICDs or pacemakers and septal myectomy. Alcohol ablation is another option for patients who are not candidates for surgery.

**Restrictive cardiomyopathy** treatment involves symptom management. Self-care is recommended in which patients monitor sodium and water intake. Pharmacologic agents may also be recommended, including diuretics, antihypertensive agents, and antiarrhythmic agents.

### *Prevention*

Cardiomyopathy can be **prevented** by managing comorbidities and environmental factors. Although patients with familial cardiomyopathy cannot prevent onset of disease, they can reduce the extent and degree of disease through self-care and proper disease management. In order to prevent onset of cardiomyopathy and decrease disease progression, individuals should avoid smoking and alcohol and drug consumption, maintain proper blood pressure, eat a diet low in saturated fats and sodium, and maintain an active lifestyle.

Patients should also undergo regular examinations by their clinical practitioner, follow the practitioner's advice regarding cardiomyopathy management, and adhere to pharmacologic treatment regimens.

## Congestive Heart Failure

### *Treatment*

Treatment of **congestive heart failure** depends on the extent and degree of disease. Patients with mild disease may only require lifestyle modifications and short-term pharmacologic treatment, whereas patients with more moderate to severe disease may require pharmacologic management and/or surgery. Lifestyle modifications include smoking cessation, diet low in saturated fats and sodium, reduced fluid intake, physical activity depending on patient's health, alcohol and drug cessation, weight loss in overweight individuals, resting, reducing stress, and treating underlying comorbidities such as diabetes and high blood pressure.

The goals of treatment include controlling excess fluid accumulation, improving cardiac function, and reducing cardiac workload.

### *Treatment Guidelines*

**Treatment guidelines** recommend that patients with congestive heart failure should not intake more than 2000 mg of sodium per day. Patients need to aggressively monitor their body weight, as rapid weight gain could be due to fluid accumulation. Therefore, if patients experience weight gain of more than 2–3 pounds over 2–3 days, they should contact their clinical practitioner immediately.

### *Pharmacologic and Surgical Approaches*

Pharmacologic agents used for the treatment of congestive heart failure include diuretics, ACE inhibitors, digoxin, beta-blockers, calcium channel blockers, anticoagulants, antiarrhythmic agents, antibiotics, and corticosteroids.

Surgical approaches include coronary artery surgery or catheter procedures, such as angioplasty or intracoronary stenting, to restore blood flow. Other options include heart transplantation, left ventricular assist devices, and pacemakers.

### *Prevention*

Congestive heart failure can be **prevented** by managing comorbidities and environmental factors. Although patients with familial congestive heart failure cannot prevent onset of disease, they can reduce the extent and degree of disease through self-care and proper disease management. In order to prevent onset of congestive heart failure or decrease disease progression, individuals should avoid smoking and alcohol and drug consumption, maintain proper blood pressure, eat a diet low in saturated fats and sodium, reduce fluid intake, treat other comorbidities, and maintain an active lifestyle.

Patients should also undergo regular examinations by their clinical practitioner, follow the practitioner's advice regarding congestive heart failure management, and adhere to pharmacologic treatment regimens.

## COR PULMONALE

### *TREATMENT*

Current treatments for **cor pulmonale** are focused on reducing symptoms and complications of disease, which are geared toward addressing the underlying cause of the disease. The type of treatment depends on whether cor pulmonale occurs acutely or evolves chronically.

The use of pharmaceutical agents such as vasodilators (nifedipine and other calcium channel blockers), diuretics (furosemide), anticoagulants (warfarin), cardiac glycosides (digoxin), methylxanthines (theophylline), and endothelin receptor antagonists (bosentan) can be used for treatment of cor pulmonale.

In some patients, the disease can progress rapidly, while in others the disease can be chronically maintained. Surgery is an option for advanced cases where heart defects are the source of failure. Also, in more severe cases, heart and/or lung transplantation may be recommended.

Supplemental oxygen may also be prescribed to increase blood oxygen levels.

### *PREVENTION*

**Prevention** of cor pulmonale includes avoidance of environmental factors that can lead to chronic pulmonary hypertension such as cigarette smoking, tobacco use, and inhalation of toxic fumes, chemicals, and/or smoke. A pulmonary specialist should monitor patients with cardiopulmonary disease in order to prevent the onset of cor pulmonale. Adolescents with serious heart murmurs caused by various cardiac defects should be monitored and treated throughout their lifespan in order to prevent onset of cor pulmonale.

Supplemental oxygen may prevent further worsening of cor pulmonale and underlying disease progression. Oxygen supplementation also improves chances of survival, decreases symptom burden, and improves patient quality of life.

## TYPE I AND TYPE II DIABETES

### *TREATMENT*

Treatment of both **type I and type II diabetes** involves management of short-term and long-term complications. Proper lifestyle modifications as well as pharmaceutical management need to be maintained in an effort to prevent long-term complications such as coronary artery disease, peripheral vascular disease, and vision problems. Patients also need to monitor their blood sugar levels on a daily basis and comply with treatment recommendations.

Patients need to make lifestyle modifications including diet, exercise, and smoking cessation. Pharmacologic management, including proper insulin or oral diabetic agent usage, is also necessary.

### *TYPE I DIABETES*

#### LIFESTYLE MODIFICATIONS AND PHARMACEUTICAL TREATMENT

For **type I diabetes**, patients need to maintain a consistent healthy weight and an exercise routine as well as to maintain compliance with insulin use. Blood sugar monitoring is of extreme importance to avoid the extreme highs and lows, both of which can be life-threatening. They also need to avoid smoking and/or tobacco use to decrease risk of cardiovascular complications.

Type I diabetes pharmacologic approaches include antidiabetic agents such as insulin lispro, insulin NPH, protamine zinc, insulin aspart, insulin glargine, and insulin glulisine. There is no cure for type I diabetes, and management of the disease requires chronic care. However, pancreatic transplantation, islet cell transplantation, and stem cell transplantation are possible cures for type I diabetes but are currently investigational and not always successful.

### *Type II Diabetes*

#### Lifestyle Modifications and Pharmaceutical Treatment

For **type II diabetes**, patients need to maintain a healthy diet, exercise, and comply with oral pharmacologic agents and insulin regimens. In some cases, type II diabetes can be cured with gastric bypass surgery in obese patients.

Pharmaceutical agents used for treatment of type II diabetes include sulfonylurea agents such as glipizide, glyburide, and glimepiride; meglitinides such as repaglinide; biguanides such as metformin; thiazolidinediones such as pioglitazone and rosiglitazone; dipeptidyl inhibitors such as sitagliptin; incretin mimetics such as exenatide; amylin analogs such as pramlintide acetate; and alpha glucosidase inhibitors such as acarbose and miglitol.

### *Prevention*

Onset of type I and type II diabetes can be attributed to both **genetic and environmental factors**. Therefore, certain steps can be taken to control environmental triggers, but nothing can be done to prevent the genetic contribution. However, type I diabetes is typically not preventable, as the disease is associated with a larger genetic contribution.

**Prevention of type II diabetes** involves maintaining a healthy diet rich in proteins, fruits, and vegetables and low in saturated fats, increasing physical activity with 2.5 hours of exercise per week, management of other comorbid conditions, and maintaining proper body fat and weight for an individual's height.

Other preventative measures for type I and type II diabetes are under investigation and not recommended by the American Diabetes Association, such as copper supplementation and niacin.

## Metabolic Syndrome

### *Treatment*

Currently, there are no set guidelines for the management **of metabolic syndrome.** However, the overall goal is to reduce an individual's risk of developing cardiovascular disease and type II diabetes. It is recommended to encourage patients to maintain proper diet and exercise, avoid smoking and tobacco use, lose excess weight, maintain proper lipid levels, maintain proper blood pressure levels, maintain proper glucose levels, and maintain proper albumin excretion and creatinine levels.

Pharmacologic agents used to treat metabolic syndrome include lipid-lowering agents, antihypertensives, anticoagulants, and diabetic agents such as oral agents and insulin.

### *Prevention*

Certain risk factors such as having a genetic predisposition for metabolic syndrome and natural aging are unpreventable. To **prevent** the onset, individuals need to maintain proper diet and exercise, avoid smoking and tobacco use, lose excess weight, maintain proper lipid levels, maintain proper blood pressure levels, maintain proper sugar levels, and maintain proper albumin excretion and creatinine levels.

Metabolic syndrome is a chronic condition that needs to be managed by lifestyle modifications and pharmacologic management of comorbid conditions. Patients should carefully watch their waistline measurement and calculate their body mass index in order to prevent abdominal obesity.

### Endothelial Dysfunction

Comorbid conditions that can lead to the development of **endothelial dysfunction** include septic shock, hypertension, hypercholesterolemia, congestive heart failure, peripheral artery disease, chronic renal failure, diabetes, and insulin resistance. Another factor that can increase the risk of developing endothelial dysfunction is smoking and/or tobacco use.

Treatment of endothelial dysfunction involves dietary changes and increased physical activity. Pharmacologic agents such as anticoagulants, antihypertensive agents, and lipid-lowering agents may be used to treat comorbid conditions and reduce an individual's risk for developing cardiovascular disease.

### Dyslipidemia

The main complication associated with **dyslipidemia** involves cardiovascular disease complications such as heart attack, stroke, and sudden death. However, aggressive treatment with lipid-lowering agents such as statins has been shown to reduce plaque formation and onset of cardiovascular disease.

Certain risk factors such as having a genetic predisposition for dyslipidemia and natural aging are not preventable. However, certain complications of dyslipidemia can be prevented by having individuals maintain a diet low in sodium and saturated fats, increase potassium intake, increase exercise and physical activity, avoid smoking and tobacco use, lose excess weight, maintain proper lipid levels, and maintain proper glucose levels.

#### *Pharmacologic Agents for Elevated LDL Levels*

**Pharmacologic agents** used for treatment depend on the type of lipid abnormality, even though multiple lipid abnormalities may present together. The goal of low-density lipoprotein levels is 100 mg/dL or below, but recent evidence suggests a lower target of 70 mg/dL. Lipid-lowering approaches include statins such as fluvastatin, lovastatin, simvastatin, pravastatin, atorvastatin, and rosuvastatin; nicotinic acid such as niacin; bile acid sequestrants such as cholestyramine, colestipol, and colesevelam; fibrates such as gemfibrozil, ciprofibrate, clofibrate, fenofibrate, and bezafibrate; cholesterol absorption agents such as ezetimibe; and combination agents such as extended-release niacin/lovastatin.

#### *Pharmacologic Approaches for Elevated TG Levels*

Pharmacologic agents used for the treatment of **elevated triglyceride levels** include fibrates such as gemfibrozil, ciprofibrate, clofibrate, fenofibrate, and bezafibrate; nicotinic acid such as niacin; and statins such as fluvastatin, lovastatin, simvastatin, pravastatin, atorvastatin, and rosuvastatin. Another approach that has been demonstrated to be effective in lowering triglyceride levels is taking high doses of omega-3 fatty acids.

## Myocardial Infarction

### Treatment

In individuals who experience an **acute myocardial infarction**, practicing clinicians should initiate oxygen, aspirin, and sublingual glyceryl trinitrate therapies to prevent further myocardium damage and/or complications. Invasive approaches for the treatment of myocardial infarction and underlying comorbid conditions include thrombolysis, percutaneous coronary intervention, angioplasty, and stent insertion. In more severe cases, with invasive plaque formation or multiple blockages, cardiopulmonary bypass surgery may be performed.

Upon myocardial infarction diagnosis, pharmacologic agents prescribed include antithrombotic agents such as aspirin; blood thinners such as heparin and enoxaparin; vasodilators such as nitroglycerin; beta-adrenergic blockers such as metoprolol and esmolol; thrombolytic agents such as alteplase, anistreplase, and tenecteplase; platelet aggregation inhibitors such as clopidogrel, eptifibatide, and tirofiban; analgesics such as morphine sulfate; and angiotensin-converting enzyme inhibitors such as captopril.

Post myocardial infarction, patients are recommended to make lifestyle modifications including a diet with low fat and low sodium foods, increased physical activity, smoking and alcohol cessation, and stress reduction. It is also recommended to comply with pharmacologic treatment regimens despite their complexity.

### Prevention

**Lifestyle modifications and pharmacologic management** can help to prevent the onset of myocardial infarction as well as recurrent myocardial infarction in patients with a previous occurrence. Patients should maintain a diet low in sodium and saturated fats, increase potassium intake, increase exercise and physical activity, avoid smoking and tobacco use, lose excess weight, maintain proper lipid levels, and control diabetes if present.

Patients with previous myocardial infarction who comply with lifestyle modification and pharmacologic management are at a much lower risk for recurrent disease. Pharmacologic agents used to prevent recurrent myocardial infarction include antiplatelet agents such as aspirin or clopidogrel, beta-blockers such as metoprolol or carvedilol, ACE inhibitor agents, and statin therapy. Other approaches include aldosterone antagonists such as eplerenone and omega-3 fatty acids.

## Stroke

### Treatment

An **acute stroke** is a medical emergency and requires immediate medical attention. Individuals experiencing an ischemic stroke should seek medical attention within three hours of onset to receive anti-coagulant and/or thrombolytic approaches to restore blood flow. Other surgical approaches include carotid endarterectomy, angioplasty, and catheter embolectomy. Pharmacologic approaches used post stroke include anti-platelet agents and anti-coagulants.

Surgical approaches are typically used to treat hemorrhagic stroke, including aneurysm coiling and arteriovenous malformation (AVM) removal.

Pharmacologic agents used to treat stroke include fibrinolytic agents such as alteplase and anti-platelet agents such as aspirin and ticlopidine.

Please note that acute lowering of blood pressure during a stroke is NOT part of the treatment, as it is important to maintain perfusion pressure to the brain.

### *Prevention*

**Preventive measures** that individuals can take to reduce the risk of stroke include maintaining proper lipid levels and blood pressure, maintaining a healthy weight and healthy diet low in sodium and saturated fats, avoiding smoking, controlling diabetes, exercising regularly, managing stress and anxiety, reducing alcohol consumption, and avoiding illicit drug use.

The American Heart Association recommends that individuals over the age of 20 undergo risk factor screening, which includes blood pressure measurement, body mass index, waist circumference, and cholesterol and glucose monitoring at least every 2–5 years.

Prevention involves primary, secondary, and tertiary prevention. Primary prevention involves reduction of factors, including smoking cessation and other behavioral measures. Secondary prevention involves reduction of risk factors in individuals at an increased risk for stroke. Tertiary prevention involves reduction of risk factors in individuals who have already experienced a transient ischemic attack or an acute stroke.



## Peripheral Arterial Disease

### *Treatment*

Treatment of **peripheral arterial disease** involves lifestyle modifications and pharmacologic management. Lifestyle changes including smoking cessation, increased physical activity, and dietary changes may improve symptoms and complications of peripheral arterial disease.

Pharmacologic agents used in peripheral arterial disease and comorbid conditions include anti-platelet agents, lipid-lowering agents, anti-hypertensive agents, diabetes agents, anti-thrombolytic agents, and symptom-relief medications. The goal of treatment is to prevent the onset of complications.

Surgical approaches used for patients with peripheral arterial disease and intermittent claudication include angioplasty. Other surgical approaches used for peripheral arterial disease include transcatheter intervention and peripheral vascular bypass.

### *Prevention*

Lifestyle modifications and pharmacologic management can prevent the onset of arteriosclerosis and peripheral arterial disease. Patients should maintain a diet low in sodium and saturated fats, increase potassium intake, increase exercise and physical activity, avoid smoking and tobacco use, lose excess weight, avoid illicit drug use, maintain proper lipid levels, maintain proper sugar levels, and control complications of diabetes.

Patients with peripheral arterial disease should practice good foot hygiene to prevent the onset of complications such as infections and gangrene. Patients should wash their feet daily and moisturize them, wear thick socks and comfortable shoes, promptly treat fungal infections, trim toenails, avoid walking barefoot, and immediately have sores and open wounds treated.

## Inflammatory Disease

### *Treatment*

The **treatment of inflammation and inflammatory disease** depends on the organ systems being affected. Treatment options include lifestyle modifications such as diet, exercise and rehabilitation, pharmacologic approaches, and surgery. The type of treatment approach depends on a patient's health status, age, extent and degree of disease, presence of other comorbid conditions, medical history, and type of pharmacologic agents already being prescribed.

Pharmacologic agents used include analgesics, anti-inflammatory agents such as nonsteroidal anti-inflammatory agents, corticosteroids, anti-malarial agents such as hydroxychloroquine and other agents including methotrexate, leflunomide, anti-tumor necrosis factor medications, cyclophosphamide, and mycophenolate. Other pharmacologic agents may be used to treat specific inflammatory conditions affecting specific organ systems.

### *Prevention of Inflammatory Cardiovascular Disease*

**Inflammation** is an important mechanism present in cardiovascular diseases such as atherosclerosis. In cardiovascular disease, acute phase inflammation occurs in the presence of C-reactive protein. Therefore, screening patients for the presence of C-reactive protein may be a proactive approach to reducing the risk of congestive heart failure, heart attack, and stroke. C-reactive protein may also be a good biomarker in predicting recurrent disease in patients with previous heart attack, stroke, and/or persistent cardiovascular disease. Recent data has demonstrated that the higher the C-reactive protein levels, the higher the risk of heart attack and/or stroke.

Atherosclerosis is actually an inflammatory response to the development of lipids in arteries, with every step of atherosclerotic disease responding to inflammatory signaling mechanisms.

## Pericarditis

### *Treatment Goals*

Treatment of **pericarditis** involves lifestyle modifications, pharmacologic approaches, and surgery. Treatment depends on the extent and degree of pericarditis as well as the patient's overall health, age, diet, physical activity, and/or presence of other comorbid conditions. In some more mild cases, pericarditis may resolve itself on its own without medical intervention. However, in cases that are more moderate to severe, pharmacologic agents and/or surgical approaches may be used based on the underlying cause of the condition.

Lifestyle modifications may include reduction of physical activity as well as increased rest and relaxation until the condition resolves.

### *Pharmacologic Agents and Surgical Approaches*

**Pharmacologic agents** include anti-inflammatory agents such as nonsteroidal anti-inflammatory agents, narcotics such as morphine or colchicine, diuretics, antifungals, antibiotics, aspirin, and corticosteroids.

**Surgical approaches** may be used in severe cases of pericarditis, including pericardiocentesis, pericardiotomy, and pericardiectomy. Pericardiocentesis is a procedure that uses a catheter to remove excess fluid from the pericardium. Pericardiectomy involves removal of the entire pericardium. This procedure is typically reserved for patients with constrictive pericarditis.

### *Prevention*

Acute and chronic pericarditis are typically not preventable, but diseases associated with pericarditis are preventable. For example, decreasing the risk of myocardial infarction or regular dialysis in patients with diabetes to avoid uremia will decrease the risk of pericarditis.

Early intervention with pericarditis may prevent onset of complications such as pericardial effusion, arrhythmias, constrictive pericarditis, and cardiac tamponade as well as decrease the risk for reoccurrence of the condition.

## Vasculitis

### *Treatment*

Treatment of **vasculitis** involves lifestyle modifications, pharmacologic approaches, and surgery. The goal of treatment is to address the underlying cause of the condition and organ systems involved. Early intervention prevents onset of complications.

Pharmacologic approaches include corticosteroids such as prednisone, prednisolone, and methylprednisolone to reduce inflammation; cytotoxic drugs such as azathioprine and cyclophosphamide to suppress inflammation; and nonsteroidal anti-inflammatory agents such as aspirin and ibuprofen to treat mild symptoms. Other pharmacologic approaches used for treatment of vasculitis include anticoagulants such as heparin and enoxaparin; immunomodulators such as immune globulin; antibiotics such as trimethoprim-sulfamethoxazole; and stronger anti-inflammatory agents such as methotrexate.

Pharmacologic agents under clinical investigation for the treatment of vasculitis include mycophenolate mofetil, tumor necrosis factor inhibitors, and rituximab.

### *Prevention*

Typically, vasculitis cannot be prevented, but early treatment and maintenance of good health promote better outcomes in patients diagnosed with the condition. Also, compliance with treatment recommendations may prevent reoccurrence and/or delay vasculitis onset if detected early.

In the United States, immunization of hepatitis B is standard of care, which may help to prevent onset of vasculitis. Avoiding IV drug use and unprotected sex decreases the risk of hepatitis C and HIV, thus decreasing the risk of vasculitis.

General preventive measures that individuals can take to reduce the risk of vasculitis and disease complications include maintaining proper lipid levels and blood pressure, maintaining healthy weight and a healthy diet low in sodium and saturated fats, avoiding smoking, controlling diabetes, obtaining adequate vitamin D and calcium, exercising regularly, managing stress and anxiety, reducing alcohol consumption, and avoiding illicit drug use.

## Endocarditis

### *Treatment*

The treatment of **endocarditis** involves the treatment of the underlying condition leading to endocarditis as well as prevention of further progression of the disease. The main goal is to prevent additional complications associated with endocarditis such as heart attack, stroke, and sudden death.

Pharmacologic agents such as intravenous antibiotics, including penicillin, gentamicin, vancomycin, rifampin, and linezolid, are used to fight infection, and nonsteroidal anti-inflammatory agents are used to reduce fever, inflammation, and associated pain. Most patients are hospitalized initially to receive intravenous antibiotics but will continue oral antibiotics for up to 6 weeks.

Heart valve replacement surgery may be an option for patients experiencing strokes due to the condition or patients with congestive heart failure and evidence of end organ system damage.

### *Prevention*

Patients at higher risk for endocarditis, including those with artificial heart valves, previous endocarditis infection, congenital heart defects, and heart transplant, are recommended preventative antibiotics before certain medical and dental procedures.

ADA and AHA guidelines were updated in 2017 to recommend that patients at high risk for endocarditis who are undergoing certain dental procedures and procedures involving the respiratory tract should be prescribed preventative antibiotics for infected tissue.

Individuals diagnosed with endocarditis should maintain good dental hygiene by brushing teeth, flossing, and maintaining gums. They should also avoid procedures that may lead to skin infections, including body piercing and tattoos. General preventive measures that individuals can take to reduce the risk of endocarditis and disease complications include maintaining proper lipid levels and blood pressure, maintaining healthy weight and a healthy diet low in sodium and saturated fats, avoiding smoking, controlling diabetes, exercising regularly, managing stress and anxiety, reducing alcohol consumption, and avoiding illicit drug use, especially intravenous drugs.

## Renal Artery Occlusion

### *Treatment*

The treatment of **renal artery occlusion** depends on the extent and degree of the condition as well as other organ systems involved. In more severe cases, where patients present with renal failure, surgical intervention may be necessary. Another alternative surgical approach is balloon angioplasty or stenting of the affected renal arteries.

Revascularization is an option in patients with bilateral stenosis, stenosis in a solitary functioning kidney, and unilateral stenosis with renal insufficiency. Revascularization is also recommended in patients with normal renal function if their degree of stenosis is more than 80% and if the degree of stenosis is 50–80% with activation of intrarenal arterial occlusion. In patients who do not meet these criteria, guidelines recommend practicing clinicians to monitor patients over a 6-month period and then reevaluate.

Pharmacologic agents used to treat associated conditions with renal artery occlusion include angiotensin-converting enzyme inhibitors such as captopril and enalapril, angiotensin II receptor antagonists such as losartan, and HMG-coenzyme A reductase inhibitors such as atorvastatin.

### *Prevention*

Smoking cessation can prevent the onset of renal artery occlusion. General preventive measures that individuals can take to reduce the risk of renal artery occlusion and disease complications include maintaining proper lipid levels and blood pressure, maintaining healthy weight and a healthy diet low in sodium and saturated fats, avoiding smoking, controlling diabetes, exercising regularly, managing stress and anxiety, reducing alcohol consumption, and avoiding illicit drug use.

In an effort to prevent further progression of renal arterial occlusion, practicing clinicians need to follow patients closely, monitoring serum creatine levels, blood pressure levels, serum potassium levels, and complete blood counts. A follow-up ultrasound should also be performed and compared to the baseline to determine progression.

## Renal Vein Thrombosis

### *Treatment*

Treatment of **renal vein thrombosis** involves lifestyle modifications, pharmacologic approaches, and possibly surgery to remove occlusion. However, surgery to remove the occluding factor is rarely performed. Lifestyle modifications include bedrest and/or limited activity for a short period to reduce embolization and new clot formation. Anti-coagulation therapy is the standard pharmacologic approach for management. However, fibrinolytic agents may also be used to dissolve the blood clot.

Pharmacologic agents used to treat renal vein thrombosis include angiotensin-converting enzyme inhibitors such as benazepril, captopril, enalapril, fosinopril, moexipril, perindopril, and lisinopril and angiotensin receptor blockers such as candesartan, eprosartan, irbesartan, losartan, telmisartan, and valsartan.

The goal of treatment is to decrease risk of new clot formation, prevent progression of current clots, and prevent embolization of formed clots to other organ systems, including heart, lungs, and/or brain.

### *Prevention*

Prevention of renal vein thrombosis is difficult, as it is a rare condition. However, adults can avoid trauma to the abdomen or back, make sure they are properly hydrated, and maintain good lifestyle habits.

Infants, toddlers, and adolescents with the flu, or who are out in very hot weather or exposed to other factors that can cause severe dehydration, should take preventive measures to avoid dehydration and potential for renal vein thrombosis.

General preventive measures that individuals can take to reduce the risk of renal vein thrombosis and disease complications include maintaining proper lipid levels and blood pressure, maintaining healthy weight and a healthy diet low in sodium and saturated fats, avoiding smoking, controlling diabetes, exercising regularly, managing stress and anxiety, reducing alcohol consumption, and avoiding illicit drug use.

## Atheroembolic Renal Disease

### *Treatment*

Treatment of **atheroembolic renal disease** is similar to atherosclerotic treatment. Pharmacologic agents used for the treatment of the disease include cholesterol medications such as statins; anti-platelet medications such as aspirin, ticlopidine, and clopidogrel; anti-coagulants such as heparin and warfarin; anti-hypertensive agents such as ACE inhibitors, beta-blockers, or calcium channel blockers; and other classes of agents for concomitant or predisposing conditions such as diabetes. Patients at high risk for atherosclerosis may also be treated prophylactically with low dose aspirin and/or statins.

Lifestyle modifications are also recommended, which include maintaining proper lipid levels, blood pressure, and glucose levels; maintaining healthy weight and a healthy diet low in sodium and saturated fats; avoiding smoking; controlling diabetes; exercising regularly; managing stress and anxiety; reducing alcohol consumption; and avoiding illicit drug use.

### *Prevention*

Lifestyle modifications can help prevent the progression of disease and initial onset of atheroembolic renal disease and/or atherosclerosis. However, pharmacologic management has not been demonstrated to improve patient outcomes or prevent onset of disease.

General **preventive measures** that individuals can take to reduce the risk of atheroembolic renal disease and disease complications include maintaining proper lipid levels, blood pressure, and glucose levels; maintaining healthy weight and a healthy diet low in sodium and saturated fats; avoiding smoking; controlling diabetes; exercising regularly; managing stress and anxiety; reducing alcohol consumption; and avoiding illicit drug use.

## Marfan Syndrome

### *Treatment*

There are no **treatments** currently available to treat **Marfan syndrome** directly. However, practicing clinicians can address complications of the condition such as cardiovascular, skeletal, and eye complications.

Pharmacologic agents used to treat Marfan syndrome with cardiovascular complications include antihypertensive agents such as beta-blockers, calcium channel blockers, angiotensin-converting enzyme inhibitors, or angiotensin receptor inhibitors. Surgical approaches include aorta composite graft repair or an aortic valve sparing technique. The extent of surgery depends on how much of the aorta is involved.

For skeletal complications, a back brace may be used to treat scoliosis. Other options for scoliosis include surgery to correct the curvature of the spine as well as posterior spinal fusion. Surgery may also be an option for a child with a concave chest that affects breathing capability.

For eye complications such as dislocated lens, patients may wear glasses or undergo intraocular lens implant surgery. Glaucoma is not curable but can be treated with eye drops, oral agents, and surgical approaches. Patients with cataracts can undergo surgery to correct the problem.

**Pharmacologic agents** used for the treatment of Marfan syndrome include beta-adrenergic inhibiting agents such as atenolol and calcium channel blockers such as verapamil hydrochloride. Other antihypertensive agents may be used in combination or as second-line therapy in patients who either fail first-line approaches or who cannot tolerate adverse events. Other pharmacologic approaches, including agents directed toward the skeletal system and other cardiovascular agents, can be used to treat other complications of the condition. However, pharmacologic agents will not cure the Marfan syndrome but will treat the complications of the syndrome. Even with pharmacologic management, progression of complications may continue. Therefore, lifestyle modifications and surgery may be other options.

### *Prevention*

Pregnancy is not recommended for women with Marfan syndrome due to risk of aortic dissection and rupture. Also, women can pass the disease to their offspring; therefore, not having children is the only way to prevent passing the disease on to offspring.

General **preventive measures** that individuals can take to reduce the risk of Marfan syndrome and disease complications include maintaining proper lipid levels, blood pressure, and glucose levels; maintaining healthy weight and a healthy diet low in sodium and saturated fats; avoiding smoking; controlling diabetes; managing stress and anxiety; reducing alcohol consumption; and avoiding illicit drug use. Physical activity is recommended based on the type of organ systems affected by Marfan syndrome.

## Atrial Septal Defect

### *Treatment*

In patients with **atrial septal defects** with few or no symptoms, treatment may not be required, especially in patients with a small defect. However, in patients with larger defects, surgical closure is recommended. Devices such as the Amplatzer device may be used to close the defect using catheterization. Minimally invasive surgical approaches may be used to prevent use of blood or blood products in certain patients.

In some cases, especially in very young or elderly patients, prophylactic antibiotics may be administered prior to surgery to prevent onset of infective endocarditis post surgery. Also, postsurgical care to prevent onset of infective endocarditis may also be recommended. Pharmacologic management does not fix the defect but can be used to alleviate some of the symptoms associated with the condition. Pharmacologic agents that may be recommended include beta-blockers such as metoprolol, propranolol, and digoxin; diuretics such as furosemide; anti-coagulants such as warfarin; and anti-platelet agents such as aspirin.

### *Prevention*

Since atrial septal defects are inherited, they cannot be prevented. Addressing the defect early in the progression of the condition may prevent complications associated with the condition, but the only way to prevent potential transmission of atrial septal defects is not to have children. However, in some cases, the disease arises from new genetic mutations during pregnancy.



## Pulmonary Embolism

### *Treatment*

Treatment of **pulmonary embolism** involves lifestyle modifications, pharmacologic management and, in more severe cases, surgery. Immediate treatment with anti-coagulation therapy is necessary for patients with suspected pulmonary embolism, as treatment decreases mortality risk.

Fibrinolytic therapy is recommended for patients who are hemodynamically unstable or those with right heart strain, exhausted cardiopulmonary reserves, or those at risk for pulmonary embolism reoccurrence. Long-term anti-coagulation therapy is considered for patients diagnosed with pulmonary embolism to prevent reoccurrence.

Pharmacologic agents used for pulmonary embolism include fibrinolytics such as reteplase, alteplase, and urokinase, as well as anticoagulants such as enoxaparin, tinzaparin, unfractionated heparin, and warfarin.

### *Prevention*

Pulmonary embolism may occur postsurgically or as a result of other cardiovascular conditions. Therefore, hospitals take a prophylactic approach to prevent pulmonary embolism. Preventative strategies include heparin or warfarin therapy, use of graduated compression stockings, use of pneumatic compression, and increased physical activity.

Preventative measures that individuals at high risk can take while traveling include increasing physical activity, exercising while seated by flexing and extending legs, using compression stockings, staying well hydrated, and using anti-coagulants for long trips.

General preventive measures that individuals can take to reduce the risk of pulmonary embolism and disease complications include maintaining proper lipid levels, blood pressure, and glucose levels; maintaining healthy weight and a healthy diet low in sodium and saturated fats; avoiding smoking; exercising regularly; controlling diabetes; managing stress and anxiety; reducing alcohol consumption; and avoiding illicit drug use.

## Deep Venous Thrombosis

### *Treatment*

The goals of treatment of **deep venous thrombosis** are to prevent pulmonary embolism and other complications associated with the condition. Treatment also aims to prevent the reoccurrence of formation of additional blood clots. Treatment involves lifestyle management, pharmacologic therapy, and, in more severe cases, surgical approaches. Pharmacologic management involves the use of anticoagulation therapy such as warfarin and/or heparin. Other pharmacologic approaches include antithrombotic agents and thrombolytics. Additional types of treatment include vena cava filter and graduated compression stockings.

Pharmacologic agents for deep venous thrombosis include anticoagulation therapy such as fondaparinux sodium, dalteparin, warfarin, enoxaparin, and tinzaparin, as well as thrombolytics such as tenecteplase, urokinase, streptokinase, and alteplase.

### *Prevention*

Preventative strategies for deep venous thrombosis and risk of pulmonary embolism include heparin or warfarin therapy, use of graduated compression stockings, use of pneumatic compression, and increased physical activity.

Preventative measures individuals at high risk can take while traveling include increasing physical activity, exercising while seated by flexing and extending legs, using compression stockings, staying well hydrated, and using anti-coagulants for long trips.

## Venous Insufficiency

### *Treatment*

The goal of treatment of **venous insufficiency** is to alleviate symptoms and address the underlying cause of the condition.

Treatment of venous insufficiency involves lifestyle modifications, pharmacologic management and, in some very severe cases, surgery. However, lifestyle modifications including bedrest to reduce leg swelling, avoiding prolonged periods of standing or sitting, and the use of graduated compression stockings are the most common and effective approaches. Other more invasive approaches include valvuloplasty, radiofrequency ablation, vein stripping with ligation, sclerotherapy, skin grafting, and endovenous laser therapy.

Pharmacologic agents used to treat venous insufficiency include sclerosing agents such as sodium tetradecyl sulfate, antibiotics for infection, and corticosteroids for associated inflammation.

Mild skin infections can be treated with antibiotics and/or steroids. Skin ulcerations can be treated with ointments, antibiotics, steroids and, in more severe cases, surgery.

### *Prevention*

Individuals with a family history of venous insufficiency should discuss prevention options with their practicing clinician. Also, individuals who are on their feet for long periods of the day with other cardiovascular comorbid conditions should consider the use of compression stockings.

General preventive measures that individuals can take to reduce the risk of venous insufficiency and disease complications include maintaining proper lipid levels, blood pressure, and glucose levels; maintaining healthy weight and a healthy diet low in sodium and saturated fats; avoiding smoking; controlling diabetes; managing stress and anxiety; reducing alcohol consumption; and avoiding illicit drug use.

## Valvular Disease

### *Treatment*

Lifestyle modifications, pharmacologic management, and surgery are approaches used to treat **valvular disease**. The goal of treatment is to reverse the underlying cause of the disease and/or alleviate symptoms in more mild cases. Treatment of valvular disease depends on the degree and extent of disease as well as the presence of other comorbid conditions and the individual's overall health.

Pharmacologic treatment does not cure the condition but does relieve the symptoms of the disease and prevent further complications. Pharmacologic approaches used for valvular disease include vasodilators such as ACE inhibitors, anti-arrhythmic agents, antibiotics, anticoagulants such as Coumadin, diuretics such as furosemide and hydrochlorothiazide, and inotrope.

Surgical approaches include percutaneous balloon valvuloplasty, valvulotomy, cardiac valve repair or replacement, and minimally invasive heart surgery.

### *Prevention*

Congenital defects and infections such as rheumatic fever are the most common causes of valvular disease. Therefore, prompt treatment of streptococcal throat infections is necessary to prevent rheumatic fever. Also, addressing cardiovascular comorbid conditions and receiving proper treatment post myocardial infarction may prevent the onset of valvular disease. Also, proper treatment of connective tissue disease is important as is avoiding risk factors for endocarditis like IV drug use.

General preventive measures that individuals can take to reduce the risk of valvular disease and disease complications include maintaining proper lipid levels, blood pressure, and glucose levels; maintaining healthy weight and a healthy diet low in sodium and saturated fats; avoiding smoking; controlling diabetes; managing stress and anxiety; reducing alcohol consumption; and avoiding illicit drug use.

## Angina Pectoris

### *Treatment*

Treatment of **angina pectoris** involves lifestyle modifications, pharmacologic management, and surgery depending on the underlying causes of the condition. The type of treatment used depends on the extent and degree of the underlying cause of angina pectoris.

Pharmacologic management of angina pectoris involves use of antiplatelet agents such as aspirin, anticoagulants like heparin, beta-adrenergic blockers, lipid-lowering agents, nitrates such as nitroglycerin, isosorbide dinitrate and isosorbide mononitrate, and calcium channel blockers such as nifedipine, amlodipine, verapamil, and diltiazem.

Lifestyle modifications include weight loss for obese patients, reduction of saturated fats and sodium in diet, increase in physical activity, cessation of smoking, stress reduction and management, and cessation of alcohol and illicit drug use.

### *Prevention*

Addressing cardiovascular comorbid conditions and receiving proper treatment post myocardial infarction may prevent the onset of angina pectoris. Also, individuals with a family history of cardiovascular disease and/or a medical history of heart disease should monitor symptoms closely.

General **preventive measures** that individuals can take to reduce the risk of angina pectoris and disease complications include maintaining proper lipid levels, blood pressure, and glucose levels; maintaining healthy weight and a healthy diet low in sodium and saturated fats; avoiding smoking; controlling diabetes; managing stress and anxiety; reducing alcohol consumption; and avoiding illicit drug use.

## Arrhythmias

### *Treatment*

The treatment of **arrhythmia** depends on the type of arrhythmia including bradycardias, supraventricular tachycardias, and ventricular tachycardias. In addressing bradycardias, practicing clinicians will assess whether an underlying condition such as thyroid dysfunction is present and treat the underlying cause to correct the problem. Another approach with undetermined bradycardias or necessary medications includes the use of a pacemaker.

In addressing tachycardias originating either in the atria or ventricles, treatment may involve the use of vagal maneuvers such as straining or coughing, anti-arrhythmic agents, cardioversion, and cardiac ablation. Implantable devices such as a pacemaker or implantable cardiac defibrillator may also be used. In more severe cases, surgery may be performed, which involves the maze procedure, ventricular aneurysm surgery, or coronary bypass surgery.

Patients diagnosed with an arrhythmia will be recommended to make lifestyle changes that include maintaining a healthy diet low in saturated fats and sodium, increasing physical activity, quitting smoking, reducing caffeine and alcohol intake, reducing stress, and avoiding stimulants. Vagal maneuvers such as gagging, holding one's breath, and coughing may be recommended as well.

**Review Video: EKG Interpretation: Ventricular Arrhythmias**
Visit mometrix.com/academy and enter code: 933152

### *Prevention*

Addressing cardiovascular comorbid conditions and receiving proper treatment post myocardial infarction may prevent the onset of arrhythmias. Also, individuals with a family history of cardiovascular disease and/or a medical history of heart disease should pay careful attention to signs and symptoms of disease.

General **preventive measures** that individuals can take to reduce the risk of arrhythmias and disease complications include maintaining proper lipid levels, blood pressure, and glucose levels; maintaining healthy weight and a healthy diet low in sodium and saturated fats; avoiding smoking; controlling diabetes; managing stress and anxiety; reducing alcohol consumption; and avoiding illicit drug use.

## Atrial Fibrillation

### *Treatment*

The goals of treatment of **atrial fibrillation** include controlling heart rate, restoring sinus rhythm, controlling ventricular response, and preventing complications such as thromboembolism and other cardiovascular complications. Treatment approaches include lifestyle modifications, pharmaceutical management, and use of assistance devices. Electrical conduction management of the heart can be maintained with synchronized electrical cardioversion and permanent atrial pacemaker. Pharmacologic management of atrial fibrillation involves the use of use of beta-adrenergic blockers; digitalis antiplatelet agents like aspirin; anticoagulants such as Coumadin and heparin; antidysrhythmic agents; and calcium channel blockers such as nifedipine, amlodipine, verapamil, and diltiazem. Other pharmacologic agents used to treat comorbid cardiovascular conditions include lipid-lowering agents and nitrates such as nitroglycerin, isosorbide dinitrate, and isosorbide mononitrate. Note that rate control (beta-blockers, etc.) with anticoagulation is equivalent to rhythm control with respect to mortality. More invasive approaches include AV node ablation, radiofrequency catheter ablation, and surgical maze procedure.

### *Prevention*

Addressing cardiovascular comorbid conditions and receiving proper treatment post myocardial infarction may prevent the onset of atrial fibrillation. Also, individuals with a family history of cardiovascular disease and/or a medical history of heart disease should pay careful attention to their symptoms.

General **preventive measures** that individuals can take to reduce the risk of atrial fibrillation and disease complications include maintaining proper lipid levels, blood pressure, and glucose levels; maintaining healthy weight and a healthy diet low in sodium and saturated fats; avoiding smoking; controlling diabetes; managing stress and anxiety; reducing alcohol consumption; and avoiding illicit drug use. Also, it is important to make sure respiratory comorbidities like chronic obstructive pulmonary disease (COPD) are under control, as this is a common source of atrial fibrillation in the elderly.

## Atrial Flutter

### *Treatment*

Lifestyle modifications, pharmacologic management, and invasive approaches are used to treat **atrial flutter**, depending on the impact on quality of life and presence of other comorbid conditions. Treatment involves slowing the heart rate and restoring cardiac rhythm as well as prevention of blood clot formation.

Pharmacologic approaches used for the treatment of atrial flutter include calcium channel blockers such as diltiazem and verapamil; beta-blockers such as metoprolol and esmolol; class I anti-arrhythmics such as procainamide and quinidine; class III anti-arrhythmics such as amiodarone, dofetilide, and ibutilide; and cardiac glycosides such as digitalis.

More invasive approaches include cardioversion and catheter ablation. Patients diagnosed with atrial flutter respond better to catheter ablation than patients diagnosed with atrial fibrillation.

Patients diagnosed with atrial flutter will be recommended to make lifestyle changes that include maintaining a healthy diet low in saturated fats and sodium, increasing physical activity, quitting smoking, reducing caffeine and alcohol intake, reducing stress, and avoiding stimulants.

### *Prevention*

Addressing cardiovascular and respiratory comorbid conditions and receiving proper treatment post myocardial infarction may prevent the onset of atrial flutter or atrial fibrillation. Also, individuals with a family history of cardiovascular disease and/or a medical history of heart disease should pay careful attention to the signs and symptoms of disease.

General **preventive measures** that individuals can take to reduce the risk of atrial flutter and disease complications include maintaining proper lipid levels, blood pressure, and glucose levels; maintaining healthy weight and a healthy diet low in sodium and saturated fats; managing stress and anxiety; reducing alcohol consumption; and avoiding illicit drug use.

## Wolff-Parkinson-White Syndrome

### *Treatment*

Lifestyle modifications, pharmacologic management, and surgery are options for treatment of **Wolff-Parkinson-White syndrome**. The goal of treatment is to reduce tachycardia and restore normal heart rhythm.

Pharmacologic approaches used to treat Wolff-Parkinson-White syndrome include anti-arrhythmic agents such as adenosine and procainamide.

The most effective and curative approach for the treatment of Wolff-Parkinson-White syndrome is radiofrequency catheter ablation. Surgical destruction of the accessory pathway may be performed effectively, but radiofrequency catheter ablation is typically the most safe and efficacious curative approach.

Patients diagnosed with Wolff-Parkinson-White syndrome will be recommended to make lifestyle changes that include maintaining a healthy diet low in saturated fats and sodium, increasing physical activity, quitting smoking, reducing caffeine and alcohol intake, reducing stress, and avoiding stimulants. Other vagal maneuvers may be recommended to reduce a patient's heart rate, including coughing and bearing down as during a bowel movement.

### *Prevention*

Wolff-Parkinson White syndrome is not preventable, but not all patients develop symptoms. Addressing cardiovascular comorbid conditions and receiving proper treatment post myocardial infarction may prevent the onset of complications associated with Wolff-Parkinson-White syndrome. Also, addressing modifiable risk factors and addressing other cardiovascular comorbid conditions promptly will reduce the likelihood of complications associated with the syndrome.

General **preventive measures** that individuals can take to reduce the risk of disease complications include maintaining proper lipid levels, blood pressure, and glucose levels; maintaining healthy weight and a healthy diet low in sodium and saturated fats; exercising regularly; avoiding smoking; controlling diabetes; managing stress and anxiety; reducing alcohol consumption; and avoiding illicit drug use.

## Ventricular Fibrillation

### *Treatment*

**Ventricular fibrillation** is a serious medical condition that should be treated as a medical emergency. If an individual is suspected of having an acute ventricular fibrillation episode, then a practicing clinician may perform cardiopulmonary resuscitation and shock the heart using an external defibrillator. The goal of treatment is to restore normal heart rhythm to reestablish proper cardiac output and blood oxygenation. The shock is given as soon as possible and, if a defibrillator is available, even before cardiopulmonary resuscitation (CPR).

Pharmacologic agents will also be administered to control the individual's heart rate and function. Pharmacologic agents used to treat ventricular fibrillation include vasopressors or sympathomimetics such as epinephrine; antidysrhythmic agents such as lidocaine, amiodarone, bretylium tosylate, and procainamide; and electrolytes such as magnesium sulfate, sodium bicarbonate, and calcium chloride. A more invasive approach includes the use of an implantable cardiac defibrillator post an acute ventricular fibrillation episode to prevent sudden cardiac death.

### *Prevention*

Addressing cardiovascular comorbid conditions and receiving proper treatment post ventricular fibrillation may prevent the onset of complications associated with the condition. Also, addressing modifiable risk factors and other cardiovascular comorbid conditions promptly will reduce the likelihood of complications associated with the condition.

General **preventive measures** that individuals can take to reduce the risk of ventricular fibrillation and complications associated with the condition include exercising regularly; maintaining proper lipid levels, blood pressure, and glucose levels; maintaining healthy weight and a healthy diet low in sodium and saturated fats; avoiding smoking; controlling diabetes; managing stress and anxiety; reducing alcohol consumption; and avoiding illicit drug use.

## Ventricular Tachycardia

### *Treatment*

Treatment of **ventricular tachycardia** depends on the degree and extent of the condition. It also varies according to the individual patient, patient's general health, and presence of other comorbid conditions. In some individuals, emergency management is necessary, and in others, no treatment is required. Treatment involves lifestyle modifications, pharmacologic management and, in more severe cases, surgical approaches.

If an individual has acute ventricular tachycardia and is pulseless or symptomatic, defibrillation is necessary. Cardiopulmonary resuscitation (CPR) is also often necessary. The goal of treatment is to restore normal heart rhythm to reestablish proper cardiac output and blood oxygenation.

Pharmacologic management of ventricular tachycardia involves treatment with antiarrhythmic agents such as lidocaine, procainamide, amiodarone, sotalol, mexiletine, acebutolol, atenolol, metoprolol, flecainide, propafenone, and quinidine.

### *Prevention*

Addressing cardiovascular comorbid conditions and receiving proper treatment post ventricular tachycardia may prevent the onset of complications associated with the condition. Also, addressing modifiable risk factors and addressing other cardiovascular comorbid conditions promptly will reduce the likelihood of complications associated with the condition.

General **preventive measures** that individuals can take to reduce the risk of ventricular tachycardia and complications associated with the condition include maintaining proper lipid levels, blood pressure, and glucose levels; maintaining healthy weight and a healthy diet low in sodium and saturated fats; exercising regularly; avoiding smoking; controlling diabetes; managing stress and anxiety; reducing alcohol consumption; and avoiding illicit drug use.

## Intermittent Claudication

### *Treatment*

Lifestyle modifications, pharmacologic management, and, in more severe cases, surgical interventions are used for the treatment of **intermittent claudication.**

Lifestyle modifications include treatment of other comorbid cardiovascular diseases, management of hypertension and high cholesterol, maintenance of proper glucose levels, increased physical activity, compliance with diabetes treatment, cessation of smoking, and/or avoidance of alcohol or illicit drug use.

Pharmacologic agents used to treat intermittent claudication include pentoxifylline and cilostazol, which act by dilating blood vessels, increasing blood flow to the extremities, and reducing clot formation. Surgical approaches used for patients with peripheral arterial disease and intermittent claudication include angioplasty and cardiopulmonary bypass surgery. Other surgical approaches used for peripheral arterial disease and intermittent claudication include transcatheter intervention and peripheral vascular bypass.

### *Prevention*

Lifestyle modifications and pharmacologic management can prevent the onset of arteriosclerosis, peripheral arterial disease, and intermittent claudication. Patients should maintain a diet low in sodium and saturated fats, increase potassium intake, increase exercise and physical activity, avoid smoking and tobacco use, lose excess weight, avoid beta-blockers and illicit drug use, maintain proper lipid levels, maintain proper glucose levels, and maintain proper albumin excretion and creatinine levels.

Patients with peripheral arterial disease and intermittent claudication should maintain their feet to prevent the onset of complications such as infections and gangrene. Patients should wash and moisturize their feet daily, wear thick socks and comfortable shoes, promptly treat fungal infections, trim toenails, avoid walking barefoot, and have sores and open wounds treated immediately.

> **Review Video: Treating Wound Infections**
> Visit mometrix.com/academy and enter code: 761736

## Hypotension

### *Treatment*

If a drop in blood pressure (**hypotension**) is acute and life threatening, vasopressors (norepinephrine) may be necessary. Treatment of the underlying cause is of primary concern, such as antibiotics for infection or defibrillation for arrhythmia. Lifestyle modifications and pharmacologic management are used to treat chronic hypotension. The type of treatment depends on the degree and extent of hypotension as well as the underlying cause of the condition. Treatment varies by the symptoms that the patient presents.

Lifestyle modifications include dietary changes like increased salt intake if no other comorbid cardiovascular conditions are present, increased fluid intake, as well as the use of graduated compression stockings. Other modifications include avoiding alcohol and illicit drug use, smoking, and prolonged heat exposure; maintaining a healthy diet; and eating small meals every few hours.

Pharmacologic agents used to treat hypotension include fludrocortisone, pyridostigmine, nonsteroidal anti-inflammatory drugs, erythropoietin, and/or caffeine.

### Prevention

Lifestyle modifications and pharmacologic management prevent the onset of hypotension. Patients should maintain a diet high in sodium if they do not have any other cardiovascular comorbidities, increase potassium intake, increase exercise and physical activity, avoid smoking and tobacco use, lose excess weight, avoid alcohol and illicit drug use, maintain proper lipid levels, maintain proper glucose levels, and maintain proper albumin excretion and creatinine levels.

The following lifestyle modifications may prevent serious complications associated with hypotension: getting up slowly when sitting (for patients with orthostatic hypotension); avoiding standing for long periods of time (for patients with neurally mediated hypotension); eating small, low carbohydrate meals; drinking plenty of fluids; avoiding alcohol and tobacco use; increasing salt intake if no other cardiovascular comorbid conditions exist; using graduated compression stockings; and maintaining daily physical activity.

## Hypertension

### Treatment

The treatment of **hypertension** involves lifestyle modification and pharmacologic management. Lifestyle modifications include weight loss, diet low in saturated fats and sodium, physical activity, smoking cessation, limiting tobacco use, and stress reduction.

The goals of pharmacologic management include reduction of blood pressure in order to prevent onset of comorbid conditions and/or complications. Pharmacologic agents include diuretics such as hydrochlorothiazide, spironolactone, amiloride, and furosemide; alpha-1-adrenergic blockers including prazosin; beta-adrenergic blockers such as atenolol; alpha/beta-adrenergic blockers such as labetalol; peripheral vasodilators such as hydralazine; calcium channel blockers such as diltiazem; angiotensin-converting enzyme inhibitors such as captopril; angiotensin II receptor antagonists such as losartan; aldosterone antagonists such as eplerenone; alpha-adrenergic agonists such as methyldopa; and renin inhibitors such as aliskiren.

Patients with diabetes and/or renal disease should be treated with pharmacologic approaches at a blood pressure of 130/80 mmHg or below due to increased risk of cardiovascular events.

### Prevention

Certain risk factors such as having a genetic predisposition for hypertension and natural aging are not preventable. However, certain lifestyle modifications can help prevent the onset of the condition by having individuals maintain a diet low in sodium and saturated fats, increase potassium intake, increase exercise and physical activity, avoid smoking and tobacco use, lose excess weight, maintain proper lipid levels, maintain proper sugar levels, and maintain proper albumin excretion and creatinine levels.

Treatment of comorbid conditions is necessary to prevent the onset of secondary hypertension. Also, individuals being prescribed oral contraceptives, NSAIDs, or other pharmacologic agents that can elevate blood pressure should monitor their blood pressure on a daily basis if they are at risk for hypertension or cardiovascular complications.

## Compartment Syndrome

### Treatment

Although lifestyle modifications and pharmacologic management may be effective for **compartment syndrome**, surgical intervention is the most effective approach to management of acute and chronic disease. The pressure and swelling in the compartment can be relieved by a long incision in the fascia of the compartment. The incision is typically left open for 48–72 hours post initial surgery, and then a second surgery is performed to close the incision. With larger incisions, skin grafts may be used to close the incision.

If a tight cast or bandage causes the problem, then the bandage and/or cast should be loosened to relieve the syndrome.

### *Prevention*

Although little can be done to prevent the onset of compartment syndrome, patient education and increased awareness is important for prompt diagnosis and treatment in individuals who have a history of the condition or other comorbid cardiovascular or respiratory risk factors.

Patients should also maintain a diet low in sodium and saturated fats, increase potassium intake, increase exercise and physical activity, avoid smoking and tobacco use, lose excess weight, avoid beta-blockers and illicit drug use, maintain proper lipid levels, maintain proper glucose levels, and maintain proper albumin excretion and creatinine levels.

## Pulmonary Edema

### *Treatment*

Lifestyle modifications, pharmacologic management, and, in more severe cases, ventilatory support, are used to treat **pulmonary edema**. In acute pulmonary edema, oxygen is immediately administered to prevent tissue damage.

Pharmacologic management depends on the underlying cause of pulmonary edema and the presence of other cardiovascular comorbid conditions. Pharmacologic agents used to treat pulmonary edema include preload reducers such as nitroglycerin; diuretics such as furosemide; morphine; afterload reducers such as nitroprusside, enalapril, and captopril; aspirin; and blood-pressure agents.

In treating patients with high altitude-induced pulmonary edema, patients should descend a few thousand feet and carry oxygen with them. Pharmacologic management with acetazolamide may be beneficial.

### *Prevention*

Although little can be done to prevent the onset of pulmonary edema, patient education and increased awareness in individuals with a history of the condition or who have other comorbid cardiovascular or respiratory risk factors is important for prompt diagnosis and treatment.

Patients should also maintain a diet low in sodium and saturated fats, increase potassium intake, increase exercise and physical activity, avoid smoking and tobacco use, get enough folic acid, manage stress, lose excess weight, avoid beta-blockers and illicit drug use, maintain proper lipid levels, maintain proper glucose levels, and maintain proper albumin excretion and creatinine levels.

If traveling or climbing at high altitudes, individuals should acclimate themselves slowly but ascend no more than 1,000–2,000 feet per day once they have reached 8,000 feet. Patients at risk for high altitude-induced pulmonary edema should also make sure to drink plenty of fluids and bring oxygen with them.

## First-Degree Atrioventricular Block

### *Treatment*

Lifestyle modifications and pharmacologic management may be used to treat **first-degree atrioventricular block**, but most patients diagnosed with the condition do not require treatment. Patients with asymptomatic first-degree atrioventricular block do not require treatment. However, patients who present with symptoms should discontinue medication that could be contributing to the atrioventricular block or seek electrophysiological consultation.

Pharmacologic agents that may be used to treat first-degree atrioventricular block include parasympathetic blockers such as atropine and sympathomimetics such as isoproterenol. Patients undergoing pharmacologic management should be monitored to make sure their condition does not progress to a higher degree of atrioventricular block.

For patients who present with severe bradycardia, syncope, and left ventricular systolic dysfunction, a pacemaker may be required.

### *Prevention*

Typically, first-degree atrioventricular blocks are not preventable unless induced by pharmacologic drugs; then the drug can be stopped or titrated down. However, it remains unclear if a particular drug will induce a first-degree atrioventricular block, as it depends on the patient. Yet, certain drugs have been known to cause the condition.

In order to prevent progression to higher degrees of atrioventricular block, patients should be monitored by their practicing clinician, especially patients with concomitant bundle-brachial blocks.

Patients should also maintain a diet low in sodium and saturated fats, increase potassium intake, increase exercise and physical activity, avoid smoking and tobacco use, get enough folic acid, manage stress, lose excess weight, avoid beta-blockers and illicit drug use, maintain proper lipid levels, maintain proper glucose levels, and maintain proper albumin excretion and creatinine levels.

## Second-Degree Atrioventricular Block Type I

### *Treatment*

The treatment of **second-degree atrioventricular block type I** depends on the presence or absence of symptoms. Treatment also varies based on the extent and degree of the condition and the presence of other comorbid cardiovascular conditions. In patients diagnosed with second-degree atrioventricular block type I with few or no symptoms, treatment may not be necessary. However, asymptomatic patients that present with intra- or infra- bundle blocks may require a pacemaker. A pacemaker may also be required for patients who present with bradycardia, heart failure, myocardial infarction, and asystole greater than or equal to 3 seconds. Additionally, patients who present with comorbid Lyme disease, drug toxicity, and hypoxia associated with sleep apnea may require treatment and modifications of drug dosing and/or lifestyle changes.

Anticholinergic agents such as atropine sulfate may be used to treat the condition, but pacemaker placement is considered standard of care when necessary.

### *Prevention*

Typically, second-degree atrioventricular blocks type I are not preventable unless induced by pharmacologic drugs, and then the drug can be stopped or titrated down.

In order to **prevent progression** to higher degrees of atrioventricular block, patients should be monitored by their practicing clinician, especially patients with concomitant bundle-branch blocks.

Patients should also maintain a diet low in sodium and saturated fats, increase potassium intake, increase exercise and physical activity, avoid smoking and tobacco use, get enough folic acid, manage stress, lose excess weight, avoid beta-blockers and illicit drug use, maintain proper lipid levels, maintain proper glucose levels, and maintain proper albumin excretion and creatinine levels.

## Second-Degree Atrioventricular Block Type II

### *Treatment*

Treatment of **second-degree atrioventricular block type II** varies according to the extent and degree of the condition and the presence of other comorbid cardiovascular conditions. The goal of treatment is to restore sinus rhythm or maintain cardiac output.

A pacemaker may be required for patients who present with bradycardia, heart failure, myocardial infarction, wide QRS complexes, and asystole greater than or equal to 3 seconds. Additionally, patients who present with comorbid Lyme disease, drug toxicity, and hypoxia associated with sleep apnea may require treatment and modifications of drug dosing and/or lifestyle.

Anticholinergic agents such as atropine sulfate may be used to treat the condition, but pacemaker placement is considered standard of care. Also, in patients with extensive symptoms, isoproterenol and dopamine may be used to achieve hemodynamic stability until a pacemaker can be placed.

### *Prevention*

Typically, second-degree atrioventricular type II blocks are not preventable unless induced by pharmacologic drugs, and then the drug can be stopped or titrated down. In order to prevent progression to higher degrees of atrioventricular block, patients should be monitored by their practicing clinician, especially patients with concomitant bundle-branch blocks.

Furthermore, family members and/or caregivers should be taught cardiopulmonary resuscitation (CPR) and how to contact emergency medical services in the event of cardiac arrest. Pacemaker education is necessary to make sure that patients do not have a problem with the battery or the device.

Patients should also maintain a diet low in sodium and saturated fats, increase potassium intake, increase exercise and physical activity, avoid smoking and tobacco use, get enough folic acid, manage stress, lose excess weight, avoid beta-blockers and illicit drug use, maintain proper lipid levels, maintain proper glucose levels, and maintain proper albumin excretion and creatinine levels.

## Third-Degree Atrioventricular Block

### *Treatment*

Lifestyle modifications, pharmacologic management, and pacemaker implantation are the key treatment approaches for **third-degree atrioventricular block.** New-onset third-degree atrioventricular block is a medical emergency, and treatment is dependent on the extent and degree of the block.

Patients undergoing treatment with pharmacologic agents that target the atrioventricular node should stop or titrate down the medication to help resolve the complete atrioventricular block.

Complete heart block associated with repeated abnormal pulse, inadequate escape rhythm, or block below the atrioventricular node should be treated immediately with a pacemaker or pacing agents.

Patients with third-degree atrioventricular block and bradycardia, other arrhythmias, and neuromuscular diseases should receive a permanent pacemaker. Individuals who undergo catheter ablation or with documented periods of asystole greater than or equal to 3 seconds should be considered for a pacemaker.

Individuals diagnosed with third-degree atrioventricular block should be on bedrest to avoid further complications. Sympathomimetic agents such as atropine and isoproterenol hydrochloride can be used to treat third-degree atrioventricular block, but pacemaker placement is standard of care in most cases.

#### *Prevention*

Typically, third-degree atrioventricular blocks are not preventable unless induced by pharmacologic drugs, and then the drug can be stopped or titrated down. Furthermore, family members and/or caregivers should learn cardiopulmonary resuscitation (CPR) and how to contact emergency medical services (EMS) in the event of cardiac arrest. Pacemaker education is necessary to make sure that patients do not have a problem with the battery or the device.

Patients should also maintain a diet low in sodium and saturated fats, increase potassium intake, increase exercise and physical activity, avoid smoking and tobacco use, get enough folic acid, manage stress, lose excess weight, avoid beta-blockers and illicit drug use, maintain proper lipid levels, maintain proper glucose levels, and maintain proper albumin excretion and creatinine levels.



### Cardiogenic Shock

#### *Treatment Goals*

Treatment of **cardiogenic shock** requires emergency and prompt attention to restore blood flow to various end organ systems. The goal of treatment is to initially treat the shock and then to treat the underlying cause of cardiogenic shock. Emergency life support treatment is required for cardiogenic shock, which aims to restore blood flow to brain, kidney, and other end organ systems. Patients experiencing cardiogenic shock will be given oxygen as well as fluids, including blood products. The goal of pharmacologic treatment is to reduce mortality and morbidity as well as to prevent further complications.

#### *Pharmacologic and Surgical Interventions*

**Pharmacologic agents** used to treat cardiogenic shock include vasopressors such as dopamine and dobutamine, phosphodiesterase enzyme inhibitors such as milrinone and inamrinone, vasodilators such as nitroglycerin, analgesics such as morphine sulfate, diuretics such as furosemide, and natriuretic peptides such as nesiritide.

More invasive **surgical approaches** used to treat cardiogenic shock include intra-aortic balloon pump and angioplasty. Other surgical approaches used to treat the underlying cause of cardiogenic shock include coronary artery bypass surgery, surgery to repair damaged cardiac valves, surgery to repair the wall between heart chambers, left ventricular assist device implantation, and heart transplant.

#### *Prevention*

Although little can be done to prevent the onset of cardiogenic shock, patient education and increased awareness is important for prompt diagnosis and treatment in individuals with a history of the condition or who have other comorbid cardiovascular or respiratory risk factors. Prevention of cardiac disease and/or myocardial infarction is the best way to prevent the onset of cardiogenic shock. Prompt treatment of myocardial infarction and/or heart disease may prevent the onset of cardiogenic shock.

Patients should also maintain a diet low in sodium and saturated fats, increase potassium intake, increase exercise and physical activity, avoid smoking and tobacco use, get enough folic acid, manage stress, lose excess weight, avoid beta-blockers and illicit drug use, maintain proper lipid levels, maintain proper sugar levels, and maintain proper albumin excretion and creatinine levels.

## Aortic Regurgitation

### *Treatment Priorities*

**Aortic regurgitation** is a condition created by valve inadequacy, affecting the flow of blood from the aorta into the left ventricle, that causes audible variances (murmur) in the heartbeat. Common causes include rheumatic heart disease and bacterial endocarditis. Whenever possible, treatment for aortic regurgitation is focused on surgical repair of the defective valve.

Heart rate and oxygen saturation levels should be monitored and medications such as inotropes, vasodilators, glycosides, and antibiotics should be administered to promote stabilization while preparing for surgery. If surgical intervention is not possible, chronic and/or end-of-life treatment plans should begin.

# Evaluation and Modification

## Important Note About This Section

Because the ANCC organizes the tested content into domains based on the type of nursing action involved rather than the disease process or body system involved, most of the content that would fall under this domain has already appeared in one of the two preceding sections. We have chosen to organize our guide in this way because we believe that this is the most coherent and useful presentation of the content for someone looking for a complete refresher on the conditions and nursing interventions most relevant to the exam and to their nursing practice.

### Common Cardiac Drug Interactions

#### *Digoxin*

Antacids, amiloride, cholestyramine, neomycin, and sulfasalazine reduce the effect of **digoxin**. Herbal remedies such as plantain and St. John's wort may also decrease effectiveness.

Albuterol, amiodarone, captopril, cyclosporine, diltiazem, erythromycin, nifedipine, omeprazole, quinidine, tetracycline, thyroxin, and verapamil can cause higher blood levels of digoxin and risk toxicity. Herbal remedies of gossypol, horsetail, licorice, oleander, Siberian ginseng, and squill (scilla) also carry a greater risk for digoxin toxicity.

Betel pal, fumitory, goldenseal, hawthorn, lily of the valley, motherwort, rue, and shepherd's purse should be avoided completely.

Therapeutic digoxin blood levels are 0.8–2.0 ng/mL. Monitor lab results and pulse prior to each administration of digoxin.

#### *Warfarin Sodium (Coumadin)*

Multiple medications will react with **Coumadin** and vary the effectiveness. Monitor PT and INR levels closely to maintain therapeutic levels. Review all medications and supplements carefully. Pay special attention to pain relievers, hormones (oral contraceptives, testosterone, estrogen, and thyroid), steroids, hypolipidemics, antidiabetics, antibiotics, and tricyclic antidepressants. Most common herbal remedies, including garlic, ginger, ginkgo, ginseng, licorice, and angelica, should not be combined with warfarin use. Alcohol use should be minimized, and any source of vitamin K (green leafy vegetables, vitamin supplements, and green tea) should be kept at a constant level.

#### *Lipitor*

Antacids, colestipol, and isradipine may decrease the effectiveness of **Lipitor**. Erythromycin, fluconazole, itraconazole, ketoconazole, and voriconazole may increase Lipitor blood levels. Lipitor also interacts unfavorably with digoxin and contraceptives, changing the effectiveness of these medications. Lipitor in combination with antifungal, cyclosporine, erythromycin, fibric acid, and niacin can increase the risk of developing muscle weakness. Herbal supplements including eucalyptus, kava, and red yeast rice can cause adverse reactions. Grapefruit juice should not be ingested while taking Lipitor. Use cautiously in the patient with a known history of heavy alcohol use and liver and/or renal disease.

## Urgent vs. Emergent Cardiovascular Conditions

**Urgent cardiovascular conditions** are not immediately life-threatening but require intervention within 24–48 hours to minimize life-threatening progression. Examples of urgent cardiovascular conditions include the following:

- **New onset shortness of breath or dizziness on exertion that resolves at rest**: May indicate worsening of a heart condition and should be investigated.
- **Changes in color or size (swelling) of extremities**: May indicate congestive heart failure (swelling) or vascular disease (color).
- **Severe intermittent claudication**: Indication of severe peripheral artery disease and possible vessel occlusion.
- **Pseudoaneurysm**: A false aneurysm that may occur post percutaneous intervention at the site of catheter injection. This may go unnoticed, but if greater than 2 cm in diameter, it may require surgical or ultrasound-guided intervention.

**Emergent cardiovascular conditions** are life-threatening and require immediate intervention in order to sustain survival. Most new onset cardiovascular symptoms are considered emergent. Examples of emergent cardiovascular conditions include indications of the following:

- **Cardiac arrest**: Requires immediate cardiac resuscitation measures.
- **Myocardial infarction**: Requires immediate percutaneous intervention/investigation and possibly open-heart surgery. May lead to cardiac arrest if untreated.
- **Stroke**: Ischemic strokes may require administration of tPA or other anticoagulation measures. Hemorrhagic strokes may require surgical evacuation.
- **Pulmonary embolism**: Requires immediate respiratory support and anticoagulation.
- **Flash pulmonary edema**: Causes respiratory distress due to pulmonary congestion, requiring respiratory support and intense diuresis.

# Patient and Community Education

## Cardiac-Vascular Risk Factors

### Modifiable and Nonmodifiable Risk Factors

**Risk factors** that the patient and their healthcare provider can exercise some control over are identified as **modifiable**. These can include smoking, excess weight, alcohol use, cholesterol levels, blood pressure, active management of diabetes, stress, and the amount of exercise the patient engages in.

Risk factors beyond the patient's control are considered **nonmodifiable** and include age, male gender, and genetic tendencies including race (Caucasian, black, or Native American) and family history.

The greatest risk is to those who have already experienced a cardiovascular event or have been previously diagnosed with a cardiovascular disease such as peripheral vascular disease, aortic aneurysm, or carotid artery disease. Others with high risk include those who have at least two of the modifiable or nonmodifiable risk factors or type II diabetes.

### NCEP Risk Calculator

Patients diagnosed with metabolic syndrome should have their **10-year risk of developing cardiovascular disease** calculated by a specialist.

The National Cholesterol Education Program (NCEP) provides a risk calculator of developing cardiovascular disease within the next 10 years:

- Individuals with a 10-year risk score higher than 20% are considered at high risk for developing cardiovascular disease.
- Individuals with a 10-year risk score of 10–20% are considered at moderately high risk for developing cardiovascular disease.
- Individuals with a 10-year risk score less than 10% are considered at moderate risk for developing cardiovascular disease.
- Individuals with a 10-year risk score of 0–1% are considered at low risk for developing cardiovascular disease.

### Cardiovascular Risk Factors

**Cardiovascular risk factors** include:

- **Ethnicity**: Prevalence of heart disease varies according to ethnicity, as follows: Non-Hispanic white adults 11.5%, non-Hispanic black adults 9.5%, Hispanic adults 7.45%, and non-Hispanic Asians adults 6.0%. However, mortality rates (according to the CDC) related to heart disease show a different story, with non-Hispanic blacks having the highest rate of death (208) per 100,000 population, followed by non-Hispanic white (168.9), Hispanics (114.1), and Asian or Pacific Islander (85.5). Non-Hispanic black adults have the highest rate of hypertension, and Hispanics and non-Hispanic black adults have high rates of obesity and diabetes, although their rate of high total cholesterol is the lowest among ethnic groups.

- **Smoking**: Chemicals in tobacco products may damage blood cells and the structure and function of both the heart and the vessels, especially if smoking is associated with other risk factors, such as hypertension and obesity. Smoking increases plaque formation and is associated with PAD.
- **Age**: Risk of heart disease increases in those over age 65 because the normal changes in the cardiovascular system associated with age may contribute to disease, especially if other risk factors are present.

## COPD

**Chronic obstructive pulmonary disease (COPD)** and chronic heart disease (CHD) share a common causative factor: smoking. Priority preventive care and education would focus on smoking cessation for the patient presenting with COPD; this will in turn lower their risk of CHD.

The patient presenting with COPD is at a greater risk for cardiac and vascular problems such as pulmonary hypertension and right ventricular heart failure (cor pulmonale). Likewise, the patient with both cardiovascular problems and COPD is faced with a higher mortality rate than the patient with only one condition. COPD also complicates and slows recovery from chronic heart disease and surgical procedures that might be used in the treatment of CHD.

### Diabetes

**Diabetes mellitus** is a significant risk factor for cardiovascular disease. The patient with diabetes should be treated as if they already have cardiovascular disease when addressing treatment and risk factor reduction. Approximately two thirds of all individuals diagnosed with diabetes will die as a result of cardiovascular disease. This is particularly alarming when considering the rapid growth trends for newly diagnosed diabetics. Highest priority is given to maintaining an HbA1c level at or below 7. Complications such as retinopathy, microalbuminuria, neuropathy, and elevated cholesterol levels can be reduced with tight blood sugar control. Careful blood sugar maintenance is also required after surgical procedures to reduce the risks of infection and delayed healing.

### Cerebrovascular Disease

Cardiovascular disease and cerebrovascular disease, most commonly chronic heart disease and carotid artery occlusive disease, are often **coexisting** because of their overlapping risk factors. Cerebrovascular accident (CVA) is the third leading cause of death in the United States and can be directly linked to atherosclerosis. The patient experiencing dysrhythmia, MI, or cardiopulmonary arrest is at increased risk for subsequent acute cerebrovascular injury. Cardiac and vascular surgeries can also result in CVAs. On the other end of the spectrum, the patient experiencing a CVA is less likely to survive if they also have chronic heart disease.

### Renovascular Disease

A history of hypertension is positively related to the development of renal disease. In turn, the presence of **renovascular disease** and its progression to end-stage renal disease (ESRD) and chronic renal failure can often lead to the development of heart failure, hypertrophic cardiomyopathy, and coronary atherosclerosis. The presence of renovascular disease complicates the risk factors of surgical interventions that might be considered for the treatment of cardiovascular disease. Highest nursing concerns will often focus on blood pressure and electrolyte and fluid balances. Medications used to treat cardiac conditions often need to be adjusted and more closely monitored to accommodate for the reduced kidney function.

# Education Topics

## Education for Patients with Acute or Chronic Illnesses

The following topics should be covered in education for the patient with acute or chronic illnesses:

- **Diagnosis**: Establish a basic understanding of the disease process, including areas of body affected, causes, prognosis, and whether or not it is contagious.
- **Complications**: Clarify possible signs and symptoms, early warning signs, and signals of disease progression and healing.
- **Management**: Define what the patient can expect from their care and recovery, including treatments, diet, activity levels, and medications.
- **Aggravating factors**: Help the patient understand what behaviors or triggers may increase their symptoms and what can be done to avoid or control them.
- **Prognosis**: Patients need both an immediate idea as well as a long-term picture of what to expect.
- **Prevention**: Establish self-care habits that can help prevent recurrence of the problem.
- **Resources**: Make sure the patient is informed of all available resources for help on their healthcare journey.

## Education for Patient/Family Experiencing Heart Failure

According to the American Heart Association (AHA), American Association of Heart Failure Nurses (AAHFN), and the Heart Failure Society of America (HFSA), the following are topics to be addressed in patient and family education for those experiencing heart failure:

- **Disease process**: Heart failure causes and disease progression should be covered. This teaching should include signs and symptoms of worsening conditions and self-monitoring techniques such as daily weights.
- **Life expectancy**: The patient should have a clear understanding of the length and quality of life they will experience as part of the disease process. End-of-life choices should be discussed, and advanced directives should be reviewed.
- **Activity levels**: Based on the current stage of the disease and diagnostic testing, parameters should be set for all activities of daily life.
- **Diet**: Detailed instruction on what constitutes a low-sodium diet is generally required; fluid restriction may also be needed.
- **Medications**: Education regarding medications should include clear and written instructions regarding dosage, timing, and frequency of each administration as well as what the expected treatment result will be, common side effects, interactions, and negative reactions.
- **Therapeutic support**: Every effort should be made to encourage compliance with treatment plans and acceptance of referrals to other health and education resources for top priority health needs such as smoking cessation and mental health.

## Necessary Teaching for Invasive Treatment Procedures

For invasive treatment procedures, the following teaching is needed:

- **Preoperative**: Provide information regarding the procedure, including who will be present in the room and each of their respective functions, what sights and sounds are typical, sensations and amount of discomfort expected both during and after the procedure, and an estimate of the amount of time required for the procedure. Review consents and other documentation, including living will/advanced directives.

- **Postoperative**: Review the procedure and its outcomes, and provide visual documentation of the procedure, including before and after images of the area(s) treated. Assess pain and instruct patient and family about expected pain levels and locations during recovery. Review expected progression of activity levels. Review what constitutes an emergency and how to contact help in the event of an emergency. Provide clear written instructions. Review all medications with clear written instructions and follow-up care plans as well as referrals to other institutes that promote further wellness interventions.

## Education Needs Prior to Discharge for Recovering CABG Patients

The education needs prior to discharge for the recovering coronary artery bypass graft (CABG) patient are discussed below:

- Notify the doctor of signs and symptoms of infection at the incision sites (leg and chest) or postpericardiotomy syndrome (fever, muscle and joint pain, weakness, and chest discomfort).
- Seek medical care immediately if the patient experiences symptoms of heart failure or myocardial infarction.
- Monitor weight and notify the doctor if there is a sudden gain.
- Verbalize explanations and tips for following prescribed diet, activity, rest, and exercise programs, including cardiac rehabilitation.
- Obtain written and verbal instructions regarding all medications, including purpose, dose, frequency, and common side effects.
- Accept referrals and information for lifestyle modifications such as smoking cessation and other support organizations.

## Postpericardiotomy Syndrome

Postpericardiotomy syndrome (PPS) is an inflammatory response most often occurring when a patient has undergone a surgical procedure involving the pericardium. Symptoms can develop 1–6 weeks after surgery. The key symptom is high fever (even if the patient has no other complaints of illness). Other symptoms might include malaise, chest or lung pain, trouble breathing, joint pain, irritability, and lack of appetite. Physical examination and testing will often exhibit friction rubs, pleural effusions, lung inflammation, and cardiac tamponade. Laboratory testing results show negative cultures but high erythrocyte sedimentation rate (ESR), C-reactive protein (CRP), and anti-heart antibodies. Treatment involves pericardial draining and anti-inflammatory medications.

## Teaching Needs for PCI

The patient and family teaching needs for percutaneous coronary intervention (PCI) are as follows:

- **Preoperative**: Information regarding the procedure, including who will be present in the room and each of their respective functions, what sights and sounds are typical, sensations and amount of discomfort expected during and after the procedure, and an estimate of the amount of time required for the procedure. Review consents and other documentation, including advanced directives.
- **Postoperative**: Review the procedure and its outcomes, and provide visual documentation of the procedure, including before and after images of the lesions. Assess pain and instruct patient and family about expected pain levels and locations (chest, back, insertion site) during recovery. Review what constitutes an emergency and how to contact help in the event of an emergency. Provide clear written instructions. Review all medications (aspirin, antiplatelets, beta-blockers, antihypertensives, antilipidemics, and nitrates) with clear written instructions. Review diet and activity expectations and progression, including

referrals to consultations for diet or lifestyle modifications and cardiac rehabilitation. Define follow-up care plans as well as referrals to other institutes that promote further wellness interventions.

### Teaching Needs for Pacemaker Placement

Patient and family teaching needs for pacemaker placement are as follows:

- **Preoperative**: Information regarding the procedure, including who will be present in the room and each of their respective functions, what sights and sounds are typical, sensations and amount of discomfort expected during and after the procedure, and an estimate of the amount of time required for the procedure. Review consents and other documentation, including advanced directives.
- **Postoperative**: Review the procedure and its outcomes. Assess pain and instruct patient and family about expected and unexpected pain levels and locations (chest, insertion site) during recovery. Review what constitutes an emergency and how to contact help in the event of an emergency. Provide clear written instructions. Review all medications (including antibiotics) with clear written instructions and follow-up care plans as well as referrals to other institutes that promote further wellness interventions. Review activity expectations and progression, including referrals to consultations for diet or lifestyle modifications and cardiac rehabilitation. Review lifestyle modifications, including carrying a pacemaker identification card and informing all healthcare providers (including dentists) of the pacemaker. Include safety precautions: may safely operate microwaves and cell phones but should avoid high-strength radiation fields such as MRI.

### Teaching Needs for Carotid Endarterectomy

Patient and family teaching needs for carotid endarterectomy are as follows:

- **Preoperative**: Information regarding the procedure, including who will be present in the room and each of their respective functions, what sights and sounds are typical, sensations and amount of discomfort expected during and after the procedure, and an estimate of the amount of time required for the procedure. Review consents and other documentation, including advanced directives.
- **Postoperative**: Review the procedure and its outcomes, providing visual documentation of the procedure. Assess pain and instruct patient and family about expected pain levels and locations (chest, back, insertion site) during recovery. Review what constitutes an emergency (including neurological impairment) and how to contact help in the event of an emergency. Provide clear written instructions. Review all medications (aspirin, clopidogrel) with clear written instructions and follow-up care plans as well as referrals to other institutes that promote further wellness interventions. Review diet and activity expectations and progression, including referrals to consultations for diet and weight loss or lifestyle modifications for hypertension, cholesterol, diabetes management, and smoking cessation.

### Areas of Education Regarding Dental Care

Good oral hygiene and regular **dental visits** should be maintained, as the presence of periodontal disease can reflect the state of the patient's cardiac health as well. Dentists need to be informed of all medications the patient is on, especially blood thinners, prior to visits. Make the dental practitioner aware of any past experiences with anxiety related to dental care, as stress-reduction protocols may need to be followed to maintain optimum cardiac health related to heart rate, rhythm, and perfusion during visits.

Cardiac patients should also receive prophylactic antibiotics before any invasive dental procedure in order to reduce the risk of contracting subacute bacterial endocarditis (SBE). SBE is often related to introduction into the bloodstream of the streptococcus bacteria naturally occurring in the mouth.

### CRISIS MANAGEMENT

A **crisis** is a change in well-being that has a definite beginning and end. It is marked by an inability to cope either because of exhaustion of normal coping mechanisms or sudden and dramatic change in circumstances. A nurse's role during times of crisis is to first ensure the safety of the individual, then improve coping strategies and assist the patient in returning to a stable level of functioning. This can be done by use of medication, therapies, controlling environmental influences, offering reassurance, suggestions for change, and support in decisions and actions toward crisis resolution.

# Self-Management Strategies

## Self-Monitoring Techniques

Self-monitoring techniques include lifestyle modifications, reducing exposure to stressful situations, alteration of thinking, and modification to reactions. Patients should maintain a well-balanced diet, increase physical activity, get adequate sleep, apply stress management techniques, and monitor blood pressure, cholesterol, and glucose levels. Reduce exposure to stressful situations by managing time and finances effectively and applying problem-solving techniques to problems that arise. Patients should try to maintain a positive attitude and decrease negative thoughts. Modifying reactions to stressful situations can help reduce stress and anxiety. Applying self-monitoring techniques can help patients improve their quality of life and reduce maladaptive behaviors.

## Health Self-Management Issues

Health self-management issues include health maintenance, disease prevention, and health promotion. Health maintenance is defined as strategies that help maintain and/or improve health over time. Health maintenance is dependent on three factors, which include health perception, motivation for behavioral change, and compliance to set goals. Disease prevention is an effort to limit the development or progression of lifestyle-related illness. **Disease prevention** can be categorized into primary, secondary, and tertiary prevention.

- **Primary prevention** measures are employed prior to disease onset and are used in health populations.
- **Secondary prevention** measures are used to screen, detect, and treat disease in earlier stages to prevent further progression or development of other complications.
- **Tertiary prevention** measures are used to prevent the onset of other complications or comorbid conditions.

Health promotion strategies include risk reduction strategies applied to the general population.

## Coping

Coping is a mechanism that is used by an individual to deal with internal and external factors that arise. It involves continuously changing one's behavioral and cognitive actions to deal with challenging circumstances. Coping is an evolving process that involves an individual changing their actions based on internal and external factors. The functions of coping include reducing stress, maintaining equilibrium, facilitating independence, enhancing personal decision making, meeting external demands, managing stressors, avoiding negative self-evaluation, and maintaining a stable psychosocial state. Coping varies from one individual to another but includes the above functions.

### Coping Styles

An individual's **approach to coping** may change based on internal and external factors. It may also change based on the situation the individual is presented with. A flexible coping style is much more effective than a rigid approach, as different situations will arise that require different modes of coping.

- **Adaptive responses** to coping includes lifestyle modification; enhancing knowledge and self-care strategies; maintaining positive goals; adjusting to changes in relationships with family, loved ones, healthcare providers, and/or co-workers; grieving over losses; dealing with role changes; adjusting to discomfort; maintaining a sense of control; maintaining hope; and confronting impending death.
- **Maladaptive responses** to coping include anxiety, anger, depression, denial, and dependence.

### Positive Coping Mechanisms

Positive coping mechanisms utilize the patient's natural responses to crisis in order to facilitate their own independence and ability to make decisions and do not compromise the patient's self-worth perceptions or mental, social, or physical stability. Positive techniques reduce tension and conflict while confronting and resolving the problem in a constructive manner. The patient who is coping positively will seek out knowledge and be involved in their own care. They will grieve appropriately and adjust to changes in health, social roles, and relationships, maintaining a sense of hope and confidence in their abilities and choices.

### Negative Coping Mechanisms

Negative responses do not allow the patient to adjust to the challenges they face. While any of these responses may occur as part of the journey to positive action, they will not be sustained over a long period of time. If negative responses continue, they may require outside intervention and treatment to assist the patient in making positive coping and self-care decisions. Negative responses can include anxiety, depression, anger, denial, noncompliance with treatment, or increased dependence on others for self-esteem and decision-making abilities. Negative coping compromises the patient's sense of independence and their mental, social, or physical stability. They increase tension and conflict without confronting and resolving the problem. The patient who is coping negatively will not seek out knowledge and be involved in their own care and cannot adjust to changes in health, social roles, and relationships while maintaining a sense of hope and confidence.

### Treatment of Maladaptive Responses to Coping

Treatment of maladaptive responses to coping includes nonpharmacologic approaches and pharmacologic approaches:

- **Nonpharmacologic strategies** include cognitive behavioral therapy, psychotherapy, electroconvulsive therapy, and/or light therapy. Pharmacologic approaches are used for cases where cognitive behavior therapy or psychotherapy is not completely effective. They are typically used in combination with these strategies.
- **Pharmacologic approaches** include selective serotonin reuptake inhibitors (SSRIs) such as fluoxetine, sertraline, paroxetine, and fluoxetine; tricyclic antidepressants such as imipramine, nortriptyline, desipramine, amitriptyline, and doxepin; benzodiazepines such as diazepam, lorazepam, and oxazepam; monoamine oxidase inhibitors (MAOIs) such as phenelzine, tranylcypromine, L-deprenyl, and moclobemide; and atypical antidepressants such as bupropion, mirtazapine, nefazodone, and trazodone.

### NURSING INTERVENTIONS TO ENHANCE COPING AND ADAPTATION

Nurses and clinical practitioners need to take a proactive approach to helping patients deal with coping and providing them with more adaptive coping strategies. Assessing and following a patient's response to illness and treatment is necessary to determine whether any interventions are needed. Practicing clinicians need to make sure that there are no maladaptive responses such as anxiety, depression, or denial that need to be addressed with nonpharmacologic or pharmacologic approaches. It is necessary to provide the patient with educational material regarding their disease and treatment. Encouraging patients to join support groups is a good approach for patients who would like to discuss their condition with other patients. Nursing and practicing clinician interventions can be changed and revised as needed, depending on the patient's psychosocial state.

## RELATIONSHIP BETWEEN CARDIOVASCULAR DISEASE AND DEPRESSION

**Depression** is a major risk factor for developing cardiovascular disease, particularly myocardial infarction. Depression affects the patient's decision-making ability as well as their interest in self-care and motivation toward healing and rehabilitation. If depression is caught and treated, it can help prevent disease development and improve quality and length of life in those with active disease processes. The first line of treatment is stress management and counseling for anxiety. Medications are carefully considered after taking into account the patient's condition and other medications and treatments. Signs and symptoms of depression should be discussed with every cardiovascular patient before discharge from a healthcare setting. Be particularly aware of symptoms of depression in postmenopausal women.

## FACTORS INFLUENCING PERCEPTION OF QUALITY OF LIFE

The factors that influence an **individual's perception of their quality of life** include health, functional status, symptoms, and life satisfaction. The acute or chronic nature of a condition influences an individual's perception of their quality of life. Health includes not only physical well-being but also mental and social well-being. Functional status is defined as an individual's ability to perform activities of daily living. Symptoms are an individual's responses to their physical, emotional, or cognitive status. Life satisfaction is defined as an individual's contentment with their quality of life, including family, health, sexuality, spirituality, friendships, job, education, housing, standard of living, and finances.

## PHYSIOLOGICAL AND PSYCHOLOGICAL RESPONSES TO STRESS

**Physiological responses to stress** include the interaction between the sympathetic nervous system, anterior and posterior pituitary gland, and adrenal gland. Physiological responses cause the release of hormones and cytokines such as norepinephrine, epinephrine, adrenocorticotropic hormone (ACTH), vasopressin, and antidiuretic hormone. These hormones and cytokines are released during the alarm stage also known as fight-or-flight.

**Psychological responses to stress** such as palpitations may result in the use of an adaptive or maladaptive coping mechanism. Psychological responses can be treated with nonpharmacologic management and/or pharmacologic agents. Coping mechanisms are best used adaptively to address psychological responses.

## General Adaptation Syndrome

General adaptation syndrome is defined as the stages associated with the body's response to a stressor. The three stages of general adaption syndrome include the alarm stage, stage of resistance or adaptation, and stage of exhaustion. The alarm stage is the initial response to a stressor, which is the fight-or-flight syndrome. The stage of resistance or adaptation is the process whereby the individual continues the fight-or-flight response. The stage of exhaustion is the point at which the stressor becomes dysfunctional and can lead to disease or illness.

## Stress Management Techniques

Stress management techniques include autogenics, cognitive restructuring, imagery, progressive muscle relaxation, meditation, and aerobic exercise. Autogenics is a technique that involves the use of repetitive verbal phases and concentrating on sensations to lead to deep relaxation. Cognitive restructuring involves the use of the mind to alter the stress response. Imagery is another method for stress reduction. Additionally, progressive muscle relaxation reduces stress by interfering with the sympathetic nervous system. Meditation is a process that leads to deep relaxation through use of mantras and concentration. Aerobic exercise reduces anxiety and stress by increasing endorphins.

# Community Resources

## Benefits of Cardiac Rehabilitation

Endorsed by both the American Heart Association (AHA) and American College of Cardiology, **cardiac rehabilitation** is an individualized program designed for patients with cardiac disease, including those recovering from myocardial infarction and treatment surgeries. Cardiac rehabilitation focuses on education, including diet and lifestyle changes, and developing an individualized exercise program that will return the cardiac patient to their highest functioning capacity and reduce the risk of further cardiac injury.

For the first 3–6 months, care is focused on gradual exercise progression and probable consults with cardiologists, health educators, dietitians, physical and occupational therapists, and psychologists/psychiatrists.

Exercise options might include both endurance and strength training. Lifestyle education and counseling focuses on disease management, risky behavior reduction, diet, and mental health.

Attending cardiac rehabilitation increases the cardiac patient's chances of survival and effective healing.

### *Roles of Cardiac Rehabilitation Nurse*

The roles of a cardiac rehabilitation nurse are as follows:

- **Clinician**: Uses the nursing process to devise individualized care plans for their patients.
- **Collaborator**: Works with other professionals to facilitate comprehensive care that meets the patient's needs.
- **Educator**: Identifies the learning needs of the patient and facilitates positive health changes through providing knowledge and encouragement toward better wellness.
- **Manager**: Identifies needs and coordinates care with other professions to provide comprehensive services and acts as an advocate for the patient's healthcare choices.
- **Researcher**: Continually seeks creative and effective ways to improve the quality of care that can be provided to the patient.

## Anticoagulation Clinic

An anticoagulation clinic may be located as a stand-alone facility or located within an existing facility, such as a physician's office or a hospital. The anticoagulation clinic is typically staffed by nurses and/or nurse practitioners and pharmacists who are experienced in working with patients receiving anticoagulation. The anticoagulation clinic monitors the medication (antivitamin K antagonists and LMWH as well as new oral anticoagulants, such as dabigatran and rivaroxaban) and treatment of patients and provides an educational resource for patients as well as emergency contact in the event the patient experiences signs of bleedings (increased bruising, nosebleeds, hematuria, blood in the stool). Patients generally have regularly scheduled visits during which the staff reviews the patient's INRs or other laboratory findings, medications, and diet to ensure that the patient's condition is stable and there are no conflicts that may interfere with the anticoagulant. Anticoagulant clinics may include a telemedicine component in order to be able to serve patients for whom coming to the clinic is difficult.

# Individualized Education Planning and Implementation

## Adult Learning

**Adult learning** is defined as a consistent change in behavior due to life experiences. The characteristics of adult learning include motivation to know more information, self-direction, life experiences that positively or negatively impact the learning process, and ability to enhance an already established knowledge base. Adult learning is most effective when an individual can relate to an immediate need, problem, or deficit. These individuals are self-directed by a need to know more information based on their current situation. They will take a proactive approach to gain more insight due to a current situation or based on a need to build on past experience.

### *Conditions for Adult Learning*

The **three conditions necessary for adult learning** include motivation to learn, ability to learn, and the learning environment. Motivation is a condition that is defined as the effect of internal and external factors that drive an individual's need to learn, change, and maintain behavior. It is a willingness of an individual to want to acquire knowledge or insight.

### *Motivation*

**Motivation** can be driven by different factors, including reinforced or rewarded behavior, need for survival, ability to recognize a previous behavior that caused a negative outcome, personality, perceived ability to achieve a specific goal, and coping style.

### *Domains*

The **domains of adult learning** include cognitive learning, affective learning, and psychomotor learning. Each type of learning impacts how an individual addresses adult learning and affects the knowledge the individual can acquire.

- **Cognitive learning** is defined as the ability to acquire knowledge or intellectual information through acquisition of facts and data, making decisions, or drawing conclusions.
- **Affective learning** is defined as the ability of an individual to change their attitude, feelings, emotions, or interests toward a particular event or idea.
- **Psychomotor learning** is defined as an individual's ability to master physical or motor skills and/or activities.

### *Impact of Environment*

**External factors** and the **environment** may affect an individual's ability to learn. Many external factors may need to be addressed in order for an individual to have the ability to learn, as these external factors may pose barriers to learning. Understanding how individuals learn most effectively is key to addressing environmental factors. Some individuals learn better on a one-on-one basis, while others learn more effectively in small groups, and still others learn better in large groups. Understanding the environmental factors that impact learning can positively or negatively influence an individual's learning process. Providing a comfortable learning environment that includes a moderate temperature, sufficient lighting, minimal noise, adequate ventilation, and comfortable furniture will facilitate the learning process.

### *Learning Ability*

**Learning ability** plays an important role in the learning process, as the ability to learn is dependent on an individual's developmental level, physical wellness, and intellectual thought process. The developmental level of learning depends on the individual's stage in life. Literacy level involves reading, comprehension, problem solving, and mathematics. Health literacy is defined as an individual's level of literacy required to function in a health environment, independent of educational literacy. Language can also influence an individual's ability to learn, especially if English is a second language. Physical wellness is defined as the level of strength, coordination, and sensory acuity to learn.

## SELF-EFFICACY THEORY OF LEARNING

**Self-efficacy learning models** are based on the core belief within the patient that change can be accomplished. This belief can be supported through educational efforts in four key ways:

- **Personal mastery** is the most vital component. Personal mastery is directly based on the patient's belief that a new skill can be mastered or a solution to a problem can be found.
- **Vicarious experience** allows the patient to observe and learn from demonstration by another, either patient or nurse. Role models with similar experiences as teaching agents are particularly helpful.
- **Verbal persuasion** provides positive reinforcement in the patient's efforts toward change and expresses the third party's (including the teacher or care provider) belief that a skill can be mastered by the patient.
- **Physiological feedback** provides tangible evaluation methods (physical appearance of a bandage, lab results, resolution of nausea, etc.) that the patient can utilize to see if their work has succeeded or failed.

## MASLOW'S HIERARCHY AND DETERMINING PRIORITIES

Understanding Maslow's hierarchy of needs can help determine priorities and timing in patient education:

1. **Basic physiological and survival needs** must always be met first. Learning cannot take place in an environment of personal emergency. Basic health needs that preserve life are addressed at this stage.
2. Patient concerns progress from there to include fears for **safety and security**, including pain control.
3. When these areas are addressed, the patient is then ready to begin **taking an active role** in their current healthcare.
4. The next step is a more active interest in **promoting current and future health and wellness**. Focus is still on problem solving and affirming positive health practices.
5. Then a desire to **reach fulfilling life goals** can be addressed.

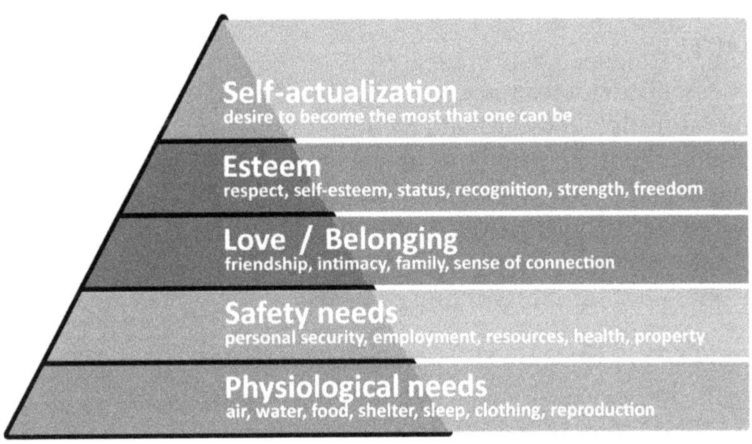


Patient and Community Education

### Effective Teaching and Learning Strategies

The role of the clinical practitioner is to **facilitate learning**, while the role of the patient is to learn. Structured learning environments are more effective than unstructured learning environments. The strategy most effective for teaching depends on the learning and what works best for that individual. Teaching strategies include lecturing, question and answer sessions, demonstrations, role playing, oral or written exams, simulation, illustrations, case studies, books, pamphlets, pictures, film, computer-assisted learning programs, and video tapes/DVDs. Clinical practitioners need to take into account the patient's learning level and adjust teaching strategies to that learning level. The practitioner should also make sure that the learning material is relevant, relatable, and organized.

### Strategies for Patient Education and Counseling

The **strategy** used should be based on the patient's perception. Practicing clinicians should inform the patient of the expected goals of these strategies and issue small goals rather than large, unattainable goals. Specific goals are much more effective than vague ones. Patients are more apt to follow specific recommendations rather than general ideas. New behaviors should be linked to old behaviors, and it is typically easier to establish new behaviors than to eliminate old habits. For the individual to achieve set goals, it is essential to follow up with the patient and have them monitor goals. Multiple members of the healthcare staff should be involved in the process, including nurses, doctors, counselors, and nutritionists.

### Methods for Individual vs. Group Teaching Sessions

The methods that are most appropriate for individual versus group teaching sessions are discussed below:

- **Lecture** can be appropriate for teaching large groups, but when used in small groups, it has better results when coupled with discussion and/or question and answer.
- **Discussion** alone is appropriate for a one-on-one instruction setting.
- **Question and answer time** should only be used in a single-learner setting when prior knowledge has been given and absorbed by the learner or as a method to assess how much learning may have taken place.
- **Demonstration and practice** work best in small groups or individual settings. Practicing skills can include return demonstration or role-playing in either setting.
- **Supportive teaching tools** such as written material or audio-visual treatments are helpful in both group and individual learning environments and provide reinforcement of material in different methods to accommodate various learning styles.

### Learning Contract

A **learning contract** establishes a formal agreement that learning will take place. A learning contract is a concrete indication of a learner's willingness to begin the learning and change process. It spells out expectations of both teacher and learner to maintain a positive and productive relationship. Goals are set and ways to evaluate progress are outlined so that both parties know what will be expected of them. Goals should be centered on patient needs and wishes and decided upon with patient input. Learning contracts can be employed in a number of healthcare settings and provide measurable outcomes for intervention evaluation.

### Strategies for Effective Evaluation and Reteaching

**Evaluation** requires the practicing clinician to assess a patient's performance and health-related outcomes and to determine competence. Evaluation is used to assess whether a patient is effectively learning and changing health-related behaviors. If the approach is not effective, practicing clinicians can alter their approach to better suit the patient's needs. Direct and indirect measurements can be used for evaluation assessment. Direct measurement involves observing the patient and recording behaviors. Indirect measurement assumes that learning has occurred, as the patient has reached a predetermined learning level. Oral questioning and written examinations are examples of indirect learning measurements.

## Assessment in the Patient Education Process

**Assessment in the patient education process** involves defining learning needs and developing a teaching plan to meet the needs of an individual. Assessment involves understanding an individual's need to learn, motivation to learn, and readiness to learn. Individuals with an internal locus of control will be more proactive in their health approach, while individuals with an external locus of control will not be as proactive in their health approach. Therefore, practicing clinicians need to take different approaches, depending on the patients' ability to take control of their own health. Practicing clinicians also need to take into account any external factors that may affect an individual's readiness to learn, including cultural or religious beliefs, perceived benefits of changing behaviors, and belief that individuals can effectively influence their own health. Other factors include physical well-being, comfort, sensory experiences, and physical and intellectual maturity.

## Distinctive Qualities of Excellent Nurse-Teachers

The following are four key distinctive qualities of an excellent nurse-teacher:

- **Confidence**: An excellent teacher provides a comfortable and appropriate learning environment and is prepared ahead of time regarding what and how to teach the individual or group, according to their needs.
- **Competence**: An excellent teacher prioritizes learning goals and material, focusing on the most critical first. They take care to ensure patient safety and confidentiality during teaching exercises.
- **Communication**: An excellent teacher speaks clearly and concisely on a level that is comfortable for the patient, provides for an interpreter or any available resources in the patient's native language, and presents materials in a variety of ways to accommodate different learning styles.
- **Caring**: The most effective teacher is able to show empathy toward the patient and their emotions and concerns. They are unhurried and willing to address any questions the patient might have while encouraging and providing positive feedback in the patient's efforts to learn.



## Evaluating the Effectiveness of Education Efforts

The standards established by JCAHO for evaluating the effectiveness of education efforts are as follows:

- Did the effort promote open and honest communication between the nurse and the participants?
- Was the patient's understanding of the concept improved after the experience?
- Was the patient actively involved in the learning and decision-making processes?
- Was the information provided pertinent to the patient's individual needs, values, abilities, and concerns at the time of the teaching event?
- Can the patient easily demonstrate the needed skills being taught?
- Is the patient aware of their responsibility related to any treatments and goals that will be employed toward a healthy lifestyle?

- Does the knowledge gained improve the patient's ability to cope with circumstances and to participate in their care?
- Will the patient be able to follow and accomplish any care goals that have been set?

## Barriers to Patient's Ability to Learn

The following are five barriers that might interfere with the patient's ability to learn:

- **Language**: Is English the patient's primary language? Are interpreters available to help the patient hear and understand the information in their native tongue?
- **Hearing impairment**: Is there a known, or suspected, hearing deficit? Is hearing equipment in use and functioning? Improve communication by facing the patient and using short sentences.
- **Sight impairment**: Is there a known, or suspected, sight deficit? Are eyeglasses clean and in use? Accommodate for the use of a magnifying glass and provide high-contrast, large-print material as needed. Offer auditory rather than written teaching supplements when available.
- **Pain**: Is the patient adequately medicated in order to pay attention and think clearly but not be drowsy?
- **Physical restriction**: Is the patient physically able to perform the tasks you are teaching them about?
- **Intellectual development**: Is the patient developmentally able to understand the concepts being presented?
- **Motivation**: Is the patient ready to learn, or is anger, denial, or another emotion impairing their readiness and receptiveness to new information?

### *Low Health Literacy*

Patient with low health literacy may:

- Express frustration or inaccurate knowledge about how and where to find needed healthcare services.
- Express frustration or difficulty following through with treatments, including medications or testing.
- Be unable to provide an accurate personal health history or fill out detailed health surveys.
- Have little or no knowledge and regard for preventative measures and the consequences of risky behaviors and may express belief in healthcare misconceptions.
- Appear disinterested in provided materials, often expressing that someone else will meet their healthcare needs.

These concerns can be addressed by:

- Ensuring that communication is provided in the patient's primary language and at a level appropriate to their developmental and learning level.
- Avoiding the use of medical jargon and complex explanations that can be misunderstood and frequently assessing the amount of learning.
- Prioritizing information according to its perceived value to the patient.
- Providing multiple learning methods and supplemental materials as needed to reinforce learning.

### *Reduced Visual Acuity and Implications for Patient Teaching*

Individuals who present with **reduced visual acuity** can learn effectively if certain teaching approaches are taken. Practicing clinicians should make sure that an individual with reduced visual acuity has clean glasses and adequate light and is wearing contacts or using magnifying glasses. In reading documents, make sure the letters are in large font and of a contrasting color. Black ink on white paper is the best for individuals with vision problems. The use of auditory tapes or CDs may also be effective in getting information across to patients with reduced visual acuity.

### *Reduced Hearing Acuity and Implications for Patient Teaching*

Individuals who present with **reduced hearing acuity** can learn effectively if certain teaching approaches are taken. A practicing clinician should speak slowly and clearly. They should get the individual's attention prior to speaking and use simple sentences. Facing the patient and standing in close proximity is most effective in teaching a patient with reduced hearing acuity. Requesting feedback from the individual will clarify whether the patient understands the clinical practitioner and whether information is coming across effectively. Additionally, if the patient is still having problems hearing the clinical practitioner, make sure that the individual's hearing aid is working properly and check to see if the patient hears more effectively in one ear versus the other.

## Conditions and Motivations That Encourage Learning

There are three domains of learning that need to be addressed: cognitive (actual knowledge of facts), affective (attitudes and feelings associated with the subject), and psychomotor (hands-on skills and actions).

Learning in these three areas is based on the patient's motivation and ability to learn as well as the environment in which they are expected to learn. A desire to learn and change is necessary, and knowledge must be presented in a manner that enables and sparks the individual's ability to learn. Knowledge and learning opportunities must be presented in an atmosphere that is respectful, encouraging, and comfortable for the patient.

# Home Monitoring

## Remote Telemetry and POC Testing

**Remote telemetry** is used to diagnose heart arrhythmias and to monitor a patient's status. For studies, a monitoring system, such as the Heartrak ECAT® (which utilizes electrodes and a battery pack) or Telepatch® (which uses patch electrodes), sends data (ECG, pulse rate) to a monitor or physician, usually for 7–30 days. The Apple Watch also now has an ECG application that can automatically transfer data when an abnormality occurs.

**Point-of-care devices** use a sample of whole blood to provide the patient's PT, aPTT, and INR for patients on warfarin anticoagulant. Some devices can measure activated clotting time (ACT) for patients on unfractionated heparin. Point-of-care tests may give qualitative results (present or absent, such as pregnancy test) or quantitative results (precise numbers, such as glucose). Quality control is critical in ensuring that test results are accurate, and those performing the tests must be well-trained. Point-of-care devices may be utilized by home health nurses or by patients or other caregivers to monitor patients' conditions or help determine appropriate dosages of medication.

## Wellness Counseling and Health Fairs

**Wellness counseling** is providing education to patients and family members in order to prevent illness. Wellness counseling may include:

- Discussion of risk factors, such as obesity and smoking
- Explanation of healthy habits, such as a well-balanced diet, weight loss, and daily exercise
- Recommendations for screenings, such as blood pressure and bone density tests, and routine immunizations
- Screening for substance abuse
- Scheduling routine physician appointments for physical examinations and follow-ups
- Education about various diseases and disorders
- Discussion of mental health issues
- Referral to community resources

**Health fairs** serve to engage the public in health issues by providing information and interactive participation. Health fairs generally include a number of information displays, such as those regarding hand hygiene and signs of common disorders, and may even include the offer of free safety equipment, such as bike helmets or knee pads. Health fairs often offer a variety of different types of health screenings, such as glucose, BP, vision and hearing, and cholesterol tests. Some health fairs may also offer routine vaccinations, such as the yearly flu vaccine, at low cost.

## Prochaska's Transtheoretical Model of Motivation and Change

**Prochaska** states that there are five stages a person must go through in order to accept the value of change and take action accordingly:

1. **Precontemplation**: The patient is resistant to change. This stage can last up to six months after a need for change has been initially identified.
2. **Contemplation**: For the next six months to a year, the patient begins to visualize what changing would actually be like.
3. **Preparation**: The patient begins taking tentative steps, such as option exploration, toward change. This stage's timeframe can vary greatly.

4. **Action**: For approximately the next six months, the patient begins taking active steps toward change; relapse and setbacks may occur, but overall, the patient remains resolved toward change.
5. **Maintenance**: For at least six months following completion of the change goal, the patient works to maintain the changes achieved. Setbacks may still occur but become less frequent.

The nurse must meet the patient at whatever stage they are currently in and promote progress toward the next stage.

## Making Successful Lifestyle and Health Changes

**Change** begins with the patient making a firm, concrete commitment to a goal or positive outcome. No change can be achieved without a decision to pursue that change.

**Goals** that are measurable, gradual and within the realistic reach for the patient must be established. A clear path needs to be visualized.

A **realistic view** of negative life events and relapses must be established that allows the patient to be forgiving of their perceived failures and maintain long-term resolve toward the change.

The patient must receive **support and encouragement** from outside sources that they trust and value.

# Cardiac/Vascular Nurse Practice Test

Want to take this practice test in an online interactive format?
Check out the online resources page, which includes interactive practice questions and much more: **mometrix.com/resources719/cardiacvas**

**1. A patient presents with pulmonary edema, tachypnea, tachycardia, hypertension, fever, and cough with frothy sanguineous sputum. What treatments are most commonly ordered initially with this clinical presentation?**

a. Oxygen, nitroglycerine, loop diuretics, and morphine.
b. Oxygen, thiazide diuretics, and angiotensin-converting enzyme inhibitors.
c. Oxygen and thiazide diuretics.
d. Oxygen, morphine, and calcium channel blockers.

**2. An 86-year-old patient with end-stage cardiac disease has a do-not-resuscitate (DNR) order as a result of an advance directive and has been explicit about her desire to avoid life-prolonging procedures. However, when she goes into cardiac arrest, her daughter demands that the nurses perform cardiopulmonary resuscitation (CPR). In this situation, the staff should do which of the following?**

a. Proceed with CPR as the patient can no longer make decisions.
b. Proceed with CPR while calling the patient's physician to request verification of the DNR order.
c. Contact the ethics committee for guidance.
d. Advise the daughter that a valid DNR order is in place and that CPR will be withheld in accordance with the patient's wishes.

**3. A patient with ventricular tachycardia at 200 bpm and multiple premature ventricular contractions loses consciousness. What treatment is most common in this situation?**

a. Antiarrhythmic medications.
b. Emergency defibrillation.
c. Digoxin.
d. Procainamide.

**4. The nurse notes that a patient who has just had cardiac surgery has decreased chest tube drainage, muffled heart sounds, tachycardia, and pulsus paradoxus. The most probable cause of these symptoms is:**

a. fluid overload.
b. cardiac failure.
c. cardiac tamponade.
d. infection.

**5. Ischemia is characterized on the electrocardiogram by:**

a. elevation of ST segments and elevated symmetrical T waves.
b. inverted T waves.
c. development of Q or QS waves.
d. abnormal Q waves or decreased elevation of R waves without alteration of ST and T waves.

**6. A patient complains of sharp pain in the substernal area or to the left of the sternum, which is referred to the neck, arms, and back. It occurs intermittently and suddenly, and increases in intensity with inspiration, coughing, swallowing, or turning of the trunk. It is somewhat relieved by sitting upright. The most likely diagnosis is:**

a. angina.
b. myocardial infarction.
c. anxiety.
d. pericarditis.

**7. If a patient has an ankle systolic pressure of 90 and a brachial systolic pressure of 120, what is the ankle-brachial index?**

a. 0.75.
b. 1.33.
c. 0.13.
d. 7.5.

**8. Which heart sound indicates atrial gallop, which is often associated with left ventricular hypertrophy, hypertension, or aortic stenosis?**

a. S1.
b. S2.
c. S3.
d. S4.

**9. Anticoagulation therapy should be given before which of the following procedures?**

a. Emergency defibrillation.
b. Direct current cardioversion.
c. Direct current and chemical cardioversion.
d. Chemical cardioversion.

**10. Is a person who drinks heavily on one occasion in danger of cardiovascular impairment?**

a. No, only chronic drinking leads to cardiovascular impairment.
b. Yes, but only if there is underlying cardiac disease.
c. Yes, but only if alcohol use is combined with drugs, such as cocaine.
d. Yes, drinking heavily on one occasion can cause cardiovascular impairment.

**11. After cardiac surgery, urinary output should be monitored to ensure adequate renal perfusion. Urinary output should be more than:**

a. 20 mL/hr.
b. 25 mL/hr.
c. 50 mL/hr.
d. 75 mL/hr.

**12. Which of the following cardiac symptoms are typical of cocaine use?**

a. Hypertension and increased heart rate.
b. Hypertension and decreased heart rate.
c. Hypotension and increased heart rate.
d. Hypotension and decreased heart rate.

**13. Venous ulcers commonly have which of the following characteristics?**

a. They are deep and circular.
b. They are superficial and irregularly shaped.
c. They are often necrotic.
d. They appear primarily on the toes and toe webs.

**14. What preparation is necessary for a patient scheduled for a radionuclide ventriculogram?**

a. No special preparation is needed.
b. Patients must fast for 4-6 hours.
c. Cardiac medications are withheld for 4 hours.
d. Patients should be on bed rest for 8 hours before the exam.

**15. Physical changes that suggest a severe cardiovascular disorder, such as pulmonary edema and congestive heart failure, include:**

a. peripheral cyanosis of the nails and skin of the nose, lips, and extremities.
b. pallor.
c. central cyanosis of the tongue and buccal mucosa.
d. xanthelasma.

**16. Angiotensin-converting enzyme inhibitors are contraindicated in patients with:**

a. hypertension.
b. diabetes mellitus.
c. heart failure.
d. renal failure.

**17. A patient on mechanical ventilation who is retaining carbon dioxide is at risk for:**

a. metabolic acidosis.
b. respiratory acidosis.
c. metabolic alkalosis.
d. respiratory alkalosis.

**18. Sexual activity after recovery from a myocardial infarction (MI) can be considered:**

a. low risk as sexual activity provides physical and psychological benefits.
b. high risk as sexual activity could precipitate another MI.
c. very high risk, especially in patients who also use nitroglycerine for angina.
d. no risk as sexual activity has no effect on cardiovascular disease.

**19. When wearing a Holter monitor, a patient should:**

a. refrain from taking cardiac medications.
b. restrict activities.
c. maintain an activity diary.
d. turn it off during the night.

**20. The best approach to be used with a 35-year-old woman who has Marfan syndrome as well as severe mitral valve prolapse and heart failure is to:**

a. delay surgery as long as possible.
b. repair the valve rather than replace it.
c. replace the valve rather than repair it.
d. avoid surgery because of life-threatening complications.

**21. When a person believes that a health action will prevent a negative outcome and then takes that action, what behavioral change model can be applied to this behavior?**

a. Theory of reasoned action.
b. Theory of planned behavior.
c. Stress appraisal and coping theory.
d. Health belief model.

**22. When assessing nicotine dependence, which action listed below indicates a serious dependence?**

a. Smoking even if bedridden with illness.
b. Smoking the first cigarette within 5 minutes of awakening.
c. Smoking 11-20 cigarettes daily.
d. Smoking in places where it is prohibited.

**23. Which teaching method listed below is probably the most effective and efficient for teaching a group of patients about lifestyle modifications related to hypertension?**

a. Computer-assisted instruction.
b. Group lecture only.
c. Group lecture and discussion.
d. One-on-one instruction.

**24. The "dietary approaches to stop hypertension" (DASH), sponsored by the National Institutes of Health and the National Heart, Lung, and Blood Institute, include a 2100-calorie diet. What percentage of this diet is total fat?**

a. 27%.
b. 55%.
c. 18%.
d. 6%.

**25. Absolute hypovolemic shock is characterized by:**

a. vasodilation.
b. external loss of fluid only.
c. internal shifting of fluid or external loss of fluid.
d. decreased colloidal osmotic pressure.

**26. Which educational tool listed below is appropriate for a patient who speaks English but is illiterate?**

a. A children's book.
b. Handouts prepared at a third-grade level.
c. Computerized instruction.
d. Video.

**27. A patient spends half the year in one state and half in another state but wants to complete an advance directive. The best approach is to:**

a. complete separate advance directives to comply with each state's regulations.
b. complete one advance directive as all states have the same regulations.
c. inform family members of specific wishes only so an advance directive is not necessary.
d. store the original advance directive in a safety deposit box.

**28. Which blood pressure (BP) listed below poses the greatest risk of cardiovascular disease for people over 50 years of age?**

a. Diastolic pressure >80 mm Hg.
b. Increased BP after exercise.
c. Systolic pressure >140 mm Hg.
d. Pulse pressure of 40 mm Hg.

**29. A patient who has been treated with unfractionated heparin over five days develops a sudden drop in platelets from 120,000 mm$^3$ to 45,000 mm$^3$, suggesting heparin-induced thrombocytopenia, which places this patient at risk for:**

a. hemorrhage.
b. thrombosis and vessel occlusion.
c. shock.
d. infection.

**30. A nursing team leader delegates a task to an unlicensed assistant. Who is responsible for the patient outcome of this task?**

a. The unlicensed assistant who completes the task.
b. Both the team leader and the unlicensed person who complete the task.
c. The team leader who delegates the task.
d. The administrative staff.

**31. Endothelial dysfunction is associated with:**

a. cardiac dysrhythmias.
b. cardiac arrest.
c. hypertension.
d. vasodilation.

**32. The goal of an exercise stress test is to raise the heart rate to what percentage predicted for age and gender?**

a. 200%.
b. 50%.
c. 80-90%.
d. >100%.

**33. Janeway lesions, splinter hemorrhages, and Roth's spots are immunological responses associated with:**

a. endocarditis.
b. pericarditis.
c. myocarditis.
d. aortic valve dysfunction.

**34. The best determinant of the effectiveness of patient education is the:**

a. patient's satisfaction.
b. patient's ability to demonstrate procedure.
c. patient's ability to explain procedure and demonstrate understanding.
d. patient's behavior modification and compliance rates.

**35. Which of the following treatments is considered appropriate palliative care?**

a. Chemotherapy for cancer.
b. Intubation with mechanical ventilation for respiratory failure.
c. Radiotherapy to relieve pain associated with bone cancer.
d. Total parenteral nutrition for patients who cannot eat.

**36. Electrocardiograph changes characteristic of hypokalemia include:**

a. tall peaked T waves with widening and increased amplitude of QRS and prolongation of the QT interval.
b. a U wave more than 1 mm high after the T wave, AV block, and flat or inverted T waves.
c. dysrhythmias with prolonged PR and QT intervals and broad flat T waves.
d. non-specific changes.

**37. Metabolic syndrome is characterized by:**

a. abdominal obesity, decreased triglyceride level, increased high-density lipoprotein (HDL) level, and hypertension.
b. hypertension, abdominal obesity, and increased HDL level.
c. abdominal obesity, increased triglycerides, decreased HDL level, elevation of blood pressure, and increased fasting blood glucose.
d. hypotension, decreased fasting blood glucose, increased triglycerides, and decreased HDL level.

**38. According to the Nursing Code of Ethics of the American Nurses Association, nurses must support a patient's autonomy and self-determination. If a 24-year-old Asian woman states a treatment preference but plans to leave the decision to family members, the nurse should:**

a. try to convince the patient to assert herself.
b. respect the patient's right to be guided by family.
c. tell the family that the patient should be the one to make the decision.
d. ask the ethics committee to intervene so that the patient is properly treated.

**39. A patient has an atrioventricular (AV) block in which there are more P waves than QRS complexes, with no clear relationship between them, and an atrial rate two to three times the pulse rate. There is also an irregular PR interval. What type of AV block is this patient likely to have?**

a. First-degree AV block.
b. Second-degree AV block, Mobitz type I.
c. Second-degree AV block, Mobitz type II.
d. Third-degree AV block.

**40. Cor pulmonale is characterized by changes in the:**

a. left atria.
b. left ventricle.
c. right atria.
d. right ventricle.

**41. The primary reason for completing professional development courses is to:**

a. comply with state requirements for licensure.
b. remain current in the field of nursing.
c. meet institutional requirements for employment.
d. fulfill requirements for a salary increase.

**42. Cognitive changes associated with aging affect learning in which of the following ways?**

a. Patients are better able to focus attention because their lives have fewer distractions (kids, jobs).
b. Explicit memories (facts) decline, but implicit memories (skills) often stay the same.
c. Older adults have the same ability to learn as young adults.
d. Patients have less difficulty with complex tasks.

**43. What adverse effects are related to immunosuppression with high doses of tacrolimus after a heart transplant?**

a. Facial dysmorphism.
b. Hypertension.
c. Hirsutism and acne.
d. Nephrotoxicity.

**44. The automatic implantable cardioverter defibrillator (AICD) delivers which of the following impulses?**

a. Continuous (asynchronous) electrical impulses to control pulse rate.
b. Dual-chamber sequential electrical impulses.
c. On-demand (synchronous) electrical impulses when the pulse increases to a preset rate.
d. On-demand electrical impulses when the pulse rate decreases to a preset rate.

**45. An episode of syncope associated with exertional exercise is a manifestation of:**

a. aortic regurgitation.
b. aortic stenosis.
c. mitral valve prolapse.
d. endocarditis.

**46. A patient with a dissecting descending thoracic aortic aneurysm will most likely complain of:**

a. severe, dull pain that builds in intensity in the anterior chest and nausea and vomiting.
b. severe, tearing, knife-like pain that builds in intensity in the anterior chest and nausea and vomiting.
c. dull, aching pain posteriorly below the scapula and nausea and vomiting.
d. severe, intense, tearing, knife-like pain posteriorly between the scapulae and nausea and vomiting.

**47. A patient who is receiving digoxin (Lanoxin) and furosemide (Lasix) daily is also prescribed tetracycline for rosacea and subsequently develops nausea, vomiting, and tachycardia. The most likely cause is:**

a. digitalis toxicity.
b. allergic response to tetracycline.
c. drug interaction.
d. superinfection.

**48. A patient is receiving warfarin (Coumadin) along with other treatment for non-valvular atrial fibrillation. The international normalized ratio range should be:**

a. 1.5-2.
b. 2-3.
c. 3-4.
d. >4.

**49. A patient with the recent implantation of a pacemaker develops severe hiccups, which indicates:**

a. irritation of the ventricular wall.
b. phrenic nerve or muscle stimulation from dislocation of leads.
c. impending cardiac tamponade.
d. allergic response to medications.

**50. A patient is being considered for thrombolytic therapy with alteplase tissue-type plasminogen activator (t-PA). Contraindications to thrombolytic therapy include which of the following?**

a. The patient has a 3.5 cm aortic aneurysm.
b. It has been two hours since the onset of symptoms.
c. The patient's blood pressure has been 180/90 mm Hg but is now controlled by medication.
d. The patient had an ischemic stroke six months previously.

**51. Which of the following medications should be discontinued for a minimum of 48 hours before cardioversion?**

a. Digoxin.
b. Warfarin.
c. Cardizem.
d. Insulin.

**52. A patient with heart failure has no symptoms at rest, but symptoms appear with physical exertion and cause some limitations of activities of daily living and slight pulmonary edema. This heart failure is classified as:**

a. class I.
b. class II.
c. class III.
d. class IV.

**53. The treatment of choice for significant pulmonary stenosis is:**

a. closed valvotomy.
b. open valvotomy.
c. balloon valvuloplasty.
d. valve replacement with homograft valve.

**54. Which of the following medications may be used after cardiac surgery to treat low cardiac output?**

a. Nitroprusside.
b. Dobutamine.
c. Dopamine.
d. Isoproterenol.

**55. When preparing written materials for patients, what reading level would be appropriate for a homogeneous group of adults in an affluent area?**

a. Grade 3 level.
b. Grade 6 level.
c. Grade 9 level.
d. Grade 12 level.

**56. Monitoring a patient for acute rejection after cardiac transplantation is primarily done by:**

a. reviewing clinical symptoms.
b. blood testing.
c. biopsy.
d. electrocardiogram.

**57. When examining the chest, where is the apex beat (pulsation) usually observed?**

a. It cannot be observed, only palpated.
b. Around the third intercostal space on the left mid-clavicular line.
c. Around the fourth intercostal space on the left mid-clavicular line.
d. Around the fifth intercostal space on the left mid-clavicular line.

**58. First-line drugs for the treatment of stage I hypertension are:**

a. loop diuretics.
b. thiazide diuretics.
c. angiotensin-converting enzyme inhibitors.
d. calcium channel blockers.

**59. Which immunizations are routinely ordered for adults 60-65 years of age and older?**

a. Influenza vaccine only.
b. Pneumococcal polysaccharide-23, influenza, and herpes zoster vaccines.
c. Hepatitis A and B vaccines.
d. Influenza and hepatitis C vaccines.

**60. Which medication order below is written correctly?**

a. Maalox 30 cc PO qhs.
b. Lasix 40.0 mg PO daily.
c. MS 4.0 mg IV q 4 hr prn.
d. Synthroid 0.88 mg PO daily at 0700.

**61. The nurse attempts to start an intravenous (IV) line on an elderly patient, but the patient refuses to cooperate. The nurse tells the patient that the nursing assistant will be called to hold him down if he does not cooperate. This nurse's response is best characterized as:**

a. coercion.
b. non-therapeutic communication.
c. abuse.
d. poor judgment.

**62. Sexual dysfunction after a heart transplant is primarily caused by:**

a. immunosuppressive drugs.
b. anxiety.
c. weakness and malaise.
d. antihypertensive drugs.

**63. A 62-year old male patient has a regular pulse of over 100 bpm with P waves occurring before the QRS complex and sometimes preceding the T wave. The QRS complex is a normal shape and duration. The PR interval is 0.12-0.20 sec, and the P:QRS ratio is 1:1. Based on these findings, the cardiac diagnosis is:**

a. sinus bradycardia.
b. sinus tachycardia.
c. sinus arrhythmia.
d. premature atrial contractions.

**64. A patient receives daily warfarin (Coumadin) after treatment for atrial fibrillation. Which of the following substances may interfere with the drug's effectiveness?**

a. One 4-ounce glass of red wine daily.
b. Caffeinated beverages.
c. A daily multivitamin.
d. Milk products.

**65. Using transesophageal Doppler ultrasonography to measure cardiac output, a short waveform with a rounded apex may indicate:**

a. decreased preload.
b. increased preload.
c. increased systemic vascular resistance.
d. left ventricular failure.

**66. Which enzyme test should be measured 8-12 hours after onset of symptoms for the diagnosis of myocardial infarction?**

a. Troponin T and I.
b. Myoglobin.
c. Lactic dehydrogenase.
d. Creatinine kinase/creatinine-myoglobin.

**67. A 48-year old male patient is referred to a cardiac care center for cardiac rehabilitation after a myocardial infarction. The cardiac care center provides:**

a. primary care.
b. secondary care.
c. tertiary care.
d. quaternary care.

**68. An absolute indication for stopping an exercise test is a:**

a. patient complaint of dyspnea that is not noticeable to the observer.
b. downsloping ST segment depression.
c. decrease in systolic blood pressure (BP) of10 mm Hg or less from baseline despite an increased workload but absent evidence of ischemia.
d. decrease in systolic BP of 10 mm Hg or more from baseline despite an increased workload and with evidence of ischemia.

**69. A 76-year-old woman with end-stage heart failure was placed on hospice care by her physician six months earlier (two 90-day periods), but she is still alive. Her family asks the nurse if the patient will be removed from hospice care. Which response by the nurse is best in this situation?**

a. "She will be removed from hospice care until her condition worsens because she has exceeded the 6-month period."
b. "She has exhausted all of her hospice care benefits and will be removed from hospice care."
c. "She can continue with hospice care as long as the physician authorizes the care every 60 days."
d. "She can continue with hospice care if the physician continues to authorize care every 90 days."

**70. Thirty hours after valvular surgery that required cardiopulmonary bypass, a 75-year-old patient, who has been apathetic and forgetful for the previous 12 hours, becomes very disoriented, confused, and combative, pulling out his intravenous lines. He is most likely suffering from:**

a. post-pump delirium and psychosis.
b. ischemic stroke.
c. a reaction to drugs.
d. hypoxia.

**71. A patient with a total cholesterol of 206, triglycerides of 105, high-density lipoprotein (HDL) of 35, and low-density lipoprotein (LDL) of 150 should have treatment with a goal to:**

a. lower total cholesterol and triglyceride levels.
b. lower total cholesterol and HDL levels.
c. lower total cholesterol and raise LDL levels.
d. lower total cholesterol and LDL levels and raise HDL levels.

**72. Which rhythm disturbance is most common after cardiac surgery?**

a. Ventricular fibrillation.
b. Ventricular tachycardia.
c. Premature ventricular contractions.
d. Atrial fibrillation, flutter, and tachycardia.

**73. Which self-monitoring skill is essential for a patient with heart failure?**

a. Intake of fats.
b. Daily weight.
c. Degree of edema.
d. Exercise.

**74. A frail 80-year old patient who lives alone requires long-term intravenous (IV) antibiotic therapy for prosthetic valve endocarditis from Staphylococcus epidermidis. His condition is stable at present. The most effective care plan includes:**

a. keeping the patient in the acute care hospital until therapy is completed.
b. sending the patient home and having home health nurses provide home intravenous antibiotic therapy.
c. instructing the patient to self-administer the antibiotic therapy.
d. transferring the patient to an extended care facility for continued treatment.

**75. A patient with severe pain is receiving pain medication routinely every six hours but usually complains of breakthrough pain in four hours, requiring an additional injection, which indicates that:**

a. the patient has a low pain tolerance and may need to be distracted.
b. the routine pain medication may need to be given every four hours or the dosage changed.
c. pain control is adequate with the additional medication.
d. pain may be intractable and cannot be controlled.

**76. Adequate perfusion requires a mean arterial pressure (MAP) of:**

a. >40 mm Hg.
b. >50 mm Hg.
c. >60 mm Hg.
d. >70 mm Hg.

**77. Patients with peripheral arterial disease and aspirin intolerance should be prescribed:**

a. clopidogrel.
b. warfarin.
c. unfractionated heparin.
d. low-molecular-weight heparin.

**78. According to the AHA/ACC Guideline for the Management of Patients with Non-ST-Elevation Acute Coronary Syndromes, for early risk stratification of patients presenting in the ED with chest pain or other symptoms indicative of acute coronary syndrome, a 12-lead ECG should be done within:**

a. 5 minutes.
b. 10 minutes.
c. 15 minutes.
d. 20 minutes.

**79. For a patient receiving a calcium channel blocker, such as diltiazem, which type of supplement may reduce effectiveness?**

a. Vitamin C.
b. B-complex vitamins.
c. Potassium.
d. Calcium.

**80. A patient preparing for discharge has been advised to make multiple lifestyle changes related to diet, medications, habits, and exercise, but the patient is upset about the changes and states repeatedly that the physician is expecting too much. The best response is:**

a. "It will get easier with time."
b. "It's difficult to make all of these changes."
c. "Let me help you map out a plan."
d. "Just take one day at a time."

**81. If a patient has a base normal control prothrombin time (PT) of 10 seconds, the maximum target PT with warfarin therapy is usually:**

a. 15 seconds.
b. 20 seconds.
c. 25 seconds.
d. 30 seconds.

**82. If a patient is taking a bile acid sequestrant, such as cholestyramine, to lower low-density lipoprotein (LDL), how long after taking the drug should the patient wait before taking other medications?**

a. Waiting is not necessary.
b. 1 to 2 hours.
c. 2 to 4 hours.
d. 4 to 6 hours.

**83. Which of the following antiplatelet drugs poses the least risk of bleeding?**

a. aspirin (ASA).
b. clopidogrel.
c. tirofiban.
d. eptifibatide.

**84. Which of the following conditions is an indication for thrombolytic therapy?**

a. NSTEMI.
b. STEMI.
c. Unstable angina.
d. Stable angina.

**85. If a patient has undergone fibrinolytic therapy per accelerated infusion of alteplase 100 mg for an acute myocardial infarction and shows 20% reduction in ST elevation after 90 minutes, the cardiac/vascular nurse anticipates:**

a. further monitoring.
b. additional thrombolysis.
c. angiography/rescue percutaneous coronary intervention (PCI).
d. administration of fondaparinux.

**86. Which of the following patients may be an acceptable candidate for catheter-directed thrombolysis (CDT) for peripheral arterial occlusion?**

a. Patient with non-life-threatening limb ischemia of 12 days.
b. Patient with limb-threatening ischemia, unknown duration.
c. Patient with non-life-threatening limb ischemia of 21 days.
d. Patient with limb-threatening ischemia of 3 days.

**87. On the ECG recording, a normal sinus rhythm is characterized by a PR interval of:**

a. 0.04 to 0.1 seconds.
b. 0.12 to 0.2 seconds.
c. 0.16 to 0.24 seconds.
d. 0.2 to 0.28 seconds.

**88. If a patient exhibits a ventricular rate of 150 bpm, the most likely cause of dysrhythmia is:**

a. accelerated idioventricular rhythm.
b. junctional tachycardia.
c. atrial fibrillation.
d. atrial flutter.

**89. After administering sublingual nitroglycerin to a patient for angina, the cardiac/vascular nurse should expect a reduction in pain within:**

a. 30 seconds to 1 minute.
b. 1 to 2 minutes.
c. 3 to 4 minutes.
d. 5 to 8 minutes.

**90. Beta-blockers are generally contraindicated for patients with a history of:**

a. liver disease.
b. asthma.
c. stroke.
d. kidney disease.

**91. *Rest potentiation* of the heart refers to:**

a. faster rate of stimulation, resulting in stronger contraction.
b. slower rate of stimulation, resulting in weaker contraction.
c. pause, resulting in stronger ensuing contraction.
d. extra beat, resulting in stronger ensuing contraction.

**92. In order to modify risk of cardiovascular disease for patients with peripheral arterial disease (PAD), the primary lifestyle change should be:**

a. emotional support.
b. improved diet.
c. increased exercise.
d. smoking cessation.

**93. At what heart rate is diastolic filling so reduced that stroke volume is diminished and coronary ischemia occurs?**

a. >140 bpm.
b. >160 bpm.
c. >180 bpm.
d. >200 bpm.

**94. Which of the following is a risk factor for coronary artery disease?**

a. Sister diagnosed with coronary artery disease at age 63.
b. Father diagnosed with coronary artery disease at age 60.
c. Mother diagnosed with coronary artery disease at age 65.
d. Brother diagnosed with coronary artery disease at age 56.

**95. When conducting the NIH Stroke Scale and evaluating "best gaze," the cardiac/vascular nurse notes a forced deviation to the side of the stroke and the patient is unable to follow the nurse's moving finger with the eyes, so the nurse carries out the oculocephalic maneuver. A normal response is:**

a. no eye movement during the maneuver.
b. eyes deviate to the side the head is turned to and then return to midline.
c. eyes deviate vertically as the head is turned and then return to previous position.
d. eyes deviate to opposite side the head is turned to and then return to midline.

**96. When assessing the adequacy of a patient's diet, the cardiac/vascular nurse recognizes that, for an elderly adult weighing 70 kg (154 lb), the average caloric requirement per day is about:**

a. 1400.
b. 1750.
c. 2000.
d. 2200.

**97. Which of the following actions by a patient most indicates a lack of readiness to learn about his heart disease and lifestyle management techniques?**

a. Patient states that the medication regimen is too confusing.
b. Patient has not read any of the written educational material left at bedside.
c. Patient turns on the TV to watch a football game when the nurse is instructing.
d. Patient remains passive, asks no questions, and shows no interest in instruction.

**98. According to the AHA/ACC Guideline for the Management of Patients with Non-ST-Elevation Acute Coronary Syndromes, patients presenting in the ED with chest pain or symptoms indicative of acute coronary syndrome should receive oxygen:**

a. in all situations.
b. if anxious and frightened.
c. with oxygen saturation <90%.
d. with oxygen saturation <94%.

**99. According to the Protection Motivation Theory, action to bring about change is precipitated by:**

a. threat.
b. education.
c. fear.
d. motivation.

**100. Considering health literacy, the cardiac/vascular nurse should expect that the average reading level of the US population is:**

a. ≤4th grade.
b. ≤5th grade.
c. ≤6th grade.
d. ≤8th grade.

**101. When administering the Tinetti Gait and Balance Instrument to an older adult, the balance assessment begins with the patient:**

a. standing in front of a chair.
b. sitting in an armed chair.
c. sitting in an armless chair.
d. standing with eyes closed.

**102. If an older adult with aortic stenosis undergoes percutaneous balloon valvuloplasty, restenosis often occurs within:**

a. 6 months.
b. 1 to 2 years.
c. 2 to 4 years.
d. 5 to 10 years.

**103. A patient with hypertension and diabetes mellitus had been a heavy smoker for 40 years before having a myocardial infarction; however, she has continued to smoke even though she states, "I know I should quit." The best response is:**

a. "Tell me about that."
b. "Your life may depend on quitting."
c. "You should join a support group."
d. "You could try the nicotine patch."

**104. Which of the following educational programs might best be conducted as a webinar?**

a. Video series regarding cardiac anatomy and physiology.
b. Orientation program for newly hired cardiac/vascular nurses.
c. Online course for cardiac/vascular nurse continuing education.
d. Interactive discussion about new techniques in cardiac rehabilitation.

**105. If a cardiac/vascular nurse working in a semi-rural area proposes a mobile clinic to better monitor, screen, and counsel patients who often cannot or do not seek medical care, the most likely impediment is:**

a. patient acceptance.
b. cost-effectiveness.
c. staffing needs.
d. clinician resistance.

**106. According to the Eighth Report of the Joint National Committee on Prevention, Detection, Evaluation, and Treatment of High Blood Pressure, systolic blood pressure is a greater cardiovascular risk factor than diastolic blood pressure after age:**

a. 40.
b. 45.
c. 50.
d. 60.

**107. A low score on the Care Transitions Measure (CTM-15) is predictive of:**

a. rehospitalization or return to emergency department.
b. stable transition to a different level of care.
c. increased risk of nonadherence to medical regimen.
d. patient adherence to medical regimen.

**108. According to Healthy People 2020 initiatives, which of the following patients should be screened for peripheral arterial disease with the ankle-brachial index (ABI)?**

a. 65-year-old obese female patient.
b. 55-year-old diabetic male patient with leg pain.
c. 60-year-old male patient after myocardial infarction.
d. 35-year-old female patient with C-6 spinal cord injury.

**109. According to the ACCF/AHA Guideline for the Management of ST-Elevation Myocardial Infarction, the pain medication of choice for patients with STEMI and acute pulmonary edema is:**

a. COX-2 inhibitors.
b. NSAIDs.
c. meperidine.
d. morphine sulfate.

**110. A patient with stage 2 Alzheimer's disease and coronary artery disease can function fairly well in her home environment but has increasing short-term memory loss and often forgets to take her medications even though her daughter calls to remind her. The best solution is likely:**

a. providing an electronic medication dispenser.
b. providing daily home health care for medication administration.
c. arranging for a neighbor to administer the medications.
d. moving the patient to an assisted living facility.

**111. A normal value for the activated partial thromboplastin time (aPTT) is:**

a. 7 to 12 seconds.
b. 10 to 14 seconds.
c. 21 to 35 seconds.
d. 30 to 45 seconds.

**112. According to the ACC/AHA Guideline on the Treatment of Blood Cholesterol to Reduce Atherosclerotic Cardiovascular Risk in Adults, the goal for LDL cholesterol reduction with treatment with high-intensity statin is:**

a. 30% to 40%.
b. ≥50%.
c. 30% to <50%.
d. 40% to 50%.

**113. If a patient with a mechanical prosthetic heart valve is on warfarin therapy and has an INR of 3.2, this probably indicates:**

a. inadequate anticoagulation.
b. slightly excess anticoagulation.
c. emergent risk of bleeding.
d. normal INR for this patient.

**114. When monitoring a patient's 12-lead ECG, the cardiac/vascular nurse would expect a lead facing an injured area of the heart to show:**

a. ST-segment elevation.
b. ST-segment inversion.
c. T-wave deflection upward.
d. R-wave regression.

**115. If C-reactive protein (CRP) is 8 mg/L in a patient with normal lipid values, this may indicate:**

a. decreased risk of cardiovascular disease.
b. increased risk of cardiovascular disease.
c. presence of myocardial injury.
d. presence of myocardial ischemia.

**116. When baroreceptors in the aortic arch and carotid arteries sense volume overload, the usual response is:**

a. decreased heart rate and vasoconstriction.
b. increased heart rate and vasoconstriction.
c. decreased heart rate and vasodilation.
d. increased heart rate and vasodilation.

**117. Which of the following is a common age-associated change in the cardiovascular system?**

a. Systolic blood pressure decreased.
b. Cardiac valves thinned.
c. Cardiac reserve increased.
d. Pacemaker cells decreased in number.

**118. If a patient with hypertension has been prescribed the DASH diet, how many servings of sweets and added sugars may the patient have per week?**

a. ≤5.
b. ≤10.
c. ≤15.
d. ≤20.

**119. Which of the following services can a patient expect from Mended Hearts?**

a. Financial assistance.
b. Visiting program (in-hospital).
c. In-home care.
d. Transportation assistance.

**120. Which of the following is part of the exclusion criteria for therapeutic hypothermia for a patient who experienced sudden cardiac arrest and resuscitation?**

a. Chemical thrombolysis.
b. Sudden cardiac arrest three hours previously.
c. Major surgery one week previously.
d. Maintenance of systolic BP of 92 to 94 mm Hg after CPR.

**121. If the cardiac/vascular nurse is serving as a preceptor for a nursing student and feels that the student lacks essential skills, the cardiac/vascular nurse should first:**

a. terminate the preceptor relationship.
b. report the student to the nursing program director.
c. ask other preceptors for advice.
d. meet with the student to outline concerns.

**122. The primary treatment focus for patients with dilated cardiomyopathy is:**

a. promoting activity.
b. controlling heart failure.
c. preparing for heart transplant.
d. preventing sudden death.

**123. A physician with whom the staff is very friendly is admitted to the cardiac unit with a myocardial infarction, and a number of nurses, who are not assigned to the patient, review his laboratory findings by reading over the shoulder of the physician's assigned nurse. This is primarily a(n):**

a. HIPAA violation.
b. standard procedure.
c. minor violation of privacy.
d. unprofessional activity.

**124. A patient experienced a severe adverse reaction to a drug while left unattended because of suboptimal staffing. This problem will likely be referred to:**

a. district attorney.
b. risk management.
c. nurses' union.
d. attorneys for the organization.

**125. A patient, Ms. Jones, who has had recent cardiac catheterization and angioplasty, presents with increasing shortness of breath, cough, and chest pain, pulse of 130, BP of 140/60, and respirations of 32 per minute. Using the SBAR communication technique, how will the cardiac/vascular nurse begin the report to the physician?**

a. "I believe Ms. Jones may have a pulmonary embolism or cardiac event."
b. "Ms. Jones has a pulse of 130, BP 140/60, and respirations of 32 per minute."
c. "Ms. Jones has had increasing shortness of breath, cough, and chest pain for the past hour."
d. "Ms. Jones recently had cardiac catheterization and angioplasty."

**126. If the cardiac/vascular nurse overhears another nurse berating a patient, telling the patient that she is "lazy and unmotivated," and refusing to assist the patient to the bathroom, the best initial response is to:**

a. immediately intervene.
b. report the other nurse to a supervisor.
c. confront the other nurse later.
d. assume the other nurse is acting in the patient's best interests.

**127. A patient is awaiting surgical intervention for a dissecting aortic aneurysm. Prior to surgery, the patient's systolic BP should be maintained at:**

a. 90 to 100 mm Hg.
b. 100 to 110 mm Hg.
c. 110 to 120 mm Hg.
d. 120 to 130 mm Hg.

**128. If the cardiac/vascular nurse proposes forming an interdisciplinary team to work on process improvement, the best members are likely to be those who:**

a. are personal friends.
b. work well with others.
c. volunteer to participate.
d. have needed knowledge/skills.

**129. Which of the following would disqualify a patient for home health care under Medicare?**

a. The patient walks one mile daily in her neighborhood.
b. The patient attends a cardiac rehabilitation program weekly.
c. The patient attends church with her daughter each week.
d. The patient attends an adult daycare program while her daughter works.

**130. A close personal friend of the cardiac/vascular nurse is a patient on the cardiac unit, and the cardiac/vascular nurse trades assignments with another nurse in order to be assigned to the patient. This constitutes a(n):**

a. HIPAA violation.
b. unprofessional act.
c. professional boundary violation.
d. acceptable procedure.

**131. A patient with bradycardia of 30 bpm is to have a temporary transcutaneous pacemaker (TCP) until a transvenous catheter can be inserted and the cause of the bradycardia determined. In preparation for the TCP, the nurse should advise the patient to expect:**

a. no discomfort.
b. slight discomfort with pacing.
c. sharp constant chest pain.
d. muscle contractions and discomfort with pacing.

**132. Osler's nodes may be found with:**

a. endocarditis.
b. heart failure.
c. pericarditis.
d. myocarditis.

**133. The mother of an 18-year-old patient with hypertrophic cardiomyopathy has been scheduled twice to attend CPR classes before her son is discharged but has failed to attend the classes, stating that the CPR class is "not necessary" and "a waste of time." According to Kübler-Ross's stages of grief, the mother is probably experiencing:**

a. depression.
b. denial.
c. anger.
d. acceptance.

**134. If a patient states, "The doctor promised that I didn't have to exercise today," and the cardiac/vascular nurse knows the physician told the patient to exercise more, the best response is:**

a. "You know that is not true."
b. "I don't believe the doctor said that at all."
c. "Why are you insisting you don't need to exercise when the doctor says you need to?"
d. "That's surprising because the doctor wrote an order for you to walk twice today."

**135. The ECG shows a heart rate of 80 bpm with regular rhythm and normal P waves and QRS complex. The PR interval is 0.5 seconds. This finding is characteristic of:**

a. first-degree atrioventricular block.
b. second-degree atrioventricular block, type I.
c. second-degree atrioventricular block, type II.
d. third-degree atrioventricular block.

**136. The primary difference between partnership councils and other forms of shared governance is that partnership councils usually include:**

a. only nursing personnel.
b. only one level of an organization.
c. all disciplines in an organization.
d. only physicians and nursing personnel.

**137. If a Middle Eastern female patient leaves all medical decisions about her treatment to her husband, this probably represents:**

a. a cultural norm.
b. an abusive relationship.
c. low health literacy.
d. apathy.

**138. A patient has coronary artery disease, and the patient's list of medications shows that the patient is currently taking clopidogrel 75 mg daily, omeprazole 20 mg daily, metoprolol 50 mg twice daily, docusate sodium one capsule daily, and atorvastatin 80 mg daily. Which drug poses the greatest risk of drug-drug interactions?**

a. clopidogrel.
b. atorvastatin.
c. metoprolol.
d. omeprazole.

**139. If a nursing diagnosis is "ineffective self-health management associated with lack of knowledge about condition and therapy," an appropriate patient goal is:**

a. "Patient exhibits improved self-health management and positive attitude toward health."
b. "Patient identifies personal needs in relation to health management."
c. "Patient can describe key elements of the disease process and therapeutic regimen."
d. "Patient expresses a willingness to undergo lifestyle changes."

**140. The primary advantage of PCI with drug-eluting stents or bare-metal stents compared with balloon angioplasty alone is:**

a. decreased restenosis.
b. decreased need for postoperative medications.
c. decreased mortality rates.
d. decreased particle embolization.

**141. A patient with an automatic implantable cardioverter defibrillator (AICD) should generally be advised to avoid:**

a. microwave ovens.
b. MRIs.
c. metal detectors.
d. anti-theft devices.

**142. For a patient with an Unna boot, the most important factor in promoting adequate compression is:**

a. elevation of the foot.
b. proper application.
c. concurrent medications.
d. ambulation.

**143. According to the ACCF/AHA/HRS Focused Update on the Management of Patients with Atrial Fibrillation, the goal for patients with atrial fibrillation is generally a ventricular rate at rest of:**

a. 60 to 80.
b. 80 to 100.
c. 90 to 115.
d. 115 to 125.

**144. According to the AACVPR's *Guidelines for Cardiac Rehabilitation and Secondary Prevention Programs*, a patient should be referred to a cardiac rehabilitation program if:**

a. the patient has adequate insurance coverage for rehabilitation.
b. the patient's mobility was limited by an acute cardiovascular event.
c. the patient is unable to adequately exercise independently.
d. the patient experienced an acute cardiovascular event.

**145. A patient has been admitted to the cardiac care unit with chest pain and atrial fibrillation. Which of the following tasks is appropriate to delegate to unlicensed assistive personnel?**

a. Apical/radial pulse rate.
b. Monitoring the IV fluids.
c. Daily weight.
d. Response to analgesia.

**146. A patient is being treated for acute heart failure. Which of the following tasks has priority?**

a. Monitor response to medications.
b. Check patient's skin for lesions.
c. Instruct patient in low-sodium diet.
d. Check that call light is within reach.

**147. Lidocaine is used primarily for treatment of:**

a. PVC suppression.
b. VT/VF.
c. Atrial fibrillation.
d. PAC suppression.

**148. A patient receiving IV morphine for treatment of severe chest pain develops opioid-induced hypotension. The best approach to treating the hypotension is to:**

a. administer naloxone (Narcan).
b. administer antihistamine.
c. administer crystalloid bolus and continue morphine.
d. hold morphine and administer crystalloid bolus.

**149. Which of the following is a characteristic of non-Q-wave myocardial infarction?**

a. MI is usually transmural.
b. Coronary occlusion is complete in 80% to 90% of patients.
c. Contraction necrosis associated with reperfusion is common.
d. Peak CK levels occur in about 24 hours.

**150. If a patient is classified as having NYHA class I heart failure, the type of symptoms the patient should expect with activities includes:**

a. no symptoms.
b. slight shortness of breath.
c. marked dyspnea and/or angina on exertion.
d. Severe symptoms even at rest.

# Answer Key and Explanations

**1. A:** The most common initial treatment of acute pulmonary edema is oxygen to relieve dyspnea, nitroglycerine to reduce preload, loop diuretics (usually furosemide-Lasix) to promote diuresis and venodilation, and morphine to reduce associated anxiety (although some physicians avoid morphine because of side effects). Angiotensin-converting enzyme inhibitors are also sometimes used to reduce afterload, but thiazide diuretics are not used to treat acute pulmonary edema. Calcium channel blockers may induce acute pulmonary edema if used with tocolytics.

**2. D:** The daughter should be advised that cardiopulmonary resuscitation must be withheld in accordance with the advance directive and desires of the mother. A valid do-not-resuscitate order is in place and does not require verification. Family members often panic at the time of death and want to institute life-saving measures against the wishes of the patient, but this does not override the patient's explicit directions. The staff should provide emotional support for the family. While this is an ethical issue, there is no time to contact an ethics committee.

**3. B:** Emergency defibrillation is usually performed in patients with ventricular tachycardia (VT) who are also unconscious. Ventricular tachycardia is characterized by three or more premature ventricular contractions in a row and a ventricular rate of 100-200 bpm. The rapid rate of contractions makes VT dangerous as the ineffective beats may render the person unconscious with no palpable pulse. A detectable rate is usually regular and the QRS complex is ≥0.12 seconds and (often) abnormally shaped. The P wave may be undetectable with an irregular PR interval if the P wave is present. The P:QRS ratio is difficult to ascertain if the P wave is missing.

**4. C:** Cardiac tamponade may result in decreased chest tube drainage, muffled heart sounds, tachycardia, pulsus paradoxus, and decreased urinary output. The pulmonary artery wedge pressure, central venous pressure, and pulmonary artery diastolic pressure equalize. The cause is fluid accumulating in the pericardial sac, compressing the heart. In some cases, it can be caused by kinks or obstructions in the drainage tube. These tubes may be gently milked to remove obstructions, but the nurse should avoid the creation of negative pressure (through stripping), which can damage the surgical site.

**5. B:** Ischemia is characterized by inverted T waves. As the cardiac muscle is damaged, the ST segment is elevated, with elevated symmetrical T waves. With a Q wave myocardial infarction, Q or QS waves develop as repolarization is altered or absent. Changes in the Q waves are usually permanent, so an old myocardial infarction (MI) is evidenced by abnormal Q waves or decreased elevation of the R waves without alterations of ST and T waves. A non-Q wave MI does not cause Q wave changes.

**6. D:** The sudden onset of intermittent substernal pain that is referred to the neck, arms, and back is typical of pericarditis. Angina pain, usually related to exertion, lasts 5-15 minutes and is substernal or retrosternal, radiating across the chest and sometimes to the inside of the arm, neck, or jaw. Myocardial pain lasts over 15 minutes and occurs spontaneously or after an episode of unstable angina. It is substernal or over the pericardium. It may spread across the chest and into the shoulders and hands. Anxiety pain lasts 2-3 minutes and tends to occur across the chest but does not radiate; however, some patients complain of numbness of the hands and mouth.

**7. A:** An ankle systolic pressure of 90 divided by a brachial systolic pressure of 120 equals 0.75. Blood pressure at the ankle should be equal to or slightly higher than that of the arm. With peripheral arterial disease, the ankle pressure falls. The degree of disease relates to the score:

- >1.2: Abnormally high, may indicate calcification of vessel wall
- 1.0-1.2: Normal
- 0.90-0.99: Lower than normal, but acceptable
- 0.80-0.89: Likely some arterial disease present
- 0.50-0.79: Moderate arterial disease, associated with intermittent claudication
- <0.50: Severe disease, ischemia

**8. D:** S4 is an extra beat (atrial gallop), occurring just before S1 and producing a triple "Tennessee" rhythm. It is often associated with left ventricular hypertrophy, hypertension, or aortic stenosis. S1 and S2 are normal heart sounds. S1 indicates the onset of systole with closure of both the tricuspid and mitral valves. S2 is the end of systole and indicates closure of the pulmonary and aortic valves. S3 is an extra beat, producing a triple rhythm ("Kentucky"), and indicates decreased ventricular compliance, often related to left ventricular failure and mitral regurgitation.

**9. C:** Anticoagulation therapy is given before direct current cardioversion and also before chemical cardioversion in most cases. There is no time to start anticoagulation when emergency defibrillation is needed. With fibrillation, blood clots may form within the heart, and when the pulse rate converts to normal, these clots can travel, increasing the risk of heart attack or stroke; thus, the patient is usually maintained on anticoagulation (commonly warfarin [Coumadin]) for up to six months after cardioversion.

**10. D:** Drinking heavily on only one occasion can result in cardiovascular impairment. While the effect of alcohol on the heart is more severe if there is underlying cardiac disease, an overdose of alcohol even with no underlying disorder weakens cardiac contractions, causing the heart rate to increase. Alcohol depresses the autonomic nervous system, which can lead to heart failure, cardiac dysrhythmias (most commonly atrial fibrillation), and cardiac arrest. Chronic drinking can severely damage the heart and blood vessels, resulting in hypertension and cardiomyopathy.

**11. B:** Urinary output after surgery varies, according to fluid intake, but should be more than 25 mL/hr. Urinary output less than 25 mL/hr indicates decreased renal function. Urine specific gravity should be maintained at 1.015-1.025, indicating the ability of the kidneys to concentrate urine in the renal tubules. Blood urea nitrogen, creatinine, urine, and serum electrolytes are monitored to ensure that the kidneys can excrete waste products. Urinary output is usually monitored every hour while the patient is in the critical care unit.

**12. A:** Most cocaine users typically demonstrate hypertension and an increased heart rate. Chest pain may mimic a myocardial infarction. Vasoconstriction occurs both within the coronary arteries and the peripheral circulation, resulting in hypertension and episodes of cardiac ischemia that may cause infarcts. In some cases, multiple infarcts may occur even with normal coronary arteries. Cardiomyopathy with enlargement of the left ventricular muscle is common in chronic users.

**13. B:** Venous ulcers are typically superficial, irregular ulcers on the medial or lateral malleolus and sometimes the anterior tibial area, causing varying degrees of pain. Surrounding skin often has a brownish discoloration. Edema is moderate to severe. Arterial ulcers are painful, deep, circular, often necrotic ulcers found on toe tips, toe webs, heels, or other pressure areas. There is often rubor on dependency but pallor on foot elevation, and skin is pale, shiny, and cool. Edema is minimal.

**14. A:** No special preparation is needed for a radionuclide ventriculogram. A sample of blood is withdrawn, labeled with a technetium 99m radionuclide, and then injected back into the patient. With electrocardiogram (ECG) guidance, images are obtained during the cardiac cycle. The video display provides images similar to that of a contrast angiogram. The radionuclide ventriculogram is used to evaluate diastolic and systolic function for patients with heart failure from valvular heart disease or to monitor the toxic effects of chemotherapeutic drugs.

**15. C:** Central cyanosis of the tongue and buccal mucosa indicates severe cardiovascular disease, such as pulmonary edema or congestive heart failure. Pallor is the result of decreased levels of oxyhemoglobin, usually resulting from anemia or decreased perfusion. Peripheral cyanosis of the nails, nose, and extremities indicates decreased circulation and can occur with heart failure or other causes of vasoconstriction (e.g., cold). Xanthelasma is a yellowish plaque, usually on the eyelids, indicating high levels of cholesterol.

**16. D:** Angiotensin-converting enzyme (ACE) inhibitors are contraindicated in patients with renal failure, as one of the most serious side effects of these drugs is renal impairment, especially in patients also taking diuretics and non-steroidal anti-inflammatory drugs. The ACE inhibitors are commonly used to treat hypertension and heart failure. They are often combined with diuretics, such as the thiazide diuretics (hydrochlorothiazide) for hypertension or furosemide (Lasix) for heart failure. The ACE inhibitors are sometimes given to patients with diabetes mellitus to prevent diabetic neuropathy.

**17. B:** Mechanical ventilation can cause hypoventilation and carbon dioxide retention, resulting in respiratory acidosis. Renal compensatory actions include retention of bicarbonate (HCO3) and increased excretion of hydrogen (H). Serum pH and PCO2 are decreased. Symptoms include flushed skin, ventricular fibrillation, and hypotension. Patients may develop drowsiness, headaches, disorientation, seizures, and coma.

**18. A:** The risks associated with sexual activity after recovery from a myocardial infarction are very low, and most heart recovery programs encourage exercise. However, before a sexual encounter, it is important to consider the following:

- The person should be well rested.
- The person should wait 1-3 hours after eating.
- A comfortable position should be used to minimize stress.
- Foreplay is important so that the heart rate increases and strengthens in preparation for intercourse.
- If the person takes nitroglycerine for angina, this medication should be taken before sexual activity.

**19. C:** While wearing a Holter monitor, patients should maintain an activity diary so that any abnormality can be linked to this activity. Conversely, the diary may demonstrate that no abnormality occurs with certain activities. Patients should continue with prescribed medications and carry out normal activities since the primary purpose of a Holter monitor is to assist in diagnosis and to determine triggers for abnormal electrocardiogram readings. The monitor should be used during the night as some cardiac abnormalities may occur during sleep.

**20. B:** The best approach for severe mitral valve prolapse with heart failure is to repair the valve rather than to replace it because of the connective tissue abnormalities associated with Marfan syndrome. These abnormalities may result in dehiscence when prosthetic valves are used. Severe mitral valve prolapse can result in complications, such as heart failure, endocarditis, and cardiac arrest, so delaying surgery increases the risk; therefore, delaying or avoiding surgery are options only for mild cases of mitral valve prolapse.

**21. D:** The health belief model is used to predict health behavior when a person takes a health action to avoid negative consequences if the person believes the action will prevent a negative outcome. The theory is based on six basic perceptions:

- Susceptibility, the belief that a person may get a negative condition
- Severity, an understanding of how serious a condition is
- Benefit, a belief that action will reduce risk
- Barriers, such as direct or psychological costs
- Action cues or strategies, such as education, to encourage action
- Self-efficacy, the confidence in the ability to take action and to achieve positive results

**22. B:** Smoking the first cigarette within 5 minutes of awakening is one of the primary signs of a high level of nicotine dependence as is smoking 31 or more cigarettes daily. Patients who are dependent on cigarettes also often smoke in areas where it is prohibited (e.g., at work) and smoke even if they are extremely ill. Patients may benefit from keeping a smoking diary to help to identify their smoking patterns.

**23. C:** The most effective and efficient method of teaching a group about lifestyle changes is the group lecture and discussion. These allow the nurse to provide information and for people with shared concerns to interact and discuss issues. Computer-assisted instruction is not effective for all patients, especially older adults, and lectures only may not address specific concerns of the patients. One-on-one instruction is good for teaching specific processes or information, but it does not allow patients to share their concerns with others.

**24. A:** The goals of the 2100-calorie DASH diet include:

- Total fat: 27%.
- Saturated fat: 6%.
- Protein: 18%
- Carbohydrates: 55%.

Cholesterol is limited to 150 mg/day and sodium to 1500-2300 mg/day. People are encouraged to eat six to eight servings of whole grains, four to five servings of fruit and vegetables, 30 g of fiber, and 6 oz of lean meat daily as well as four to five servings of nuts, seeds, or legumes each week. Sweets and added sugars are limited to five or fewer servings each week.

**25. C:** Hypovolemic shock occurs when there is inadequate intravascular fluid. The loss is absolute if caused by internal shifting of fluid or external loss of fluid, such as with massive hemorrhage, thermal injuries, severe vomiting and diarrhea, or a ruptured spleen. The loss is relative if related to vasodilation, increased capillary membrane permeability from sepsis or injuries, and decreased colloidal membrane permeability from loss of sodium or from diseases, such as hypopituitarism or cirrhosis.

**26. D:** Videos are appropriate educational tools for illiterate patients. Material should be at an adult level, so a children's book is not appropriate, and material at a third-grade level may be too difficult for someone who cannot read. Computerized instruction almost always involves some reading for instructions, so this also may not be appropriate. Allowing patients and their families to watch a video demonstration can help them to grasp the fundamentals before they must apply them. Videos are much more effective than written materials for those with low literacy or poor English skills.

**27. A:** Each state has separate regulations regarding advance directives, so the patient should check state regulations and fill out two advance directives if necessary. Most require two witnesses, but some do not. Some states invalidate an advance directive if the person is pregnant. Telling family members is not adequate as these people may not be available or may be unwilling to carry out the patient's wishes. Advance directives should not be placed in a safety deposit box where access is limited.

**28. C:** The greatest risk of cardiovascular disease for people over 50 years of age is from a systolic blood pressure (BP) of 140 mm Hg or more rather than an increased diastolic pressure. However, increased diastolic pressure (>80 mm Hg) is a greater risk factor for people younger than 50 years of age. Pulse pressure of 40 mm Hg is normal for people at rest. Patients should avoid caffeine, exercise, and smoking for 30 minutes before a BP examination.

**29. B:** Heparin-induced thrombocytopenia can cause a thrombosis syndrome that increases the patient's risk for thrombosis and vessel occlusion rather than hemorrhage. A platelet count below 50,000 $mm^3$ indicates a type II reaction (rather than transient type I reaction), an autoimmune reaction to heparin; the reaction causes heparin-antibody complexes to form and also causes a release of platelet factor 4, which in turn attracts heparin molecules that adhere to platelets and endothelial lining, stimulating thrombin and platelet clumping. Discontinuation of the heparin and treatment with direct thrombin inhibitors (lepirudin [Refludan], argatroban [Argatroban]) are indicated.

**30. C:** A nurse who delegates a task to an unlicensed assistant is accountable for patient outcomes and for supervision of the person to whom the task was delegated. The scope of nursing includes delegation of tasks to unlicensed assistive personnel, providing those personnel have adequate training and knowledge. Delegation can be used to manage the workload and to provide adequate and safe care. Delegation should be done in a manner that reduces liability by providing adequate communication.

**31. C:** Endothelial dysfunction is a key factor in the development of atherosclerosis and hypertension. The ability of arteries and arterioles to dilate is impaired. As the impairment of the endothelium becomes greater, the blood pressure rises. The endothelium mediates hemostasis, coagulation, fibrinolysis, cell proliferation, and cell wall inflammatory mechanisms. Endothelial dysfunction is associated with hyperlipidemia, smoking, diabetes, and lack of exercise. Research has not yet indicated if endothelial dysfunction is the direct cause of hypertension or the result.

**32. C:** The goal of the exercise stress test is to raise the heart rate to 80-90% of that predicted for age and gender. Cardiac stress testing is done to determine if the coronary arteries dilate adequately during exercise. Normal coronary arteries dilate four times the resting diameter when under stress, so testing is more accurate when exercising than when resting to determine if there is compromised blood flow. The Bruce protocol, in which the speed and grade of the treadmill increases every three minutes, is most common. Chemical stress tests, using adenosine or dipyridamole (Persantine), may be used for those who cannot exercise.

**33. A:** Janeway lesions, splinter hemorrhages, Roth's spots, petechiae on oral mucosa, and glomerulonephritis are immunological responses associated with endocarditis, which is an infection of the endothelial surface and valves of the heart caused by invasion of the tissue by a pathogen, usually after surgery, intravenous (IV) catheterization, or IV drug abuse. Other manifestations include low-grade fever, anorexia, weight loss, malaise, splenomegaly, and anemia. Patients with pericarditis present with chest pain, mild fever, increased erythrocyte sedimentation rate, white blood cell count, and friction rub. It may cause aortic valve dysfunction or mitral valve insufficiency. Patients with myocarditis may present asymptomatically or with fatigue, dyspnea, and palpitations, but also with sudden cardiac arrest.

**34. D:** Behavior modification and compliance rates are the best determinants of the effectiveness of patient education. Patients may be satisfied, may understand, and may be able to provide a demonstration, but if they do not use what they have learned, the education has not been effective. Behavior modification involves thorough observation and measurement, identifying behavior that needs to be changed, and then planning and instituting interventions. Compliance rates should be determined by observation on multiple occasions.

**35. C:** Palliative care provides comfort rather than curative treatment although sometimes treatment that may be considered curative—such as radiotherapy—may be used to relieve pain or symptoms. Palliative care is meant to improve the quality of life and relieve suffering but to neither prolong life nor hasten death. Palliative care provides adequate pain management and relief of symptoms (such as nausea and shortness of breath). Chemotherapy, intubation, ventilation, and total parenteral nutrition are not generally considered palliative care.

**36. B:** Changes on an electrocardiogram (ECG), such as a U wave more than 1 mm high after the T wave, AV block, and flat or inverted T waves, are characteristic of hypokalemia. Tall peaked T waves with widening and increased amplitude of QRS and prolongation of the QT interval are characteristic of hyperkalemia. Dysrhythmias with prolonged PR and QT intervals and broad flat T waves are characteristic of hypomagnesemia. Other electrolyte imbalances are not reflected by specific ECG changes although hypermagnesemia can lead to cardiac arrest, and hypercalcemia can cause dysrhythmias (similar to those of digitalis toxicity).

**37. C:** Metabolic syndrome (insulin resistance) puts people at risk for the development of diabetes mellitus and cardiovascular disease; it is characterized by abdominal obesity (>35 inches in women and >40 inches in men), increased triglycerides (≥150), decreased HDL level (<40 in men and <50 in women), elevation of blood pressure (≥130/85 mm Hg), and increased fasting glucose (≥110). Other indicators include elevation of C-reactive protein, evidence of a proinflammatory state, high levels of fibrinogen, and evidence of a prothrombotic state.

**38. B:** Under the Nursing Code of Ethics of the American Nurses Association, autonomy and self-determination are viewed within the broader context of diverse cultures. The idea of individualism is less important in some cultures, so the nurse must respect and appreciate the patient's right to be guided by her family. Trying to convince the patient to assert herself may just lead to emotional conflict. This is not an appropriate concern for the ethics committee, as the woman is not being forced to comply with family decisions but chooses to do so.

**39. D:** In third-degree atrioventricular (AV) block, there are more P waves than QRS complexes, with no clear relationship between them, and an atrial rate two to three times the pulse rate, with an irregular PR interval. If the sinoatrial node malfunctions, the AV node fires at a lower rate, and if the AV node malfunctions, the pacemaker site in the ventricles takes over at a bradycardic rate: thus, with complete AV block, the heart still contracts but often ineffectually. The atrial P (sinus rhythm or atrial fibrillation) and the ventricular QRS (ventricular escape rhythm) are stimulated by different impulses, so there is AV dissociation. The heart cannot compensate with exertion.

**40. D:** Cor pulmonale (also known as pulmonary heart disease) is characterized by changes in the right ventricle because of a pulmonary disorder, such as chronic obstructive pulmonary disease. Cor pulmonale begins with endothelial dysfunction, resulting in vasoconstriction and vessel wall thickening, with sustained pulmonary hypertension, resulting in right ventricular hypertrophy in chronic cor pulmonale and right ventricular dilation in acute cor pulmonale. The end result is right-sided heart failure.

**41. B:** The primary reason for completing continuing education courses is to remain current in the field of nursing. It is every nurse's responsibility to be informed and aware of changes in practice. Many states require continuing education for licensure, and some institutions require continuing education for employment. Taking courses to meet requirements for salary increase is a personal reason that does not obviate professional responsibility for learning.

**42. B:** Cognitive changes associated with aging may result in the decline of explicit memories (facts) while implicit memories (skills) remain intact. Older adults may have difficulty in completing complex tasks that require processing of new information and may become easily distracted and less able to focus attention. Working memory declines, making it more difficult for older adults to complete mental processes that require keeping facts in memory (e.g., calculating costs); they may also have difficulty retrieving words, such as the names of people or objects.

**43. D:** High doses of tacrolimus (an immunosuppressive macrolide antibiotic) can result in nephrotoxicity (similar to cyclosporine) with elevated blood urea nitrogen and creatinine. Other effects include hyperkalemia, insomnia, and malaise. Tacrolimus is often used instead of cyclosporine because it is generally well tolerated and is also effective for rescue therapy during cardiac rejection. Hypertension is an adverse effect of cyclosporine and corticosteroids. Facial dysmorphism is related to cyclosporine use. Hirsutism and acne are common adverse effects of corticosteroids.

**44. C:** The automatic implantable cardioverter defibrillator (AICD), used to control tachycardia and fibrillation, provides on-demand (synchronous) small electrical impulses to the atrial or ventricular myocardium to slow the heart when the pulse rate increases to a preset rate. If fibrillation occurs, a high-energy shock is delivered. It takes 5-15 seconds for the device to detect abnormalities in the pulse rate, and more than one shock may be required, so fainting may occur. Some devices can function as both a pacemaker and an ICD for patients with episodes of both bradycardia and tachycardia.

**45. B:** Syncope associated with exertional exercise is a manifestation of aortic stenosis. With aortic stenosis, exercise results in reduced cerebral blood flow because of peripheral dilation without increased cardiac output. In some cases, the hypotension related to syncope may result in ventricular fibrillation or ventricular tachycardia and death. Syncope, a sudden brief loss of consciousness, may also be caused by carotid sinus sensitivity (vasovagal syndrome) or dysrhythmias (tachycardia, bradycardia). In older adults, syncope often occurs with postural hypotension, sometimes related to medications or alcohol.

**46. D:** Symptoms typical of a dissecting descending aortic aneurysm include severe, intense, knife-like pain posteriorly between the scapulae and nausea and vomiting. In addition, patients may be cold and clammy. Dissection of the ascending thoracic aorta results in similar symptoms, but the pain is in the anterior chest. Pain with dissection does not generally increase in intensity, as it is severe at onset when the tearing occurs. Peripheral arteries may be involved, which can cause numbness, tingling, and evidence of vascular insufficiency in the affected limb.

**47. A:** The most likely cause of nausea, vomiting, and tachycardia is digitalis toxicity. Most cases of digitalis toxicity can be traced to drug interactions. In this case, both furosemide (Lasix) and tetracycline can cause digitalis toxicity when taken with digoxin (Lanoxin). Digoxin levels should be monitored to ensure that therapeutic levels (0.5-2.0 ng/mL) are maintained. Early signs of digitalis toxicity include fatigue, lethargy, depression, nausea, and vomiting. Sudden changes in heart rhythm, atrioventricular or sinoatrial block, new ventricular dysrhythmias, or tachycardia may occur. Digoxin immune FAB (Digibind) may be given to inactivate digoxin, if necessary.

**48. B:** While the international normalized ratio (INR) is individualized, depending on baseline readings, a normal INR is usually about 1. Patients receiving warfarin (Coumadin) for atrial fibrillation are usually maintained at an INR of 2-3. The INR for prophylaxis for deep vein thrombosis is 1.5-2 and for pulmonary emboli and mechanical heart values is 3-4. The higher the number, the greater the anticoagulation effect, so a level over 4 may put the patient at risk for hemorrhage.

**49. B:** Hiccups are an indication that a pacemaker lead has become dislodged and is causing phrenic nerve or muscle stimulation. Other complications include infection; bleeding; hematoma; puncture of the subclavian vein or internal mammary artery, causing hemothorax; irritation of the ventricular wall by the endocardial electrode, causing ectopic beats or tachycardia; malfunction or perforation of the myocardium from dislodgement of a transvenous lead; and cardiac tamponade, resulting from removal of epicardial wires used for temporary pacing.

**50. A:** Contraindications to thrombolytic therapy include an aortic aneurysm, hemorrhagic stroke, recent surgery, or bleeding. While ideally thrombolytic therapy should be administered within 90 minutes of the onset of symptoms, some thrombolytics (tenecteplase) may be given within 6 hours and some within 12 hours. A history of any type of stroke within two months precludes thrombolytic therapy. Severe hypertension (>210/130 mm Hg) that is uncontrolled by medications or that occurs with retinal-vascular disease is also a contraindication. Relative contraindications include age over 75 years, pregnancy, pericarditis, and endocarditis.

**51. A:** Digoxin should be withheld for a minimum of 48 hours before cardioversion. Anticoagulation, usually with warfarin (Coumadin), is prescribed at least three weeks before cardioversion to prevent emboli. Sometimes drug therapy is used in conjunction with cardioversion: for example, antiarrhythmics (Cardizem, Cordarone) may be given before the procedure to slow the heart rate. Insulin should not be withheld for 48 hours, but the patient must fast before cardioversion and may be asked to delay the insulin injection on the morning of the procedure.

**52. B:** Symptoms that do not occur with rest but with physical exertion, limitations with the activities of daily living (ADLs), and slight pulmonary edema are typical of class II heart failure:

- Class I: Asymptomatic during normal activities and no pulmonary congestion or peripheral hypotension. Prognosis is good.
- Class II: No symptoms at rest but symptoms appear with physical exertion, limiting ADLs. Slight pulmonary edema may be evident. Prognosis is good.
- Class III: Obvious limitations of ADLs and discomfort on any exertion. Prognosis is fair.
- Class IV: Symptoms are present. Prognosis is poor.

**53. C:** Balloon valvuloplasty is the treatment of choice for significant pulmonary stenosis, resulting in a narrowing of the valve or the area above or below the valve. Closed valvotomy (without cardiopulmonary bypass) is no longer done, but open valvotomy with cardiopulmonary bypass may be needed if the balloon valvuloplasty is unsuccessful and symptoms recur. Valve replacement with a homograft valve is sometimes required, usually as an intervention after previous failure to correct the disorder.

**54. B:** Dobutamine is used to treat low cardiac output after cardiac surgery. Nitroprusside decreases blood pressure and afterload. Dopamine is used to treat shock and hypotension for patients who require volume resuscitation. Isoproterenol is used to stimulate the heart in patients with severe bradycardia. Other drugs include nitroglycerine, which is used to prevent spasm in arterial grafts and to reduce preload and afterload, and epinephrine, which is used to treat low cardiac output related to shock. Milrinone is also used to treat low cardiac output. Phenylephrine, norepinephrine, and vasopressin increase systemic vascular resistance and blood pressure and are used to treat shock.

**55. B:** The best reading level for a group of adults from an affluent area is grade six. The average American reads effectively at the sixth- to eighth-grade level, regardless of education achieved, and research shows that even people with high reading skills learn health information most effectively when the material is presented at the sixth- to eighth-grade reading level. Grade-three reading level is too simple for native English speakers but might be appropriate for an immigrant population with limited English.

**56. C:** While clinical symptoms, blood tests, and electrocardiogram monitoring are all important, biopsy remains the primary tool to diagnose acute rejection after cardiac transplantation. Acute rejection can occur with few clinical symptoms even when using cyclosporine or tacrolimus to prevent rejection, so routine biopsies are done for the first three months after surgery. The first biopsy is generally done in two weeks and then once weekly for the first month; biopsies are then tapered to every other week, then once monthly after the initial 3-month period, and then every 4-12 months, depending on the institutional protocol.

**57. D:** The apex beat (pulsation) can be observed in about half of patients at about the fifth intercostal space along the left mid-clavicular line. The pulsation is caused by thrusting of the left ventricle. The pulsation is easy to observe in patients with thin chest walls. If the heart is enlarged, the pulsation may be observed at the second intercostal space. Aiming a flashlight at a tangential angle across the chest can help cast a shadow that facilitates observation. If no pulsation is evident, the apex beat can be palpated in the same area.

**58. B:** Thiazide diuretics are the first-line drugs used to treat stage I hypertension. Stage II hypertension is usually treated with a two-drug combination of a thiazide diuretic with an angiotensin-converting enzyme (ACE) inhibitor, ARB, beta-blocker, or calcium-channel blocker. If there are compelling indications, such as heart failure, post myocardial infarction, coronary disease risk, diabetes, or chronic kidney disease, then a wide range of drugs may be needed, including diuretics, beta-blockers, ACE inhibitors, ARB, calcium channel blockers, or aldosterone antagonists, depending on the condition.

**59. B:** Pneumococcal polysaccharide-23 (single dose), influenza (annual), and herpes zoster (single dose) immunizations are recommended for all adults 60-65 years of age and older. The hepatitis B vaccine is recommended for older adults with end-stage renal disease (including those receiving dialysis), chronic liver disease, or HIV/AIDS and those in correctional facilities or substance abuse facilities. The hepatitis A vaccine is recommended for those at risk because of lifestyle (e.g., men who have sex with men, substance abusers) or medical conditions (e.g., liver disease). International travelers may receive hepatitis A and B vaccines, depending on the destination. There is no hepatitis C vaccine.

**60. D:** Synthroid 0.88 mg PO daily at 0700 is the correct medication order because of the following: (1) the medication is spelled out; (2) the decimal has a leading zero; (3) PO is clearly written; and (4) "daily" is used instead of "qd," which can be misinterpreted as "QID" if the nurse uses periods or does not write clearly. Additionally, a 24-hour time designation is used. "Maalox 30 cc" should be "Maalox 30 mL" because "cc" may be misread as "U" for "unit." Instead of "qhs," which can be misread as "qhr," "nightly" should be used. "Lasix 40.0 mg" should be "Lasix 40 mg" because the trailing zero may cause someone to read the order as "400 mg." "MS" could be misread as "magnesium sulfate."

**61. A:** Threatening to force a patient to undergo a treatment is a form of coercion. Nurses can easily intimidate patients into having procedures or treatments they do not want. Regardless of age, patients have the right to choose and refuse treatment. Forcing patients to do something against their will can be considered as borderline abuse. Furthermore, this can sometimes degenerate into actual abuse if physical coercion is involved. If patients are cognitively impaired, other family members may be designated to make decisions, but every effort should be made to gain the patient's cooperation.

**62. D:** Sexual dysfunction, including impotence, is quite common after heart transplant surgery and most often relates to antihypertensive drugs. Hypertension is a chronic problem after a heart transplant, especially with some immunosuppressive drugs, such as cyclosporine, and patients may require two or more drugs to control blood pressure. The patient should be given assistance or counseling to deal with sexual dysfunction, both before and after surgery. In some cases, alternative drugs may be used.

**63. B:** Sinus tachycardia is characterized by a pulse of 100 bpm and above. The rapid pulse decreases diastolic filling time and reduces cardiac output with resultant hypotension and pulmonary edema. Bradycardia is characterized by a pulse of 60 bpm and less. Sinus arrhythmia is characterized by cyclic changes in pulse during respiration and is common in children and young adults; however, it may also occur with vagal stimulation from suctioning, vomiting, or defecating. Premature atrial contractions are essentially extra beats caused by an electrical impulse to the atrium before the sinus node impulse, resulting in an irregular pulse.

**64. B:** Caffeinated beverages (e.g., tea, coffee, hot chocolate) may increase the effects of warfarin (Coumadin). Alcohol intake should be limited to no more than three drinks daily. A daily multivitamin should not affect warfarin, but some herbal medications can affect clotting time. Milk products should not affect warfarin, but foods that are high in vitamin K (e.g., broccoli; green leafy vegetables, such as kale, turnip greens, and beet greens; cauliflower; legumes; soybean oil; canola oil) may affect the medication and should be limited.

**65. D:** Using transesophageal Doppler ultrasonography to measure cardiac output, a short waveform with a rounded apex may indicate left ventricular failure. Decreased preload (hypovolemia) is indicated by a pointed wave with a narrow base. As preload increases with fluid administration, the base widens. Increased systemic vascular resistance (high afterload) is indicated by a pointed short waveform with a narrow base, with both height and base increasing with vasodilation, which reduces afterload.

**66. A:** Troponin levels (cTnT and cTnI) should be measured 8-12 hours after the onset of symptoms. Earlier testing may result in false negatives. Levels rise within 3-4 hours and peak at 4-24 hours but do not return to normal for 1-3 weeks. Myoglobin (MB) begins to rise within 1-3 hours and peaks at 4-12 hours, returning to normal usually in about 12-36 hours, but it is nonspecific for cardiac damage. Measurement of low-density lipoprotein levels is not usually ordered because troponin tests are more specific. Creatinine kinase (CK) levels rise in 3-6 hours, peaking at 24-36 hours, and return to normal in 3 days. The more specific CK-MB (found only in cardiac cells) increases at 4-8 hours and peaks at 12-24 hours, returning to normal in 3-4 days. CK/CK-MB should be tested on admission and in 24 hours.

**67. C:** A cardiac care center provides tertiary care, as it is a specialized center with a variety of programs to meet the needs of the cardiac patient. Primary care is usually provided by the first physician the patient sees, such as a general practitioner or an internist. Secondary care is provided by a specialist, such as a cardiologist, to whom the patient is referred. Quaternary care is provided by those who are highly specialized in very specific and limited areas of medicine or involved in special experimental programs.

**68. D:** The absolute indication for stopping an exercise test is a decrease in blood pressure of 10 mm Hg or more from baseline, despite increased workload, with evidence of ischemia. The other choices are relative indications and depend upon the patient's general condition and the assessment of the observer. Other absolute indications include moderate-to-severe angina, cyanosis or pallor, nervous system symptoms (dizziness, ataxia), sustained ventricular tachycardia, ST segment elevation of 10 mm or more in leads without Q waves (other than V1 or VR), and the patient's wish to stop the test.

**69. C:** Initially, a physician must certify that a patient who is eligible for Medicare A is terminal with a life expectancy 6 months or less (two 90-day periods), but if the patient remains alive, the physician can extend coverage by authorizing care every 60 days. The goal is to maintain the patient in the home environment with home health aides, homemakers, durable goods, pain management, case management, counseling, and social worker assistance. Routine intermittent home care must comprise 80% of the total care with in-home continuous care and inpatient hospice care available for short periods.

**70. A:** The patient described in the question is demonstrating symptoms of post-pump delirium psychosis (PPD). Patients may exhibit symptoms ranging from memory loss, alterations of personality, and apathy to clinical psychosis. Risk factors include increasing age, poor cardiac status preoperatively or postoperatively, co-morbidities, hypoxia, sepsis, CPB for more than 2-3 hours, and valvular surgery. Postoperative infection, sleep deprivation, and medications can also be factors. Usually, PPD occurs 48 hours or less postoperatively and lasts 2-5 days.

**71. D:** The treatment goal would be to lower total cholesterol to 200 or less and LDL to 130 or less and raise the HDL to 40 or more. Treatment usually includes an increase in exercise, such as daily walking; dietary modifications, such as a decrease in saturated fats; and anti-lipid medications, such as the statins. Normal cholesterol ranges include:

- Total cholesterol: 120-200 mg/dL; borderline high is 200-239 mg/dL.
- Triglyceride: 0-150 mg/dL; borderline high is 150-199 mg/dL.
- HDL: 40-70 mg/dL. This is the "good" cholesterol.
- LDL: 50-129 mg dL; borderline high is 130-159 mg/dL. This is the "bad" cholesterol.

**72. D:** Atrial arrhythmias, including fibrillation, flutter, and tachycardia, are very common after cardiac surgery, occurring in over half of patients with valvular surgery. Arrhythmias occur usually in the first 2-3 postoperative days and are often transient but may recur. Arrhythmias are usually related to surgical manipulation. Treatment includes digoxin, β-blockers, calcium channel blockers, and amiodarone (often given preoperatively for seven days to reduce the incidence of postoperative arrhythmias. Electrical cardioversion may be indicated after 24 hours if sinus rhythm remains abnormal.

**73. B:** The self-monitoring skill that is most essential for a patient with heart failure is daily weight as increased weight can indicate fluid overload and edema before it becomes evident (usually after about 5 L of retained fluid or a 10-pound weight increase). Patients may also need to monitor sodium intake. Self-management skills require an initial discussion of needs and presentation of scenarios to help the patient determine appropriate responses and practice self-management.

**74. D:** While home intravenous (IV) antibiotic therapy is appropriate for many patients, the patient in the question is frail and elderly and not a good candidate for home treatment, so transferring the patient to an extended care facility is probably the best option. Extended treatment in an acute care hospital is probably not necessary since the patient's condition is stable. A few patients may be able to self-administer IV medications if they have adequate instruction and family or other support, but the patient in the question is frail, elderly, and lives alone.

**75. B:** If a patient asks for pain medication after four hours when it has been prescribed for every six hours, the pain control is not adequate to prevent breakthrough pain, and the routine medication may need to be increased in dosage or frequency. While tolerance to pain varies, pain is what the individual perceives it to be, and distraction is rarely effective in relieving severe pain. Since breakthrough pain commonly occurs, this most likely reflects inadequate control. Patients have a right to pain control, and almost all pain can be controlled with proper analgesia.

**76. C:** Adequate perfusion requires a mean arterial pressure (MAP) of >60 mm Hg because ischemia of the internal organs will occur if the MAP falls below this level for an extended period. MAP is the average pressure within the arterial system. Because the duration of diastole is about twice that of systole, the formula to calculate the MAP is systolic BP plus 2 times the diastolic BP divided by 3:

$$MAP = \frac{Diastole \times 2 + Systole}{3}$$

**77. A:** Patients with peripheral arterial disease and aspirin intolerance should be prescribed clopidogrel. Antiplatelet therapy is essential to reducing the risk of cardiovascular disease events, but heparin and warfarin are not recommended as preventive medications. Clopidogrel requires activation by CYP2C19, and tests are available to determine if patients have normal CYP2C19 function. NSAIDs should be avoided with clopidogrel as the combination may increase risk of GI bleeding. Platelet aggregation does not return to normal after discontinuation of clopidogrel for about five days.

**78. B:** According to the AHA/ACC Guideline for the Management of Patients with Non-ST-Elevation Acute Coronary Syndromes, for early risk stratification of patients presenting in the ED with chest pain or other symptoms indicative of acute coronary syndrome, a 12-lead ECG should be done within 10 minutes of arrival at the ED. If this initial ECG is negative and the symptoms persist, then repeat 12-lead ECGs should be done every 15 to 30 minutes for the first hour. Additionally, serial troponin I or T (with contemporary assay) should be completed every 3 to 6 hours.

**79. D:** For a patient receiving a calcium channel blocker (CCB), such as diltiazem, calcium supplements may reduce effectiveness. CCBs are class IV antidysrhythmics, primarily used for SVT but also frequently used to reduce hypertension and to relieve angina. CCBs block the inward flow of calcium ions into the calcium channels in the heart's conduction tissue. Patients must be advised to avoid calcium supplements and calcium-based antacids, such as Tums. Vitamin D supplements may also interfere with absorption.

**80. B:** If a patient preparing for discharge has been advised to make multiple lifestyle changes in relation to diet, medications, habits, and exercise but the patient is upset about the changes and states repeatedly that the physician is expecting too much, the best response is: "It's difficult to make all of these changes." When a patient is venting and upset, often the best response is to be empathetic, showing that the person's concerns are understood and appreciated. Giving advice to a patient when they are in a resistant frame of mind could merely further resistance.

**81. C:** If a patient has a base normal control prothrombin time (PT) of 10 seconds, the maximum target PT with warfarin therapy is usually 25 seconds. The normal time is 10 to 14 seconds, and with warfarin, the PT should be 1 to 2.5 times the base control value. Prothrombin (factor II) is produced by the liver, and the PT can be used to evaluate extrinsic coagulation factors (V, VII, and X), fibrinogen, and prothrombin, and may be used to monitor oral anticoagulation therapy as well.

**82. D:** If a patient is taking a bile acid sequestrant, such as cholestyramine, to lower LDL, a patient should wait 4 to 6 hours after taking the drug before taking other medications because pronounced drug interactions with multiple drugs may occur. Alternately, other medications may be taken 1 to 2 hours prior to the bile acid sequestrant. Cholestyramine especially poses a problem because it may be prescribed twice daily. The drug is administered in powdered form, must be mixed with liquid, and should be taken with a meal.

**83. A:** While all antiplatelet drugs pose some risk of bleeding, ASA poses the least risk. However, it can result in gastrointestinal bleeding, a risk somewhat mitigated by taking ASA with food or using enteric-coated formulations. Clopidogrel poses a greater risk of gastrointestinal bleeding and intracranial bleeding. The drugs with the greatest risk are the intravenous glycoprotein IIb/IIIa inhibitors, including tirofiban and eptifibatide. All patients should be assessed for risk of bleeding before administration of antiplatelet drugs.

**84. B:** ST-elevation MI (STEMI) is an indication for thrombolytic therapy as is new left bundle branch block (LBBB). When a vessel is completely occluded for an extended period of time, the thrombin and fibrin become increasingly concentrated, and a STEMI usually develops, characterized by both ST-elevation and T-wave inversion. In about 90% of STEMIs, pathologic Q waves develop. Thrombolysis should ideally be carried out within 30 minutes to be most effective; however, there is benefit within the first 12 hours and in some cases up to 24 hours.

**85. C:** If a patient has undergone thrombolysis per accelerated infusion of alteplase 100 mg (maximum dose) for an acute myocardial infarction and shows 20% reduction in ST elevation after 90 minutes, the cardiac/vascular nurse anticipates angiography and rescue PCI because ST elevation should decrease by at least 50% within this timeframe. Fibrinolytic therapy is often administered instead of PCI if PCI is not available at the hospital or within an acceptable period of time, so arrangements should be made to transfer the patient to another facility if necessary.

**86. A:** The patient that may be an acceptable candidate for catheter-directed thrombolysis (CDT) for peripheral arterial occlusion is the one with non-life-threatening limb ischemia of 12 days. Thrombolysis may be indicated (depending on risk factors) if the ischemia has been present for fewer than 14 days. CDT is not indicated for limb-threatening ischemia because lysis of the occluding clot may take between 6 and 72 hours. These patients should undergo emergent embolectomy.

**87. B:** On the ECG recording, a normal sinus rhythm is characterized by a PR interval of 0.12 to 0.2 seconds. Normal rate is 60 to 100 bpm, with rates below 60 considered bradycardic and rates above 100 considered tachycardic. The PR interval usually remains normal with both sinus bradycardia and sinus tachycardia. P waves should precede each QRS complex and should be consistent in shape. The duration of the QRS complex should range from 0.04 to 0.1 seconds.

**88. D:** If a patient exhibits a ventricular rate of 150 bpm, the most likely cause of dysrhythmia is atrial flutter. While the atrial rate with atrial flutter may vary from 250 to 450 bpm, around 300 bpm is the most common. The AV node generally blocks about 50% of the atrial impulses in order to prevent too rapid contractions, resulting in a ventricular rate of about 150 bpm. This would be categorized as atrial flutter with 2:1 conduction.

**89. C:** After administering sublingual nitroglycerin to a patient for angina, the cardiac/vascular nurse should expect a reduction in pain within 3 to 4 minutes. If no relief occurs, the drug may be administered every five minutes for a total of three doses. Sublingual or buccal preparations are usually given for acute angina because they are absorbed into the bloodstream quickly but IV nitroglycerine may be given in the hospital.

**90. B:** Beta-blockers are generally contraindicated for patients with a history of asthma and COPD because they may cause bronchospasm and may block the effects of bronchodilators. Some patients may develop cough-variant asthma as an adverse effect of beta-blockers. Other contraindications include severe sinus bradycardia and second- or third-degree heart block because beta-blockers slow conduction. Beta-blockers should also be avoided in the presence of cardiogenic shock or acute heart failure. Beta-blockers may interact with a number of different medications.

**91. C:** *Rest potentiation* of the heart refers to a pause resulting in a stronger ensuing contraction, assuming an intact organism. After an extra beat, the ensuing contraction is stronger, an effect referred to as *postextrasystolic potentiation*. The force of contraction is influenced by the heart rate, a phenomenon referred to as the Treppe or staircase phenomenon, so the faster the rate of stimulation, the stronger the contraction, and the slower the rate of stimulation, the weaker the contraction.

**92. D:** In order to modify risk of cardiovascular disease for patients with peripheral arterial disease (PAD), the primary lifestyle change should be smoking cessation. Patients are at high risk for MI, cerebrovascular accident (CVA), and cardiovascular disease-associated death. Smoking cessation is especially important because of the vasoconstrictive and inflammatory properties of tobacco. Because of the addictiveness of tobacco products, patients may require comprehensive assistance, such as medications, education, and support groups, in order to succeed in smoking cessation.

**93. C:** At a heart rate of >180 bpm, diastolic filling is so reduced that stroke volume is diminished and coronary ischemia occurs. This may occur at much lower rates if heart failure or cardiac pathology is present. Generally, an increased heart rate results in increased cardiac output and the strength of contraction increases with the heart rate. Normal cardiac output is 5.5 L/min (70 kg male patient) but can increase to 18 L/min with exercise in order to meet body demands.

**94. A:** An increased risk factor for coronary artery disease is a sister who developed the disorder at age 63. Family history of coronary artery disease is a risk factor for developing the disease. Risk increases if a father or brother developed the disease before age 55 or if a mother or sister developed it before age 65, as onset is usually later in females than males. Other risk factors include advanced age, male gender, smoking, hypertension, hyperlipidemia, obesity, lack of exercise, and stress.

**95. D:** If deviation is present when assessing best gaze, then the oculocephalic maneuver can be carried out to determine if one or both eyes has reflexive movement. The cardiac/vascular nurse must grasp the patient's head on each side and turn it quickly side to side while observing the eyes.

A normal response is for the eyes to deviate to the opposite side the head is turned to and then to return toward midline. If there is no movement, then the best gaze is scored as 2 (out of a 0 to 2 range) because the oculocephalic maneuver did not overcome the deviation.

**96. B:** When assessing the adequacy of a patient's diet, the cardiac/vascular nurse recognized that, for an elderly adult weighing 70 kg (154 lb.), the average caloric requirement per day is about 1750 calories. On average, elderly adults require approximately 25 calories per kg of body weight, while a healthy younger adult requires 30 calories per kg. Obese adults who need to lose weight should have an intake ranging from 20 to 25 calories per kg.

**97. D:** If a patient remains passive, asks no questions, and shows no interest during instruction, then the patient is not exhibiting readiness to learn; the patient is not engaged in any way. If a patient indicates confusion about the medication regimen, this indicates the patient is seeking more information. Patients who are not visual learners or who lack literacy skills may avoid written materials, and if a patient turns on the TV to watch a football game when the nurse is instructing, this may simply indicate that the nurse has not chosen a good time for instruction.

**98. C:** According to the AHA/ACC Guideline for the Management of Patients with Non-ST-Elevation Acute Coronary Syndromes, patients presenting in the ED with chest pain or symptoms indicative of acute coronary syndrome should receive oxygen with oxygen saturation <90%, respiratory distress, or indications of hypoxemia. Patients should also receive sublingual nitrates every five minutes for up to three doses, and IV morphine to control pain. NSAIDs other than aspirin should be avoided. Beta-blockers should be started within 24 hours.

**99. A:** According to the Protection Motivation Theory, action to bring about change is precipitated by a threat, such as hypertension that threatens health. This threat serves as a stimulus for protection motivation. The patient cognitively assesses sources of information (internal and external) and the extent of a threat and develops coping mechanisms that include action to bring about change. According to this theory, protective coping strategies develop based on the patient's perception of the severity of the threat, the probability the threat will occur, the ability of preventive measures to allay the threat, and the degree of self-efficacy.

**100. D:** In assessing health literacy, the cardiac/vascular nurse should expect that the average reading level of the US population is ≤8th grade. However, almost half of Americans lack the basic skills in reading and comprehension needed to carry out every day literacy tasks, and many adults read at levels that are two to four grade levels below their level of completed formal education. Thus, the cardiac/vascular nurse must assess each patient individually and cannot make assumptions based on formal education history alone.

**101. C:** When administering the Tinetti Gait and Balance Instrument to an older adult, the balance assessment begins with the patient sitting in an armless chair. The patient is assessed for the ability to lean or slide in the chair, arise, stand immediately without stagger, remain standing, stand with feet close together while pushed, stand with eyes closed, turn full circle, and then sit down. The higher the score, the better the performance. Sixteen is the total maximum number of points for the balance portion of the assessment.

**102. B:** If an older adult with aortic stenosis undergoes percutaneous balloon valvuloplasty, restenosis often occurs within 1 to 2 years. Balloon valvuloplasty is most commonly used for patients who are not candidates for open surgical procedures, but patients must be monitored closely following the valvuloplasty. Complications may include bleeding/hematoma at insertion site (usually the femoral artery), damage to valve leaflets (rare), worsening of condition, embolism (rare), and cardiac abnormalities, such as arrhythmias or ischemia.

**103. A:** If a patient with hypertension and diabetes mellitus was a heavy smoker for 40 years before suffering a myocardial infarction, but she has continued to smoke even though she states, "I know I should quit," the best response is, "Tell me about that." This is a patient-centered response that encourages the patient to reflect and respects the patient's autonomy. It is clear the patient knows the importance of smoking cessation, so repeating advice to quit or making further suggestions may only engender a negative response—reasons why the patient cannot quit.

**104. D:** The educational program that might best be conducted as a webinar is the interactive discussion about new techniques in cardiac rehabilitation because the key feature of a webinar is interactivity, so participation is synchronous (in real time). Orientation program and online courses are generally set up as asynchronous so that they can be accessed at any time. A webinar is generally not needed for a video series because videos are not, by nature, interactive.

**105. B:** If a cardiac/vascular nurse working in a semi-rural area proposes a mobile clinic to better monitor, screen, and counsel patients who often cannot or do not seek medical care, the most likely impediment is cost-effectiveness. While a mobile unit may seem an ideal solution, both the initial cost and ongoing costs are high, and demonstrating cost savings, such as fewer rehospitalizations, can be difficult, especially if the patient population is low. Mobile clinics are often funded by grants to target specific populations.

**106. C:** According to the Eighth Report of the Joint National Committee on Prevention, Detection, Evaluation, and Treatment of High Blood Pressure, systolic blood pressure is a greater cardiovascular risk factor than diastolic blood pressure after age 50. Before age 50, diastolic hypertension with or without systolic hypertension is the most common, but this changes at about age 50 when the diastolic blood pressure stabilizes. However, the systolic blood pressure continues to rise, so controlling systolic blood pressure in patients older than 50 is essential to reducing risk of cardiovascular events/mortality and stroke.

**107. A:** A low score on the Care Transitions Measure (CTM-15) is predictive of rehospitalization or return to the emergency department. The CTM-15 has 15 statements that patients score using a Likert scale (strongly disagree, disagree, agree, strongly disagree, or don't know/don't remember, not applicable). Statements focus on in-hospital care, discharge planning, follow-up care, and patient medications, and ask patients to rate their understanding, satisfaction, and confidence in their own ability to manage their health care.

**108. B:** According to the Healthy People 2020 initiatives, a 55-year-old diabetic male patient with leg pain should be screened for peripheral arterial disease with the ankle-brachial index (ABI) because the patient is symptomatic (leg pain) and has a disorder that increases risk (diabetes). General screening of the adult population is not recommended in the absence of symptoms because evidence-based research shows no advantage, and false positives may result in increased cost and patient anxiety.

**109. D:** According to the ACCF/AHA Guideline for the Management of ST-Elevation Myocardial Infarction, the pain medication of choice for patients with STEMI and acute pulmonary edema is morphine sulfate, which should relieve the pain, respiratory distress, and associated anxiety. Atropine can be administered if necessary if the morphine induces bradycardia, and naloxone may be necessary if excessive sedation occurs. Both NSAIDs and COX-2 inhibitors increase risk of severe complications, such as reinfarction and death, and should be avoided.

**110. A:** If a patient with stage 2 Alzheimer's disease and coronary artery disease can function fairly well in her home environment but has increasing short-term memory loss and often forgets to take her medications (even though her daughter calls to remind her), the best solution is likely providing an electronic medication dispenser. Some dispensers require filling only once a week or once a month and have various methods to remind patients to take medications, including beeps, alarms, and verbal messages.

**111. C:** A normal value for the activated partial thromboplastin time (aPTT) is 21 to 35 seconds (may vary somewhat according to reference lab). This test is commonly used to monitor heparin dosage. The aPTT is prolonged with deficiencies of clotting factors, vitamin K deficiency, and administration of unfractionated heparin or direct thrombin inhibitors (hirudin, dabigatran, and argatroban). Warfarin usually only prolongs the aPTT by a few seconds, although with overdose the prolongation may be pronounced.

**112. B:** According to the ACC/AHA Guideline on the Treatment of Blood Cholesterol to Reduce Atherosclerotic Cardiovascular Risk in Adults, the goal for LDL cholesterol reduction with treatment with high-intensity statin is ≥50% from baseline. For patients treated with moderate-intensity statins, the goal is 30% to <50% reduction from baseline. If baseline is not known, then reduction should generally be <100 mg/dL. Patients should be monitored every 3 to 12 months to assess adherence and lifestyle changes.

**113. D:** If a patient with mechanical prosthetic heart value is on warfarin therapy and has an INR of 3.2, this probably indicates a normal INR for this patient because patients with mechanical prosthetic heart valves are usually maintained at an INR of 2.5 to 3.5. This is higher than for patients without prosthetic valves because those patients are usually maintained at 2 to 3. The INR is not used for screening purposes but is routinely used to monitor oral anticoagulation therapy.

**114. A:** When monitoring a patient's 12-lead ECG, the cardiac/vascular nurse would expect a lead facing an injured area of the heart to show ST-segment elevation and those leads facing away from the injured area to show ST-segment depression. Abnormal variations in the ST segment include elevation of more than 1 mm above the baseline and depression of more than 0.5 mm below the baseline. T-waves may vary for many reasons; very tall or inverted T-waves may indicate myocardial ischemia. Abnormal Q waves commonly occur with myocardial necrosis.

**115. B:** If C-reactive protein (CRP) is >3 mg/L (especially >10 mg/L) in a patient with normal (or abnormal) lipid values, this may indicate increased risk of cardiovascular and peripheral arterial disease. CRP is a glycoprotein produced in the liver in response to acute inflammation and serves as a nonspecific marker for inflammation. CRP is often ordered along with an ESR. Lowest risk is at <1 mg/L, and moderate risk is at 1 to 3 mg/L. CRP may better predict risk of cardiac disease in females than LDL levels.

**116. C:** When baroreceptors in the aortic arch and carotid arteries sense volume overload or increased pressure in the arteries, the usual response is decreased heart rate and vasodilation. When pressure in the arterial system stimulates these receptors, information is transmitted to the vasomotor center of the brainstem, and this inhibits the sympathetic nervous system so that the parasympathetic nervous system causes the heart rate to temporarily decrease and vasodilation to occur. Decreased pressure in the arteries causes the opposite effect, increased heart rate and vasoconstriction.

**117. D:** A common age-associated change in the cardiovascular system is decreased number of pacemaker cells in the SA node to the point that patients older than 75 years may have only one-tenth the normal number of pacemaker cells. While this number of cells may be adequate, the decrease of pacemaker cells increases the risk of sinus dysrhythmias. Other changes include decreased cardiac reserve, decreased cardiac output, decreased stroke volume, and decreased contractility of the heart because of increased collagen and decreased elastin in the heart muscle.

**118. A:** On the DASH diet, a patient may have ≤5 servings of sweets and added sugars per week. One serving is equal to 1 tablespoon of sugar, jelly, or jam, one-half cup of sorbet or gelatin, or 1 cup of lemonade. Patients should have 4 to 5 servings per week of nuts, seeds, and legumes, as well as 7 to 8 servings/day of whole grains, 4 to 5 servings/day of vegetables and fruits, 2 to 3 servings/day of low-fat or fat-free dairy foods, 2 or fewer servings/day of lean meats, poultry, and fish, and 2 to 3 servings/day of fats and oils.

**119. B:** Mended Hearts is a national support organization for patients with cardiovascular disease and their families/caregivers. Programs include the visiting program in which volunteers visit patients in the hospital and make contact per the Internet and telephone. Some chapters have regular meetings that provide emotional and educational support. Mended Hearts publishes *Heartbeat* magazine for members as well as a variety of other educational resources, including newsletters and online information, such as information about clinical trials.

**120. C:** Exclusion criteria for therapeutic hypothermia for a patient who experienced sudden cardiac arrest and resuscitation is major surgery within the previous two weeks because of increased risk of bleeding and infection associated with hypothermia. Other factors that may increase risk to the patient during hypothermia include preexisting bleeding diathesis (although not thrombolysis) and systemic infections. Additionally, therapeutic hypothermia is usually avoided in patients with a DNR order. Various cooling methods can be used to reduce the body temperature to 32-34 °C over a 3- to 4-hour period.

**121. D:** If the cardiac/vascular nurse is serving as a preceptor for a nursing student and feels that the student lacks essential skills, the cardiac/vascular nurse should first meet with the student to outline concerns. While the student may, in fact, lack essential skills, the student may also feel stressed or intimidated and be afraid to demonstrate skills effectively. The cardiac/vascular nurse should avoid using an accusatory or critical approach but should focus on what the nurse has observed.

**122. B:** The primary treatment focus for patients with dilated cardiomyopathy is controlling heart failure by improving myocardial contractility and decreasing afterload. Patients may take a variety of medications, including diuretics, nitrates, ACE inhibitors, beta-blockers, antidysrhythmics, and anticoagulants. However, dilated cardiomyopathy does not readily respond to medications, and patients may experience repeated episodes of heart failure. Some patients may receive a ventricular-assist device, especially while awaiting transplant.

**123. A:** If a physician with whom the staff is very friendly is admitted to the cardiac unit with a myocardial infarction, and a number of nurses, who are not assigned to the patient, review his laboratory findings by reading over the shoulder of the physician's assigned nurse (shoulder surfing), this is primarily a HIPAA violation and is a major violation of privacy, as well as an unprofessional activity. Both the nurse accessing the patient's file and those looking over the nurse's shoulder are in violation of the law and may be disciplined or fired.

**124. B:** If a patient experienced a severe adverse reaction to a drug while left unattended because of suboptimal staffing, this problem will likely be referred to risk management, which will determine liability issues and further courses of action. Depending on policies in place in the organization, the patient/family may or may not be apprised of the staffing problem or may not understand the implications. Incident reports are generally not included in the patient's record but are filed separately.

**125. C:** Using the SBAR communication technique, the cardiac/vascular nurse will begin the report about Ms. Jones to the physician in this order:

- (S) Situation: "Ms. Jones has had increasing shortness of breath, cough, and chest pain for the past hour."
- (B) Background: "Ms. Jones recently had cardiac catheterization and angioplasty, and Ms. Jones has a pulse of 130, BP 140/60, and respirations of 32 per minute."
- (A) Assessment: "I believe that Ms. Jones may have a pulmonary embolism or cardiac event."
- (R) Recommendation: "I recommend immediate oxygen and physician examination."

**126. A:** As a patient advocate, any time a cardiac/vascular nurse observes a patient being mistreated, the best initial response is to immediately intervene, such as by stepping in and offering to assist the patient. The cardiac/vascular nurse should avoid reprimanding the other nurse in the patient's presence but may confront the nurse later and/or report the nurse's behavior to a supervisor. There is no circumstance in which being verbally abusive to a patient is acceptable.

**127. C:** If a patient is awaiting surgical intervention for a dissecting aortic aneurysm, prior to surgery, the patient's systolic blood pressure should be maintained at 110 to 120 to ensure adequate perfusion of the patient's organs while preventing undue pressure on the dissection. The patient should receive medications to reduce pain and anxiety as these symptoms may increase the blood pressure. Antihypertensive agents should be administered under close supervision with constant monitoring of ECG recordings and vital signs.

**128. D:** If the cardiac/vascular nurse proposes forming an interdisciplinary team to work on process improvement, the best members are likely to be those who have needed knowledge/skills. While the temptation is often to form a team of friends or like-minded staff members, if they lack the necessary expertise, the team may not be productive, and friends may be reluctant to offer a different perspective. When forming a team for any purpose, the cardiac/vascular nurse should look for the best-qualified members.

**129. A:** Because Medicare restricts coverage for home health care to patients who are essentially homebound, a patient who is able to walk for one mile around her neighborhood would not be classified as homebound. A patient may, with effort and/or assistance, walk for a short distance (such as down the block), may visit physicians, and may attend rehabilitation programs and adult daycare programs and still qualify. Patients may also attend church or other religious programs with assistance.

**130. C:** If a close personal friend of the cardiac/vascular nurse is a patient on the cardiac unit, and the cardiac/vascular nurse trades assignments with another nurse in order to be assigned to the patient, this constitutes a professional boundary violation. It is very important for a nurse to treat all patients with the same degree of professional consideration and care, but it is very difficult to avoid showing preference when a personal relationship, such as family or friend, is involved.

**131. D:** If a patient with bradycardia of 30 bpm is to have a temporary transcutaneous pacemaker (TCP) until a transvenous catheter can be inserted and the cause of the bradycardia determined, in preparation for the TCP, the nurse should advise the patient to expect muscle contraction and discomfort with pacing. Most patients find these contractions uncomfortable and, if possible, should receive analgesia and/or sedation prior to application of the TCP to minimize discomfort.

**132. A:** Osler's nodes may be found with bacterial endocarditis, which is most commonly caused by *Staphylococcus aureus* or *Streptococcus viridans.* Osler's nodes are small painful red/purple lesions occurring on the fingertips or toes. Endocarditis is characterized by vegetations that adhere to the valves or endocardium. In about half of patients with vegetations, embolization will occur. Endocarditis is most commonly caused by aging, aortic stenosis, IV drug use, prosthetic valves, intravascular devices, or (about 20%) rheumatic fever.

**133. B:** If the mother of an 18-year-old patient with hypertrophic cardiomyopathy has been scheduled twice to attend CPR classes before her son is discharged but has failed to attend the classes, stating that the CPR class is "not necessary" and "a waste of time," according to Kübler-Ross's stages of grief, the mother is probably experiencing denial. Other stages in the grief process include anger, bargaining, depression, and acceptance. While some people go through all stages, some do not, and some become fixed at one stage.

**134. D:** If a patient makes a statement that is untrue or a distortion of reality, such as "The doctor promised that I didn't have to exercise today," the cardiac/vascular nurse should avoid directly agreeing or disagreeing but should comment on the distortion of fact in a way that presents the truth without being judgmental: "That's surprising because the doctor wrote an order for you to walk twice today." It is important to avoid arguing with the patient because patients retain the right to refuse treatment.

**135. A:** If the ECG shows a heart rate of 80 bpm with regular rhythm and normal P waves and QRS complex with a PR interval of 0.5 seconds, this finding is characteristic of first-degree atrioventricular block. It presents much like the normal sinus rhythm except that the PR interval is extended (normal is 0.12 to 0.2), sometimes up to a full second or longer. The delay in conduction occurs in the AV node, but generally all impulses are conducted.

**136. C:** The primary difference between partnership councils and other forms of shared governance is that partnership councils (an evolution of shared governance that usually included only nursing personnel) include all disciplines and all levels and areas within an organization. One organization may have many partnership councils, such as at the unit level and department level with one member (usually the chairperson) as representative to a central council. The central council often serves as an advisory board to the administration and/or board of directors.

**137. A:** If a Middle Eastern female patient leaves all medical decisions about her treatment to her husband, this probably represents a cultural norm of patriarchal societies. Because the male traditionally makes decisions in Middle Eastern countries, when decisions about treatment are necessary, the discussion should be directed to the male, such as a spouse, son, or father, rather than directly to the female patient. It is important to remember that these practices are meant to protect and support the female even though they are counter to Western practice.

**138. D:** If a patient with coronary artery disease has a medication list that shows the patient is currently taking clopidogrel 75 mg daily, omeprazole 20 mg daily, metoprolol 50 mg twice daily, docusate sodium one capsule daily, and atorvastatin 80 mg daily, the drug that may pose the greatest risk of drug-drug interactions is omeprazole. Omeprazole may decrease the antiplatelet effect of clopidogrel by up to 50%, increasing the risk of a cardiovascular event. Omeprazole may also increase the effects of atorvastatin as well as the risk of adverse effects.

**139. C:** If a nursing diagnosis is "ineffective self-health management associated with lack of knowledge about condition and therapy," an appropriate patient goal is, "Patient can describe key elements of the disease process and therapeutic regimen." Self-health management must begin with knowledge and understanding about the patient's condition and therapeutic regimen, which should include the treatment plan, preventive measures (including lifestyle changes), medications, and any other treatments, such as diet and exercise.

**140. A:** The primary advantage of PCI with drug-eluting stents (DES) or bare-metal stents (BMS) is decreased restenosis and need for revascularization techniques with a DES more effective than BMS, although even BMS decreases restenosis by about 50% compared with balloon angioplasty. About 9 out of 10 PCI procedures now utilize stents. CABG is done much less frequently, and PCI with stents has almost completely replaced directional coronary atherectomy (DCA), which has higher rates of complications. Rotational atherectomy is still occasionally used for patients with severe calcifications that prevent balloon inflation.

**141. B:** A patient with an automatic implantable cardioverter-defibrillator should generally be advised to avoid MRIs because of the potential for harm to the patient or the device. However, some centers have successfully done MRIs on patients with ICDs when the MRI was deemed essential, such as with suspected brain tumors. While in some cases the threshold for pacing changed or the device required reprogramming, no deaths or severe injuries have been associated with MRIs in patients with ICDs. Patients should avoid prolonged exposure to metal detectors and anti-theft devices, but microwave ovens should cause no problem.

**142. D:** For a patient with an Unna boot, the most important factor in promoting adequate compression is ambulation because the pumping action of the calf muscles is necessary to increase compression. Nonambulatory patients should not have an Unna boot applied. Proper application is also necessary because improper application may further impair circulation. Patients should be advised to elevate the leg with the Unna boot above the level of the heart for 10 to 15 minutes two or three times daily, and to assess the color and swelling of the leg and the toes and report tingling, numbness, or pain.

**143. A:** According to the ACCF/AHA/HRS Focused Update on the Management of Patients with Atrial Fibrillation, the goal for patients with atrial fibrillation is generally a ventricular rate at rest of 60 to 80 bpm and a ventricular rate of 90 to 115 bpm during moderate activity; however, targeted rates should be individualized depending on the patient's age and condition. Patients treated for atrial fibrillation are usually maintained on warfarin as a preventive measure. Patients unable to tolerate warfarin may be treated with clopidogrel and ASA.

**144. D:** According to the AACVPR's *Guidelines for Cardiac Rehabilitation and Secondary Prevention Programs*, patients should be referred to a cardiac rehabilitation program if they experience an acute cardiovascular event, such as acute coronary syndrome or acute myocardial infarction. Once the patient is discharged, outpatient cardiac rehabilitation is usually done for a period of up to 36 weeks. Cardiac rehabilitation services can help ensure that patients adhere to treatment regimens and have access to needed resources.

**145. C:** If a patient has been admitted to the cardiac care unit with chest pain and atrial fibrillation, unlicensed assistive personnel can take daily weight. The cardiac/vascular nurse should assess the apical/radial pulse rate to evaluate the atrial fibrillation and should monitor the IV fluids. Additionally, the cardiac/vascular nurse should monitor the response to medications, such as analgesia. Assessment is outside the scope of practice of unlicensed assistive personnel.

**146. A:** If a patient is being treated for acute heart failure, the task that has priority is monitoring response to medications because acute heart failure is a life-threatening condition; physiological functioning is critical. The cardiac/vascular nurse must ensure that the patient's oxygenation is above 90% and that perfusion is adequate. The patient should be assessed for skin lesions once stabilized and the nurse should always check that the call light is within reach before leaving a patient unattended. Instruction in low-sodium diet has the lowest priority because this is information the patient will need for discharge.

**147. B:** Lidocaine is used primarily for treatment of ventricular tachycardia/fibrillation (VT/VF), both of which can be life-threatening dysrhythmias. Lidocaine can also be used for premature ventricular contraction (PVC) suppression, but PVC suppression is usually not recommended. Typically, for VT, lidocaine 1 mg/kg is administered IV as a bolus over 3 minutes and then followed by a 2 to 4 mg/min infusion. A repeat bolus of 0.5 mg/kg may be administered after 10 minutes. For VF or pulseless VT, lidocaine is administered as a 1.5 mg/kg bolus, repeated if necessary, and followed by infusion of 2 to 4 mg/min.

**148. D:** Opioid-induced hypotension does not respond to reversal agents, such as naloxone, so the medication should be held and a crystalloid bolus administered to reverse the hypotension. When pain medication resumes, smaller, more frequent doses or a different medication should be used and fluid status optimized. Antihistamines (such as diphenhydramine) may be administered to help alleviate opioid-induced pruritus. If the itching is intractable and not responsive to the antihistamine, naloxone may be administered.

**149. C:** Non-Q-wave myocardial infarctions are characterized by contraction necrosis associated with reperfusion, which usually occurs spontaneously because infarct area tends to be small with complete coronary occlusion occurring in only 20% to 30% of cases and mortality rates of about 2% to 3%. The non-Q-wave MI is usually non-transmural. Peak CK levels occur in 12 to 13 hours. Reinfarction is common, so 2-year survival rates are similar to Q-wave MIs, which have a higher initial mortality rate of about 10%.

**150. A:** If a patient is classified as having NYHA class I heart failure, the patient should expect no symptoms with activities because, while there are some changes in the heart, these changes remain asymptomatic. With class II, the patient may experience some shortness of breath and/or angina with activities of daily living. With class III, the patient will experience marked symptoms, such as dyspnea and angina while doing routine activities or walking a short distance and will only feel comfort at rest. With class IV, the patient will have severe symptoms even at rest.

# How to Overcome Test Anxiety

Just the thought of taking a test is enough to make most people a little nervous. A test is an important event that can have a long-term impact on your future, so it's important to take it seriously and it's natural to feel anxious about performing well. But just because anxiety is normal, that doesn't mean that it's helpful in test taking, or that you should simply accept it as part of your life. Anxiety can have a variety of effects. These effects can be mild, like making you feel slightly nervous, or severe, like blocking your ability to focus or remember even a simple detail.

If you experience test anxiety—whether severe or mild—it's important to know how to beat it. To discover this, first you need to understand what causes test anxiety.

## Causes of Test Anxiety

While we often think of anxiety as an uncontrollable emotional state, it can actually be caused by simple, practical things. One of the most common causes of test anxiety is that a person does not feel adequately prepared for their test. This feeling can be the result of many different issues such as poor study habits or lack of organization, but the most common culprit is time management. Starting to study too late, failing to organize your study time to cover all of the material, or being distracted while you study will mean that you're not well prepared for the test. This may lead to cramming the night before, which will cause you to be physically and mentally exhausted for the test. Poor time management also contributes to feelings of stress, fear, and hopelessness as you realize you are not well prepared but don't know what to do about it.

Other times, test anxiety is not related to your preparation for the test but comes from unresolved fear. This may be a past failure on a test, or poor performance on tests in general. It may come from comparing yourself to others who seem to be performing better or from the stress of living up to expectations. Anxiety may be driven by fears of the future—how failure on this test would affect your educational and career goals. These fears are often completely irrational, but they can still negatively impact your test performance.

## Elements of Test Anxiety

As mentioned earlier, test anxiety is considered to be an emotional state, but it has physical and mental components as well. Sometimes you may not even realize that you are suffering from test anxiety until you notice the physical symptoms. These can include trembling hands, rapid heartbeat, sweating, nausea, and tense muscles. Extreme anxiety may lead to fainting or vomiting. Obviously, any of these symptoms can have a negative impact on testing. It is important to recognize them as soon as they begin to occur so that you can address the problem before it damages your performance.

The mental components of test anxiety include trouble focusing and inability to remember learned information. During a test, your mind is on high alert, which can help you recall information and stay focused for an extended period of time. However, anxiety interferes with your mind's natural processes, causing you to blank out, even on the questions you know well. The strain of testing during anxiety makes it difficult to stay focused, especially on a test that may take several hours. Extreme anxiety can take a huge mental toll, making it difficult not only to recall test information but even to understand the test questions or pull your thoughts together.

## Effects of Test Anxiety

Test anxiety is like a disease—if left untreated, it will get progressively worse. Anxiety leads to poor performance, and this reinforces the feelings of fear and failure, which in turn lead to poor performances on subsequent tests. It can grow from a mild nervousness to a crippling condition. If allowed to progress, test anxiety can have a big impact on your schooling, and consequently on your future.

Test anxiety can spread to other parts of your life. Anxiety on tests can become anxiety in any stressful situation, and blanking on a test can turn into panicking in a job situation. But fortunately, you don't have to let anxiety rule your testing and determine your grades. There are a number of relatively simple steps you can take to move past anxiety and function normally on a test and in the rest of life.



## Physical Steps for Beating Test Anxiety

While test anxiety is a serious problem, the good news is that it can be overcome. It doesn't have to control your ability to think and remember information. While it may take time, you can begin taking steps today to beat anxiety.

Just as your first hint that you may be struggling with anxiety comes from the physical symptoms, the first step to treating it is also physical. Rest is crucial for having a clear, strong mind. If you are tired, it is much easier to give in to anxiety. But if you establish good sleep habits, your body and mind will be ready to perform optimally, without the strain of exhaustion. Additionally, sleeping well helps you to retain information better, so you're more likely to recall the answers when you see the test questions.

Getting good sleep means more than going to bed on time. It's important to allow your brain time to relax. Take study breaks from time to time so it doesn't get overworked, and don't study right before bed. Take time to rest your mind before trying to rest your body, or you may find it difficult to fall asleep.

Along with sleep, other aspects of physical health are important in preparing for a test. Good nutrition is vital for good brain function. Sugary foods and drinks may give a burst of energy but this burst is followed by a crash, both physically and emotionally. Instead, fuel your body with protein and vitamin-rich foods.

Also, drink plenty of water. Dehydration can lead to headaches and exhaustion, especially if your brain is already under stress from the rigors of the test. Particularly if your test is a long one, drink water during the breaks. And if possible, take an energy-boosting snack to eat between sections.

Along with sleep and diet, a third important part of physical health is exercise. Maintaining a steady workout schedule is helpful, but even taking 5-minute study breaks to walk can help get your blood pumping faster and clear your head. Exercise also releases endorphins, which contribute to a positive feeling and can help combat test anxiety.

When you nurture your physical health, you are also contributing to your mental health. If your body is healthy, your mind is much more likely to be healthy as well. So take time to rest, nourish your body with healthy food and water, and get moving as much as possible. Taking these physical steps will make you stronger and more able to take the mental steps necessary to overcome test anxiety.

## Mental Steps for Beating Test Anxiety

Working on the mental side of test anxiety can be more challenging, but as with the physical side, there are clear steps you can take to overcome it. As mentioned earlier, test anxiety often stems from lack of preparation, so the obvious solution is to prepare for the test. Effective studying may be the most important weapon you have for beating test anxiety, but you can and should employ several other mental tools to combat fear.

First, boost your confidence by reminding yourself of past success—tests or projects that you aced. If you're putting as much effort into preparing for this test as you did for those, there's no reason you should expect to fail here. Work hard to prepare; then trust your preparation.

Second, surround yourself with encouraging people. It can be helpful to find a study group, but be sure that the people you're around will encourage a positive attitude. If you spend time with others who are anxious or cynical, this will only contribute to your own anxiety. Look for others who are motivated to study hard from a desire to succeed, not from a fear of failure.

Third, reward yourself. A test is physically and mentally tiring, even without anxiety, and it can be helpful to have something to look forward to. Plan an activity following the test, regardless of the outcome, such as going to a movie or getting ice cream.

When you are taking the test, if you find yourself beginning to feel anxious, remind yourself that you know the material. Visualize successfully completing the test. Then take a few deep, relaxing breaths and return to it. Work through the questions carefully but with confidence, knowing that you are capable of succeeding.

Developing a healthy mental approach to test taking will also aid in other areas of life. Test anxiety affects more than just the actual test—it can be damaging to your mental health and even contribute to depression. It's important to beat test anxiety before it becomes a problem for more than testing.

## Study Strategy

Being prepared for the test is necessary to combat anxiety, but what does being prepared look like? You may study for hours on end and still not feel prepared. What you need is a strategy for test prep. The next few pages outline our recommended steps to help you plan out and conquer the challenge of preparation.

### Step 1: Scope Out the Test

Learn everything you can about the format (multiple choice, essay, etc.) and what will be on the test. Gather any study materials, course outlines, or sample exams that may be available. Not only will this help you to prepare, but knowing what to expect can help to alleviate test anxiety.

### Step 2: Map Out the Material

Look through the textbook or study guide and make note of how many chapters or sections it has. Then divide these over the time you have. For example, if a book has 15 chapters and you have five days to study, you need to cover three chapters each day. Even better, if you have the time, leave an extra day at the end for overall review after you have gone through the material in depth.

If time is limited, you may need to prioritize the material. Look through it and make note of which sections you think you already have a good grasp on, and which need review. While you are studying, skim quickly through the familiar sections and take more time on the challenging parts.

Write out your plan so you don't get lost as you go. Having a written plan also helps you feel more in control of the study, so anxiety is less likely to arise from feeling overwhelmed at the amount to cover.

## Step 3: Gather Your Tools

Decide what study method works best for you. Do you prefer to highlight in the book as you study and then go back over the highlighted portions? Or do you type out notes of the important information? Or is it helpful to make flashcards that you can carry with you? Assemble the pens, index cards, highlighters, post-it notes, and any other materials you may need so you won't be distracted by getting up to find things while you study.

If you're having a hard time retaining the information or organizing your notes, experiment with different methods. For example, try color-coding by subject with colored pens, highlighters, or post-it notes. If you learn better by hearing, try recording yourself reading your notes so you can listen while in the car, working out, or simply sitting at your desk. Ask a friend to quiz you from your flashcards, or try teaching someone the material to solidify it in your mind.

## Step 4: Create Your Environment

It's important to avoid distractions while you study. This includes both the obvious distractions like visitors and the subtle distractions like an uncomfortable chair (or a too-comfortable couch that makes you want to fall asleep). Set up the best study environment possible: good lighting and a comfortable work area. If background music helps you focus, you may want to turn it on, but otherwise keep the room quiet. If you are using a computer to take notes, be sure you don't have any other windows open, especially applications like social media, games, or anything else that could distract you. Silence your phone and turn off notifications. Be sure to keep water close by so you stay hydrated while you study (but avoid unhealthy drinks and snacks).

Also, take into account the best time of day to study. Are you freshest first thing in the morning? Try to set aside some time then to work through the material. Is your mind clearer in the afternoon or evening? Schedule your study session then. Another method is to study at the same time of day that you will take the test, so that your brain gets used to working on the material at that time and will be ready to focus at test time.

## Step 5: Study!

Once you have done all the study preparation, it's time to settle into the actual studying. Sit down, take a few moments to settle your mind so you can focus, and begin to follow your study plan. Don't give in to distractions or let yourself procrastinate. This is your time to prepare so you'll be ready to fearlessly approach the test. Make the most of the time and stay focused.

Of course, you don't want to burn out. If you study too long you may find that you're not retaining the information very well. Take regular study breaks. For example, taking five minutes out of every hour to walk briskly, breathing deeply and swinging your arms, can help your mind stay fresh.

As you get to the end of each chapter or section, it's a good idea to do a quick review. Remind yourself of what you learned and work on any difficult parts. When you feel that you've mastered the material, move on to the next part. At the end of your study session, briefly skim through your notes again.

But while review is helpful, cramming last minute is NOT. If at all possible, work ahead so that you won't need to fit all your study into the last day. Cramming overloads your brain with more information than it can process and retain, and your tired mind may struggle to recall even previously learned information when it is overwhelmed with last-minute study. Also, the urgent nature of cramming and the stress placed on your brain contribute to anxiety. You'll be more likely to go to the test feeling unprepared and having trouble thinking clearly.

So don't cram, and don't stay up late before the test, even just to review your notes at a leisurely pace. Your brain needs rest more than it needs to go over the information again. In fact, plan to finish your studies by noon or early afternoon the day before the test. Give your brain the rest of the day to relax or focus on other things, and get a good night's sleep. Then you will be fresh for the test and better able to recall what you've studied.

### Step 6: Take a Practice Test

Many courses offer sample tests, either online or in the study materials. This is an excellent resource to check whether you have mastered the material, as well as to prepare for the test format and environment.

Check the test format ahead of time: the number of questions, the type (multiple choice, free response, etc.), and the time limit. Then create a plan for working through them. For example, if you have 30 minutes to take a 60-question test, your limit is 30 seconds per question. Spend less time on the questions you know well so that you can take more time on the difficult ones.

If you have time to take several practice tests, take the first one open book, with no time limit. Work through the questions at your own pace and make sure you fully understand them. Gradually work up to taking a test under test conditions: sit at a desk with all study materials put away and set a timer. Pace yourself to make sure you finish the test with time to spare and go back to check your answers if you have time.

After each test, check your answers. On the questions you missed, be sure you understand why you missed them. Did you misread the question (tests can use tricky wording)? Did you forget the information? Or was it something you hadn't learned? Go back and study any shaky areas that the practice tests reveal.

Taking these tests not only helps with your grade, but also aids in combating test anxiety. If you're already used to the test conditions, you're less likely to worry about it, and working through tests until you're scoring well gives you a confidence boost. Go through the practice tests until you feel comfortable, and then you can go into the test knowing that you're ready for it.

## Test Tips

On test day, you should be confident, knowing that you've prepared well and are ready to answer the questions. But aside from preparation, there are several test day strategies you can employ to maximize your performance.

First, as stated before, get a good night's sleep the night before the test (and for several nights before that, if possible). Go into the test with a fresh, alert mind rather than staying up late to study.

Try not to change too much about your normal routine on the day of the test. It's important to eat a nutritious breakfast, but if you normally don't eat breakfast at all, consider eating just a protein bar. If you're a coffee drinker, go ahead and have your normal coffee. Just make sure you time it so that the caffeine doesn't wear off right in the middle of your test. Avoid sugary beverages, and drink enough water to stay hydrated but not so much that you need a restroom break 10 minutes into the test. If your test isn't first thing in the morning, consider going for a walk or doing a light workout before the test to get your blood flowing.

Allow yourself enough time to get ready, and leave for the test with plenty of time to spare so you won't have the anxiety of scrambling to arrive in time. Another reason to be early is to select a good seat. It's helpful to sit away from doors and windows, which can be distracting. Find a good seat, get out your supplies, and settle your mind before the test begins.

When the test begins, start by going over the instructions carefully, even if you already know what to expect. Make sure you avoid any careless mistakes by following the directions.

Then begin working through the questions, pacing yourself as you've practiced. If you're not sure on an answer, don't spend too much time on it, and don't let it shake your confidence. Either skip it and come back later, or eliminate as many wrong answers as possible and guess among the remaining ones. Don't dwell on these questions as you continue—put them out of your mind and focus on what lies ahead.

Be sure to read all of the answer choices, even if you're sure the first one is the right answer. Sometimes you'll find a better one if you keep reading. But don't second-guess yourself if you do immediately know the answer. Your gut instinct is usually right. Don't let test anxiety rob you of the information you know.

If you have time at the end of the test (and if the test format allows), go back and review your answers. Be cautious about changing any, since your first instinct tends to be correct, but make sure you didn't misread any of the questions or accidentally mark the wrong answer choice. Look over any you skipped and make an educated guess.

At the end, leave the test feeling confident. You've done your best, so don't waste time worrying about your performance or wishing you could change anything. Instead, celebrate the successful completion of this test. And finally, use this test to learn how to deal with anxiety even better next time.

**Review Video: Test Anxiety**
Visit mometrix.com/academy and enter code: 100340

## Important Qualification

Not all anxiety is created equal. If your test anxiety is causing major issues in your life beyond the classroom or testing center, or if you are experiencing troubling physical symptoms related to your anxiety, it may be a sign of a serious physiological or psychological condition. If this sounds like your situation, we strongly encourage you to seek professional help.

## Online Resources

Due to our efforts to try to keep this book to a manageable length, we've created a link that will give you access to all of your online resources:

**mometrix.com/resources719/cardiacvas**

# It's Your Moment, Let's Celebrate It!

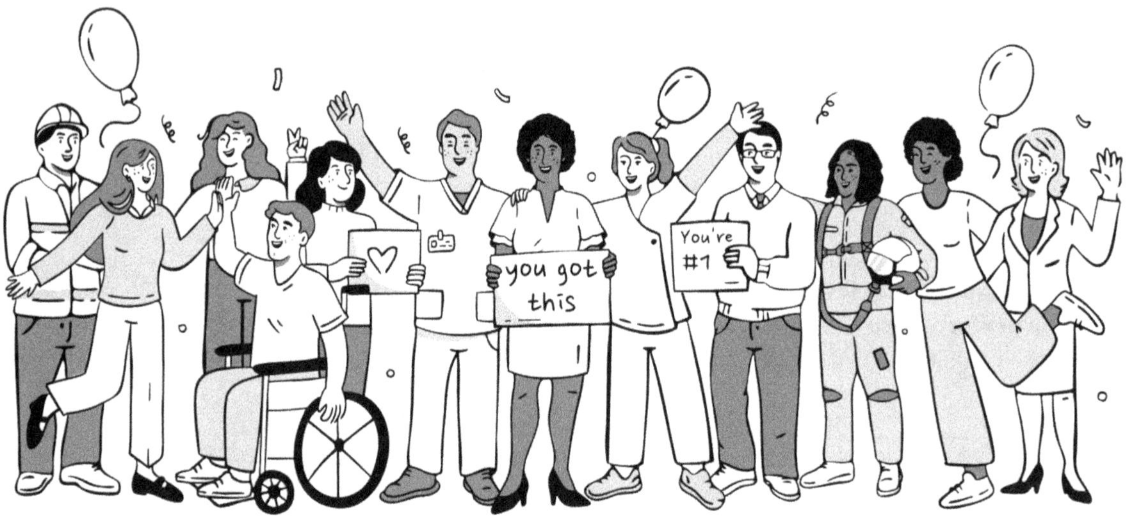


**Share your story @mometrixtestpreparation**

www.ingramcontent.com/pod-product-compliance
Lightning Source LLC
LaVergne TN
LVHW062148200926
848484LV00007B/1879